Primary Care
Mentor

Your Clerkship &
Shelf Exam Companion

Primary Care

Mentor
Your Clerkship & Shelf Exam Companion

Marianne M. Green, MD
Associate Dean for Medical Education and Competency
Achievement and Assistant Professor of Medicine
Division of General Internal Medicine
Northwestern University Feinberg School of Medicine
Chicago, Illinois

Jennifer A. Bierman, MD
Division of General Internal Medicine
Northwestern University Feinberg School of Medicine
Chicago, Illinois

James J. Foody, MD
Professor of Medicine
Vice Chairman of Medicine for Clinical Affairs
Division of General Internal Medicine
Northwestern University Feinberg School of Medicine
Chicago, Illinois

Russell G. Robertson, MD
Professor and Chair
Department of Family Medicine
Northwestern University Feinberg School of Medicine
Chicago, Illinois

Gary J. Martin, MD
Raymond J. Langenbach, MD Professor of Medicine and
Vice Chair for Faculty Affairs and Education, Department of Medicine
Northwestern University Feinberg School of Medicine
Chicago, Illinois

F. A. DAVIS COMPANY • Philadelphia

F. A. Davis Company
1915 Arch Street
Philadelphia, PA 19103
www.fadavis.com

Printed in the United States of America

Last digit indicates print number: 10 9 8 7 6 5 4 3 2 1

Senior Acquisitions Editor: Andy McPhee
Developmental Editor: Andy Pellegrini
Manager of Content Development: George W. Lang
Manager of Art and Design: Carolyn O'Brien

As new scientific information becomes available through basic and clinical research, recommended treatments and drug therapies undergo changes. The author(s) and publisher have done everything possible to make this book accurate, up to date, and in accord with accepted standards at the time of publication. The author(s), editors, and publisher are not responsible for errors or omissions or for consequences from application of the book, and make no warranty, expressed or implied, in regard to the contents of the book. Any practice described in this book should be applied by the reader in accordance with professional standards of care used in regard to the unique circumstances that may apply in each situation. The reader is advised always to check product information (package inserts) for changes and new information regarding dose and contraindications before administering any drug. Caution is especially urged when using new or infrequently ordered drugs.

Library of Congress Cataloging-in-Publication Data

Primary care mentor : your clerkship & shelf exam companion / [edited by] Marianne M. Green ... [et al.].
    p. ; cm.
  ISBN 978-0-8036-2125-1 (pbk. : alk. paper) 1. Primary care (Medicine)—Outlines, syllabi, etc. 2. Clinical clerkship—Outlines, syllabi, etc. I. Green, Marianne M.
  [DNLM: 1. Ambulatory Care—Handbooks. 2. Clinical Clerkship—Handbooks.
3. Diagnostic Techniques and Procedures—Handbooks. WB 39 P9525 2009]
  RC59.P75 2009
  616.0076—dc22

                                                                    2009001350

To the patients, whose lives we endeavor to improve

To the students, residents, and fellows who have stimulated our development as teachers

To our families, for everything

FOREWORD

The final 2 years of medical school are a critical period of physician development. Students make the final leap across the chasm separating educated layperson from medical professional. Fortified by 2 years of medical school instruction in basic and medical sciences and armed with fledgling clinical skills, students suddenly find themselves thrust into the "real" world—a world where "practice" subjects are replaced by bona fide patients with real medical needs and expectations. It is a world that no longer revolves around the student, a world with neither a structured curriculum nor controlled clinical settings. It is a time of discovery, a time when "teaching moments" do not occur on a schedule, when a day's lessons are not known until they occur, and when students really begin to appreciate just how much more there is to learn.

Although hospital-based rotations may appear to students, on the surface, to be the most demanding of all, in reality students play an apprentice role in this setting—being handed a working diagnosis at the time of a patient's admission and learning principally by observing and following in the steps of others. A far greater challenge lies in the ambulatory arena, where students are placed in the role of physician and can find themselves in a "sink-or-swim" situation. This challenge is only heightened in the primary care setting, where students must also grapple with the uncertainties of first contact and undifferentiated symptoms. This can be a humbling time because students are ill-prepared to attend to the broad clinical agenda that is the hallmark of primary care. Not surprisingly, many students find themselves growing increasingly frustrated and discouraged as they struggle to see the "forest for the trees."

Although numerous primary care texts directed at practicing clinicians exist, ready references in primary care designed for novice clinicians are sorely lacking. Stepping up to help fill this void is *Primary Care Mentor*. This carefully crafted compendium, edited by five master clinician-teachers, was developed specifically to provide guidance and direction to medical student clerks making their initial ventures into primary care. Each chapter in this thoughtfully written manual is presented in a structured outline format to provide the reader with a succinct, no-frills, nuts-and-bolts approach to the subject covered.

Including insightful introductory information on patient communications skills and clinical epidemiology are 37 chapters covering a wide array of topics, ranging from preventive medicine to common symptoms and complaints to chronic conditions seen in primary care. In addition to providing the working knowledge needed to approach problems, each chapter is replete with clinical pearls, instructive figures, and handy tables. Each chapter concludes with a Mentor Tips Digest highlighting major teaching points, a list of key references and recommended readings, and a set of self-test questions designed to help learners gauge their understanding of the material presented.

In reviewing this book, I could not help but think back to an early lesson taught to me and my classmates on our first day of medical school. In an effort to provide us with a glimpse of what the next 4 years held in store, a sagacious professor shared his version of the "There must be a pony...." vignette. He began by telling us that medical school could be likened to entering a room full of horse manure. Pessimists in the class would immediately be repulsed by the excrement, whine about the smell, strive to stay away from it, and plea to be let out. He said optimists would joyously throw themselves into the muck and, using their bare hands, cheerfully burrow and shovel through it with glee. "Why?" one might ask. Because optimists would figure that with so much horse manure in the room, there just had to be a pony in there!

Although this book won't spare novice clinicians from having to shovel their way through the challenges of primary care, it certainly figures to make them feel more optimistic.

Martin A. Quan, MD
Professor of Clinical Family Medicine
Director of Continuing Medical Education
David Geffen School of Medicine
University of California Los Angeles

PREFACE

Primary care medicine continues to advance, furthering its mission of maximizing the health of patients throughout their lives. In order to give the next generation of clinicians the very best possible study tools, we have created *Primary Care Mentor: Your Clerkship & Shelf Companion* for the primary care clerkship rotation and shelf examinations.

This book will also be helpful to mid-level providers, residents in primary care fields, and even attending physicians who want to update and review their knowledge base. *Primary Care Mentor* is a collaborative effort between internal medicine and family medicine faculty, with additional input from relevant subspecialists.

We sincerely believe the information contained in this book will help students who go on to any medical specialty. It covers common problems they will encounter as students and on into their practice. Primary care is a rewarding area. Being able to provide comprehensive care to patients and having longitudinal relationships with them energizes us as physicians and is a cost-effective strategy for providing health care to the nation. We hope this book helps in your quest to practice medicine, wherever it might be.

Marianne M. Green, MD

Jennifer A. Bierman, MD

James J. Foody, MD

Russell G. Robertson, MD

Gary J. Martin, MD

CONTRIBUTORS

Stephen L. Adams, MD
Professor of Medicine
Division of Sports Medicine
Northwestern University Feinberg School of Medicine
Chicago, Illinois
Chapter 13: Musculoskeletal Pain

Martin J. Arron, MD, MBA
Vice President for Ambulatory Operations
Beth Israel Medical Center
New York, New York
Chapter 15: Fatigue

Jennifer A. Bierman, MD
Assistant Professor of Medicine
Division of General Internal Medicine
Northwestern University Feinberg School of Medicine
Chicago, Illinois
*Chapter 1: Office Management and the Principles of Diagnosis
   and Management of Ambulatory Patients*
Chapter 32: Hormone Replacement Therapy

John E. Butter, MD
Assistant Professor of Medicine
Division of General Internal Medicine
Northwestern University Feinberg School of Medicine
Chicago, Illinois
Chapter 8: Dizziness

Raymond H. Curry, MD
Dean for Education
Professor of Medicine
Division of General Internal Medicine
Northwestern University Feinberg School of Medicine
Chicago, Illinois
Chapter 2: Communicating with Patients

Aarati D. Didwania, MD
Assistant Professor of Medicine
Division of General Internal Medicine
Northwestern University Feinberg School of Medicine
Chicago, Illinois
Chapter 31: Preconception Care

Deborah L. Edberg, MD
Assistant Professor
Department of Family Medicine
Northwestern University Feinberg School of Medicine
Chicago, Illinois
Chapter 33: Menstrual Disorders

James J. Foody, MD
Professor of Medicine
Vice Chairman of Medicine for Clinical Affairs
Division of General Internal Medicine
Northwestern University Feinberg School of Medicine
Chicago, Illinois
Chapter 6: Headache
Chapter 36: Osteoporosis
Chapter self-test questions and testbank

Jordana Friedman, MD
Assistant Professor of Medicine
Division of General Internal Medicine
Northwestern University Feinberg School of Medicine
Chicago, Illinois
Chapter 36: Osteoporosis

Ellen J. Gelles, MD
Assistant Professor of Medicine
Division of General Internal Medicine

Case Western Reserve University School of Medicine
Cleveland, Ohio
Chapter 35: Pap Smear and Cervical Cancer Screening

Joseph P. Gibes, MD
Instructor, Department of Family Medicine
Northwestern University Feinberg School of Medicine
Chicago, Illinois
Chapter 28: Otitis Media in Children
Chapter 33: Menstrual Disorders

Robert M. Golub, MD
Associate Professor of Medicine
Division of General Internal Medicine
Northwestern University Feinberg School of Medicine
Chicago, Illinois
*Chapter 3: Clinical Epidemiology and Principles of Quantitative
    Decision Making*

Marianne M. Green, MD
Associate Dean for Medical Education and Competency Achievement
    and Assistant Professor of Medicine
Division of General Internal Medicine
Northwestern University Feinberg School of Medicine
Chicago, Illinois
Chapter 13: Musculoskeletal Pain
Chapter 34: Female Genital Symptoms

Heather Heiman, MD
Assistant Professor of Medicine
Division of General Internal Medicine
Northwestern University Feinberg School of Medicine
Chicago, Illinois
Chapter 10: Sinusitis, Bronchitis, and Pharyngitis

Mitchell S. King, MD
Associate Professor of Family Medicine
Associate Dean for Academic Affairs
University of Illinois College of Medicine at Chicago
Chicago, Illinois
Chapter 11: Abdominal Pain

Elizabeth Nguyen Kirchoff, DO
Resident
McGaw Northwestern Family Medicine Residency
Chicago, Illinois
Chapter 28: Otitis Media in Children

Michael Kornfeld, MD
Instructor, Department of Medicine
Division of Hospital Medicine
Northwestern University Feinberg School of Medicine
Chicago, Illinois
Chapter 5: Preoperative Evaluation

Robert F. Kushner, MD
Professor, Department of Medicine
Division of General Internal Medicine
Northwestern University Feinberg School of Medicine
Chicago, Illinois
Chapter 25: Obesity

Cynthia A. Lagone, MD
Clinical Instructor, Department of Medicine
Division of General Internal Medicine
Northwestern University Feinberg School of Medicine
Chicago, Illinois
Chapter 14: Dermatology in Primary Care

Martin S. Lipsky, MD
Regional Dean and Professor
Department of Family Medicine
University of Illinois College of Medicine at Rockford
Rockford, Illinois
Chapter 12: Diarrhea
Chapter 23: Diabetes
Chapter 29: Geriatric Conditions

Janice A. Litza, MD
Assistant Professor
Department of Family Medicine
Northwestern University Feinberg School of Medicine
Chicago, Illinois
Chapter 26: Well-Child Visit

Melissa Yvette Liu, MD
Chief Resident
McGaw Northwestern Family Medicine Residency
Chicago, Illinois
Chapter 33: Menstrual Disorders

Gregory Makoul, PhD
Chief Academic Officer
Senior Vice President for Innovation and Quality Integration
Saint Francis Hospital and Medical Center
Hartford, Connecticut
Chapter 2: Communicating with Patients

Gary J. Martin, MD
Raymond J. Langenbach, MD Professor of Medicine and Vice Chair for Faculty Affairs and Education, Department of Medicine
Northwestern University Feinberg School of Medicine
Chicago, Illinois
Chapter 4: Prevention and Screening
Chapter 6: Headache
Chapter 9: Chest Pain
Chapter 18: Somatization
Chapter 19: Congestive Heart Failure
Chapter 24: Hyperlipidemia
Chapter 29: Geriatric Conditions

Helen Gartner Martin, MD
Assistant Professor of Medicine
Division of Pulmonary and Critical Care Medicine
Northwestern University Feinberg School of Medicine
Chicago, Illinois
Chapter 7: Common Sleep Disorders

Kevin T. McVary, MD
Director, Center for Sexual Health and Director Prostate Diseases
Minimally Invasive Program
Associate Professor of Urology
Northwestern University Feinberg School of Medicine
Chicago, Illinois
Chapter 16: Erectile Dysfunction

Michael J. Moore, MD
Assistant Professor of Medicine
Division of Pulmonary and Critical Care Medicine
Northwestern University Feinberg School of Medicine
Chicago, Illinois
Chapter 21: Asthma
Chapter 22: Chronic Obstructive Pulmonary Disease

David B. Neely, MD
Director, Undergraduate Education
Assistant Professor of Medicine
Division of General Internal Medicine
Northwestern University Feinberg School of Medicine
Chicago, Illinois
Chapter 20: Hypertension

Kevin O'Leary, MD
Assistant Professor of Medicine
Division of Hospital Medicine
Northwestern University Feinberg School of Medicine
Chicago, Illinois
Chapter 5: Preoperative Evaluation

Sandra A. Pagan, MD, MPA
Resident
McGaw Northwestern Family Medicine Residency
Chicago, Illinois
Chapter 27: Fever in Children

Karin G. Patterson, DO
Clinical Faculty
St. Vincent's Family Medicine Residency Program
Indianapolis, Indiana
Chapter 27: Fever in Children

Michael J. Polizzotto, MD
Assistant Professor of Family Medicine
University of Illinois College of Medicine at Rockford
Rockford, Illinois
Chapter 12: Diarrhea

Eduard Porosnicu, MD

Director, Palliative Care Service
Clinical Assistant Professor of Medicine
State University of New York Downstate Medical Center
Brooklyn, New York
Chapter 15: Fatigue

Aparna Priyanath, MD

Assistant Professor of Medicine
Division of General Internal Medicine
Northwestern University Feinberg School of Medicine
Chicago, Illinois
Chapter 30: Benign Breast Disease

Douglas R. Reifler, MD

Associate Professor of Medicine
Division of General Internal Medicine
Northwestern University Feinberg School of Medicine
Chicago, Illinois
Chapter 17: Anxiety and Depression

Russell G. Robertson, MD

Professor and Chair
Department of Family Medicine
Northwestern University Feinberg School of Medicine
Chicago, Illinois
Editorial review

Phillip E. Roemer, MD

Assistant Professor of Medicine
Division of General Internal Medicine
Northwestern University Feinberg School of Medicine
Chicago, Illinois
Chapter 2: Communicating with Patients

Adam D. Rosenfeld, DO

Resident
McGaw Northwestern Family Medicine Residency
Chicago, Illinois
Chapter 26: Well-Child Visit

Jeffrey S. Royce, MD
Director, Swedish-American Center for Headache Care
Clinical Assistant Professor of Family Medicine
University of Illinois College of Medicine at Rockford
Rockford, Illinois
Chapter 23: Diabetes

Herbert Sier, MD
Associate Chief of Geriatric Medicine
Assistant Professor of Medicine
Division of Geriatrics
Northwestern University Feinberg School of Medicine
Chicago, Illinois
Chapter 29: Geriatric Conditions

Lenore F. Soglin, MD
Instructor, Department of Medicine
Division of General Internal Medicine
Northwestern University Feinberg School of Medicine
Chicago, Illinois
Chapter 37: Intimate Partner Violence

Christopher Varona, DO
Resident
McGaw Northwestern Family Medicine Residency
Chicago, Illinois
Chapter 28: Otitis Media in Children

CONTENTS

PART three

DIAGNOSIS AND MANAGEMENT OF COMMON CHRONIC ILLNESSES 269

PART four

DIAGNOSIS AND MANAGEMENT OF AGE-RELATED CONDITIONS 359

PART five

WOMEN'S HEALTH   409

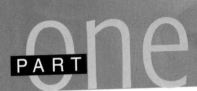

PART one

OVERVIEW OF PRIMARY CARE

1 CHAPTER

OFFICE MANAGEMENT AND THE PRINCIPLES OF DIAGNOSIS AND MANAGEMENT OF AMBULATORY PATIENTS

Jennifer A. Bierman, MD

I. Introduction to Ambulatory Medicine
    A. The majority of medical care is received in the outpatient setting.
    B. The ambulatory physician is what most patients consider their "doctor."

II. Differences in Inpatient Versus Ambulatory Care
    A. Inpatient care focuses on curing or resolving an acute condition, such as an exacerbation of congestive heart failure.
    B. Ambulatory care may focus on curing or resolving an acute medical problem such as treating a bacterial sinus infection.

C. Further goals of ambulatory care include:
   1. Providing longitudinal care of a patient's chronic medical problems; e.g., diabetes over years, not days
   2. Preventing further health problems
      a. Primary prevention by screening for and treating hypertension to prevent Coronary Heart Disease
      b. Secondary prevention by lowering the cholesterol of a patient who is post myocardial infarction (MI) with medication to prevent a future MI.
   3. Improving the patient's quality of life
D. Diagnosis
   1. Inpatient care typically involves a disease process that is already differentiated, and the focus is on treating that process; e.g., intravenous (IV) antibiotics for pneumonia.
   2. Ambulatory care typically involves undifferentiated symptoms; e.g., fatigue, cough. The goal is to make a correct diagnosis in a cost-conscious manner, which often leads to symptoms being treated presumptively.

III. Principles of Diagnosis and Treatment
A. Clinical presentation
   1. Patients may present with symptoms that need a diagnosis and treatment plan.
   2. Patients may present for the management of a known health problem.
   3. Patients may present for a prevention visit.
B. History and physical
   1. Diagnosis-specific
   2. Interview should focus on the presenting symptoms
      i. Using a mnemonic is helpful to focus the history of present illness (HPI) and to minimize the chance of omitting important information.
      ii. Example: OLDCARTS
         O Onset of symptoms
         L Location
         D Duration
         C Characteristics
         A Aggravating and alleviating factors
         R Radiation
         T Treatment
         S Significance

3. Physical examination needs to be focused on organ system related to the complaint.
   i. Use your initial differential diagnosis to focus your physical examination.
4. Manage a chronic disease
   a. Interview should:
      i. Explore how the disease affects the individual
         (1) Does an asthmatic patient have any nighttime symptoms?
         (2) Does a diabetic patient have any hypoglycemic episodes?
      ii. Determine the patient's response to previous treatments
      iii. Monitor compliance with prescribed treatments
      iv. Monitor for side effects of treatment
   b. Physical examination
      i. It may be very brief, e.g, in a known hypertensive patient, may include only checking blood pressure (BP) and listening to the heart
   c. Review the chart for results of recent tests, and identify recent treatments the patient may have undergone.
   d. Order needed testing.
   e. Change the treatment plan as needed, and ensure the patient understands the plan.
      i. Patient understanding and compliance are essential in the ambulatory setting

 Use the teach-back technique by having the patient tell you the plan to ensure understanding.

5. Prevention
   a. The interview needs to focus on a complete review of systems (ROS), family history, and any risk factors the patient may have, especially related to heart disease, cancer, infections.
   b. The physical examination should be complete.
   c. Know the indications for routine health maintenance testing (e.g., Pap smears, mammograms, colonoscopies, immunizations), and schedule appropriately.
   d. Counsel patients on the role of a healthy diet and exercise program for their long-term health.

C. Diagnostic and therapeutic plan

    1. Pace of ambulatory care can be hectic.

        a. Each return patient is seen and managed in 10–20 minutes. New patients are often given longer appointments.

    2. Physicians need to assemble clinical information from the history, physical examination, and old records efficiently.

    3. The differential diagnoses should be grouped into 1) most likely, 2) most worrisome, and 3) least likely.

    4. A plan needs to be formulated in a stepwise fashion regarding diagnosis and treatment.

        a. Serial testing versus parallel testing

            i. In the inpatient setting parallel testing is often undertaken.

                (1) Patients are often very ill, and determining a diagnosis quickly is imperative.

                (2) Hospital care is very expensive, and there is pressure to limit the length of stay for each patient.

                (3) Ordering several tests at once is an efficient way to achieve both these goals.

                    (A) For example, a patient with chest pain and shortness of breath undergoes simultaneous testing for cardiac ischemia and pulmonary embolus.

            ii. In the outpatient setting, serial testing is often undertaken.

                (1) Cost-effective care is a priority.

                (2) A test or treatment plan is ordered, and the results are analyzed prior to further testing.

                (3) Diagnostic studies that are minimally invasive are preferred.

                (4) Symptoms are often treated empirically, based on a presumptive diagnosis.

                    (A) For example, a young female with 1 day of dysuria without fever may be treated with antibiotics for presumed cystitis without any further testing.

                (5) A treatment failure or worsening of symptoms may then prompt further testing.

D. Management

    1. Reevaluate the patient after initial testing and treatment.

    2. Educate and advise patients on their symptoms, disease process, and goals of therapy.

IV. Role of Students

A. Learn to focus on a specific complaint.

1. Interview and examine patients in a concise manner appropriate to specific complaints.

2. Formulate a diagnostic hypothesis without laboratory or radiologic testing.

3. Learn to treat symptoms when appropriate.

4. Learn to follow a patient's response to treatment.

   a. Monitor for side effects to medications.

   b. Monitor for compliance.

   c. Learn to adjust treatment based on the above factors.

B. Prevention

1. Know how to modify risk factors for chronic diseases.

   a. This is especially important for risks related to heart disease, stroke, cancer, and infections.

2. Learn to counsel patients effectively to promote behavioral change.

   a. Effectively counsel a patient on smoking cessation.

   b. Give appropriate dietary and exercise advice.

   c. Effectively and empathetically give advice on how to limit sexually transmitted infections.

   d. Improve patient's compliance with health maintenance issues.

C. Time management

1. Learn the benefits of reviewing a patient's chart to improve efficiency and quality of the visit.

2. Learn to set the agenda based on office visit type: 1) chronic disease management; 2) new problem; or 3) prevention issue.

3. Learn to help an office run efficiently.

   a. Having a student in the office slows down the flow of patients and can upset patients.

      i. A student typically adds an hour of work to the attending physician's day.

      ii. Most physicians are not paid or are paid nominally to have a student in their office.

      iii. Patients present to see their doctor and are often fearful when a student is present.

   b. There are ways to alleviate time pressures and patient's fears.

      i. Alleviate tension with patients by letting them know that the attending physician is present and will see them.

        (1) Say, e.g., "Hi. My name is John Doe. I am a medical student working with Dr. X. Dr X asked me to get started and he/she will be in shortly."

        (2) This statement can allay the patients' fears and let them know that they will see their doctor.

    ii. Perform bedside presentations as often as possible.

        (1) Patients enjoy learning from this interaction.

        (2) It improves "face time" with the attending physician and avoids the need to repeat the HPI for the attending physician.

        (3) It saves time overall.

    iii. Offer to move on to the next patient while the attending physician is finishing charting.

    iv. Orient yourself to the triage and rooming nurses to help facilitate patient flow.

V. Learn What It Means to Be Someone's "Doctor"

A. Observe the attending physician's interactions with patients the physician has known for many years.

  1. Observe to see how the attending physician makes a personal connection with patients.

    a. The physician may relate by talking about common hobbies, sports.

    b. The physician may review the chart to refresh his/her memory about the patient's recent life stressors. Employment changes and marriage issues are important themes.

> Understand the broader context of your contact with patients: their work, their family life, their chronic illnesses (if any).

B. Learn the role of work and family life in a patient's long-term health.

  1. Review a patient's chart to see how work and family life stressors have affected health.

    a. Job losses may lead to difficulty purchasing needed medications or inability to see a physician for periods of time.

    b. Family stressors (especially the illness of a loved one) can affect a patient's compliance with a medical regimen.

2. Review a patient's chart to see how medical illnesses have affected employment and family life.
   a. Sometimes patients need to modify their job, given their illness.
   b. A patient on dialysis may not be able to continue with a job that requires travel.

MENTOR TIPS DIGEST

- Use the teach-back technique by having the patient tell you the plan to ensure understanding.
- Learn what it means to be someone's "doctor." Understand the broader context of your contact with patients: their work, their family life, their chronic illnesses (if any).

Chapter Self-Test Questions

Fill in the answers. When you're done, check your answers in Appendix A.

1. List 2–3 life stressors that may negatively affect a patient's management of his/her chronic illness.

_____

_____

_____

2. Patients can be nervous about medical students because patients want to know that they will still see their doctor. Write an example of how you can introduce yourself in a way that allays patient fears:

_____

_____

_____

3. List 2–3 differences in general approach between outpatient care and inpatient care.

_____

_____

_____

2
CHAPTER

COMMUNICATING WITH PATIENTS

Phillip E. Roemer, MD, Gregory Makoul, PhD, and Raymond H. Curry, MD

I. Overview

A. Communication: a transactional process in which messages are filtered through the perceptions, emotions, and experiences of those involved

B. Increasing volume of medical literature strongly suggests that effective communication is associated with improved patient outcomes

  1. An accurate diagnosis is more frequently made when the history is obtained effectively and directly from the patient.

  2. Effective communication leads to improved adherence to the treatment plan and, in some studies, better physiologic outcomes (e.g., blood pressure control).

  3. Effective communication empowers patients and allows them to take responsibility for their health.

C. Physician education in communication skills shown to result in better patient satisfaction and even reduction in malpractice suits

D. Better communication makes patient-physician encounter more productive and rewarding for both the patient and physician

II..Structured Framework Is Key to Effective Interview

A. SEGUE is an acronym that outlines the transition through the stages in the patient interview. Box 2.1 shows the basic meaning. The text below discusses each idea in more detail.

  1. Set the stage

  a. When entering the room, greet your patient appropriately, which, unless you know the patient well, generally involves saying both the patient's name and your name. For instance,

BOX 2.1
The SEGUE Approach to Communicating With Patients

Set the stage
Elicit information
Give information
Understand the patient's perspective (and show the patient that you understand)
End the encounter

if Dr. Robert Franklin is meeting Ms. Jane Smith, we suggest that he say: "Jane Smith? Hi, I'm Bob Franklin." Adopting this strategy of using parallel identity terms communicates respect and reciprocity.

b. Be sure to provide for a private setting by shutting the door/drawing the curtain and asking the patient if others in the room may stay. There are several strategies for establishing the reason for the visit, including "What can I do for you?" "How can I help you today?" "What brings you in today?"

c. Listening skills

 Allow the patient to speak without interruption, especially at the beginning of the encounter.

i. This listening usually takes only a minute or two and provides the best opportunity for patients to make sure you have heard what they came to say.

ii. Your careful listening during this phase can also be an invaluable opportunity to discern nuances of the patient's perceptions and expectations and other aspects of their affective and psychological state.

d. Determining an agenda

 Outline an agenda for the visit during the first few minutes.

      i. "What else can I do for you?" "Is there anything else you would like to discuss?" This efficiently establishes an outline for the visit and allows the patient to highlight concerns, which can then be prioritized early in the encounter. Otherwise, patients may delay additional concerns until the end of the encounter when you may not be able to handle them effectively. Accomplishing this task will facilitate a more organized encounter.

2. *E*licit information

   a. It is important to obtain information both about the patient's condition (i.e., symptoms) and the patient's perceptions of the health problem.

      i. What does the patient believe is causing the symptoms?

      ii. What are the patient's major concerns about the problem (even unspoken concerns)? e.g., with headaches: "Are you concerned about what they might mean?" "Well, one of my coworkers was just diagnosed with a brain tumor."

      iii. Explore the physical and physiologic factors contributing to the patient's symptoms. "Do certain kinds of food cause or worsen your headaches?" "Do the headaches correlate with your menstrual cycle?"

      iv. Explore psychosocial and emotional factors influencing the patient's condition. "Is your headache worse during certain times of the day or week? Is it related to work?" Assess how the problem affects the patient's life. "How do your headaches limit your activities at home and work?"

      v. Has the patient already attempted to address the problem? Review antecedent treatments to better determine the patient's perspective on the condition. "What have you tried to relieve your headaches?" What treatments are acceptable to the patient? For example, many people prefer not to take even over-the-counter medications. What is the patient willing to do to improve the situation (e.g., exercising regularly to better control diabetes or reducing fat intake in order to lower cholesterol)? There are many effective strategies for eliciting information, as discussed below.

b. Asking open-ended questions allows patients to tell you in their own words what is wrong.

  i. The use of close-ended questions is also appropriate when you need to focus on a specific point. "Do you ever experience nausea?" "How many cigarettes do you smoke daily?"

  ii. Avoid leading questions. "You don't have any chest pain, do you?" Answers formulated by the patient are much more accurate and unbiased.

  iii. Listen attentively at all times, and allow the patient uninterrupted time to speak.

  iv. Repeatedly check and clarify information. "So let me recap to make sure I understand: You have been experiencing pressure in the middle of your chest on and off for the last 6 weeks associated with nausea and shortness of breath?"

 Listen carefully and actively.

  (1) Give the patient your undivided attention. Patients' satisfaction and sense of well-being have been shown to correlate more closely with the quality of the attention given them by the physician than with the quantity of time devoted to the encounter.

3. *G*ive information

  a. Communication involves sending, giving, or exchanging (information, ideas, etc.). The physician's role includes giving information as well as obtaining it. Information is better provided if it is presented at the level of understanding of the patient. Explain in layman's terms the rationale behind your diagnosis and recommendations for further testing and treatment

  b. Review findings of the physical examination and laboratory tests in the context of the patient's situation. "The pain in your upper belly and the findings from your recent tests strongly suggest that you have something called gastroesophageal reflux disease."

c. Encourage patients to ask questions about their problem. "Doctor, what causes reflux disease?"

d. Teach the patient about the body and the condition. "A valve between your stomach and esophagus, the tube that leads from your mouth to your stomach, leaks and allows stomach acid to back up into the esophagus causing your heartburn pain." Use written diagrams to more concretely describe a patient's problem

e. Review recommendations for improving the patient's situation. "There are several strategies for helping your condition. Let's review these, and I will also provide you with some written information. In addition, I believe this medication should help."

f. Explain the likely benefits of treatment options. "This antacid medication should reduce the acid in your stomach and the acid that then refluxes into your esophagus, reducing the pain you are experiencing."

g. Explain likely and possible side effects of treatment. "Most people tolerate this medication without problems. Possible side effects include cramping and diarrhea."

h. Acknowledge other possible diagnoses and symptoms with which to be concerned. This encourages an interactive encounter and allows the patient more control. "If your cough does not improve using these treatments for acid reflux, then we should consider other possible problems such as asthma or other gastrointestinal disorders. Please contact me if you do not have any improvement over the next 2 weeks."

4. *U*nderstand the patient's perspective (and show the patient that you understand)

a. Most important: acknowledge the patient's accomplishments, progress, and challenges. "It's great that you've been able to stop smoking. Keep it up!"

b. Try to make a link between the patient's perspective of the situation and your recommendations. "You mentioned that your headache seems to worsen when you are pressured at work. Can you think of any opportunities for reducing your stress level at work, such as relaxing or exercising during your breaks?"

      c. Discuss improvement or worsening of patient's situation in the context of your findings. Acknowledge challenges to improving the patient's circumstances, e.g., financial barriers. Explore your patient's expectations and goals for treatment and/or prevention.

  5. *E*nd the encounter

      a. At the end of the encounter, ask if there is anything else the patient would like to discuss. Major concerns will have been addressed early on when setting the agenda for the visit.

      b. Review the next steps with the patient. Schedule next visits or tests. It is very important to provide hope as well as expectations in more serious situations and when bad news is given. "There are effective options for approaching this kind of cancer, and many people have been treated successfully."

B. Utilizing effective strategies for communication

  1. One way to facilitate better communications is to make a personal connection. This provides a more comfortable environment for communication. "I understand how stressful caring for your children can be. I also have two little ones at home."

  2. Pay attention to nonverbal messages you are sending the patient as well as those you receive from the patient. A judgmental tone of voice will often reduce a patient's willingness to speak freely with you. Patients will often communicate how they feel without speaking or before they speak. For example, a patient pacing the room with arms folded may suggest angry feelings or anxiety.

  3. Maintain a respectful tone at all times. This conveys to the patient that you care and that you are serious about helping. Express caring, concern, and empathy with your words, voice inflections, and body posture. Patient's reactions to your recommendations often reflect *how* you say something rather than *what* you say.

C. Difficult encounters

> It is especially important in difficult encounters to stop and think for a moment about the communication skills and strategies you can use to facilitate the interaction.

1. Angry patient—need to "defuse" intense feelings
   a. Acknowledge the patient's apparent feelings.
   b. Determine the reason for anger.
   c. Provide an explanation, if pertinent.
   d. If the patient has reason to be angry with you, apologize.
   e. Reinforce your commitment to help.
2. Breaking bad news
   a. Provide a comfortable and private setting in which to meet.
   b. Establish how much information the patient has about the current condition, and provide updates before communicating the bad news.
   c. Provide the news in a clear and concise way.
   d. Allow for questions, and give information in small bits.
   e. Discuss the next steps.
   f. Offer hope in some form.
   g. Plan for follow-up.
3. Taking a sexual history
   a. Start by telling the patient why you are asking the questions—health risks or sexual health/function.
   b. Do not assume anything regarding sexual orientation or practices.
   c. Remember to be nonjudgmental when asking questions and receiving answers.
4. Talking to patients from different cultures
   a. It is better to ask questions than resort to stereotypes—get the patient's perspective on the problem and its cause.
   b. Be sure to confirm your interpretations.
   c. Check the patient's understanding and acceptance of your recommendations.

MENTOR TIPS DIGEST

- Allow the patient to speak without interruption, especially at the beginning of the encounter.
- Outline an agenda for the visit during the first few minutes.

- Listen carefully and actively.
- It is especially important in difficult encounters to stop and think for a moment about the communication skills and strategies you can use to facilitate the interaction.

Resources

Makoul G. The SEGUE Framework for teaching and assessing communication skills. Patient Education & Counseling 45:23–34, 2001.
Reviews several years of experience with the SEGUE Framework, the most widely used model for teaching and assessing communication skills in North America.

Makoul G (for the Bayer-Fetzer Conference on Physician-Patient Communication in Medical Education). Essential elements of communication in medical encounters: The Kalamazoo consensus statement. Academic Medicine 76:390–393, 2001.
Reports consensus of leading educators and researchers regarding communication tasks that should be accomplished in medical encounters.

Platt FW, Gordon GH. Field Guide to the Difficult Patient Interview. Philadelphia: Lippincott, Williams & Wilkins, 2004.

Chapter Self-Test Questions

Circle the correct answer. After you have responded to the questions, check your answers in Appendix A.

1. Fill in the expanded meaning of the SEGUE acronym.

S _____

E _____

G _____

U _____

E _____

2. When asking questions of a patient, one style of question that is usually *not* appropriate is a style in which you are more or less coaching the patient to give you the answer that you expect. This style of question is called what?

_____.

3. Sometimes patients' biggest concern is something they are hesitant to bring up, e.g., presenting with headaches. You may ask, "Are you concerned about what they might mean?" What do you think this patient may be worried about, more than minor pain relief?

_____

See the testbank CD for more self-test questions.

3

CLINICAL EPIDEMIOLOGY AND PRINCIPLES OF QUANTITATIVE DECISION MAKING*

Robert M. Golub, MD

I. Consider These Two Problems

A. Problem 1: In the emergency room you are seeing a 32-year-old female who yesterday developed pleuritic chest pain and shortness of breath. She has had a painful, warm, and swollen left calf for the last 3 days, with tenderness and edema on examination. She takes oral contraceptives (OCPs) and smokes. In addition to the leg findings, her examination is notable for a heart rate of 112; when she was in the office for a Pap smear 2 weeks ago her heart rate was 88. Several questions arise:

1. What is the likelihood that she has had a pulmonary embolism (PE)?
2. Does taking an OCP or smoking make her predisposed to a PE?
3. Would a D-dimer test help to make the diagnosis?
4. What is the best treatment for her?
5. If she has had a PE, what problems can she expect in the future?

B. Problem 2: Should you be advocating screening mammograms for your patients between the ages of 40 and 50 years?

---

*Data used in examples have been excerpted from the medical literature. However, they have been adapted for teaching purposes; the risk measures calculated in these examples are therefore different from those reported in the articles, and the reader should refer back to the original study for the true risk measures as well as confidence intervals.

II. Overview

A. These are the types of questions that you face in making decisions with all of your patients. The approaches that you use to answer them in the best way come from the discipline of **clinical epidemiology**, which is the application of epidemiologic principles and methods to problems encountered in clinical medicine.

B. The core idea is that issues such as diagnosis and treatment outcome are uncertain for individual patients, are therefore expressed as probabilities, and are best estimated by referring to past experience with groups of similar patients. In other words, information is taken from (ideally large) studies and applied one-on-one with each patient. This requires understanding and being able to use certain basic quantitative methods.

C. These decisions should be made using the approach of **evidence-based medicine.** This involves:

   1. Framing the question in a precise way that will facilitate finding needed information.

   2. Accessing that information efficiently (e.g., searching primary literature, reading textbooks, speaking to local experts).

   3. Evaluating the quality of that information critically, using methodical approaches to determine its validity.

   4. Determining how to apply valid information to the specific circumstances of the individual patient.

D. This chapter briefly considers the key concepts of clinical epidemiology as they relate to these common questions, the types of measures you will encounter, and how to apply them. A textbook of clinical epidemiology, such as that by Fletcher and Fletcher,[1] will provide more background. Methodical approaches to critiquing the studies you will be reading are essential, but they go beyond the scope of this book; a number of texts address these well, such as that by Guyatt and Drummond.[2,3]

III. Topics of Clinical Epidemiology and Medical Decision
Making. Problem 1 illustrates the categories of typical epidemiologic questions. To understand the measures used with each, it is helpful to divide them into questions of frequency, diagnosis, and association.

A. How common is a condition? *(frequency and prevalence)*

   1. For Problem 1, in deciding whether to pursue the diagnostic possibility of a PE, you should be interested in knowing the probability that someone who presents like this patient has a PE. When considering the likelihood of disease in a patient, the starting point is usually the **prevalence** of the disease in the relevant population, which is defined as:

$$\frac{\text{number of people with a condition}}{\text{number of people at risk for having a condition}}$$

2. The best way to estimate this prevalence is a **cross-sectional study** that looks at a population of people similar to the patient to find out what percentage had a PE and what percentage had another diagnosis. In looking for prevalence studies, try to find ones in which the denominator (population at risk) matches your patient as closely as possible. For example, look for studies that were done only on people who presented as outpatients with pleuritic pain, or only on women, or only on women who smoke and take OCPs. Unfortunately, this is not always possible, and in applying studies in which the population is different from your patient you have to use your judgment to adjust the probability up or down.

3. It is important not to confuse **prevalence** (which is a snapshot of a population at a single point in time) with **incidence**, which is a measure of the number of new cases in a population that occur over a specified length of time and is discussed later in the chapter.

B. **Does my patient have a particular disease?** (choice and interpretation of *diagnostic* tests) To decide whether a particular diagnostic test is useful to do, you need to combine three pieces of information: the **treatment threshold** for the diagnosis under consideration, the **test characteristics** of the diagnostic test under consideration, and your patient's **pre-test probability** (the likelihood of disease before getting new information).

1. **The treatment threshold and the threshold model**

   a. In thinking about diagnostic tests, it is useful to conceptualize your patient having the disease as a probability falling along a continuum between 0 (absolute certainty that she does *not* have it) and 1 (absolute certainty that she *does* have it) (Fig. 3.1A). As you gain new information about the patient, whether from additional history, physical examination findings, or test results, the patient moves right or left along the continuum as you become more certain she does or does not have the disease of interest (Fig. 3.1B). One is almost never 100% sure about presence or absence of disease because information is rarely perfect. Given this, how certain do you need to be that someone has a disease before you are willing to label the patient with it and to take the necessary action? Because this could involve mistakenly treating some people who in fact do not have disease or failing to treat some people who do have it, you must consider the tradeoffs between the benefits and risks of treatment for those with and without disease.

b. In general, if the benefit of treatment is high and/or the risks are low, you are willing to treat someone even if there is a low probability the patient has the disease. Conversely, if the benefit of treatment is relatively low and/or the risks are high, you require a high probability that the patient has the disease before deciding to treat. These tradeoffs are incorporated in the **treatment threshold:** the lowest probability that someone could have a disease whereby, *in the absence of any further available information,* you would be willing to treat the patient as if he or she did (Fig 3.1C) (Chapter 9 of Sox et al[4]). If you can estimate the relative risks and benefits, the formula for the treatment threshold is:

$$\frac{\dfrac{risk}{benefit}}{1 + \dfrac{risk}{benefit}}$$

c. For example, if you consider the risk of complication from anticoagulation against the benefit of preventing a future possibly fatal PE, a reasonable risk/benefit ratio might be 1/5. This would result in a treatment threshold of 0.17. This means that, in the absence of further information, if you believed your patient's probability of a PE was any less than 0.17 you should not anticoagulate, despite the possibility of missing someone with a PE; alternately, if probability is *any* greater than 0.17 (even 0.18), you *should* anticoagulate, recognizing that you may be unnecessarily anticoagulating some people without a PE.

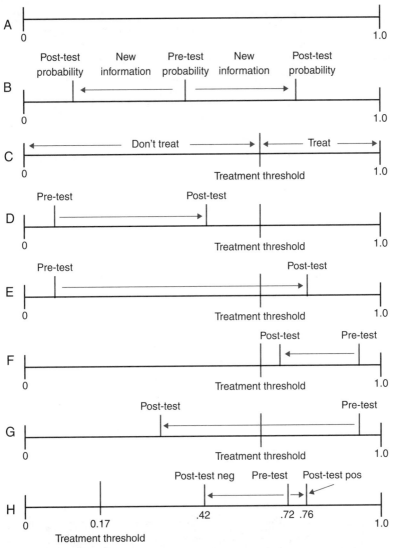

FIGURE 3.1 The threshold model for choice and interpretation of test results.

d. To decide whether to order a test or to interpret the test results, you can then use the **threshold model** that says that you should only perform a test if it could potentially move you from a pre-test probability on one side of the threshold to a **post-test probability** (the probability of a disease after you have gained new information) on the other side of the threshold. For example, the test shown in Figure 3.1D, in which the patient's pre-test probability is less than the threshold, should not be done because a positive result would not make you certain enough of the diagnosis to change how you would label the patient. However, the test in Figure 3.1E will change this if it is positive, and therefore it is reasonable to perform. If you start with a pre-test probability above the threshold, you are interested in whether a negative test will cross the threshold. Figure 3.1F shows a test in which that will not happen; thus, the test should not be used. In Figure 3.1G, the test will change how you treat the patient and can give useful information.

   e. To use this approach, you need to be able to calculate post-test probability. Before you can do that, you have to know the **test's characteristics** (which tell you how accurate the test is) and your patient's **pre-test probability.**

2. Test characteristics

   a. Most tests in medicine are not perfect; those that are tend to be invasive, expensive, or autopsies (usually not the ideal diagnostic approach). The accuracy of an imperfect test is measured in two ways: **sensitivity/specificity** and **likelihood ratios**.

      i. **Sensitivity and specificity** are determined by a **cross-sectional** study of a population with and without disease, as determined by everyone getting a **gold-standard test** (a test that is considered to define presence or absence of disease) and everyone getting the **index test** (the particular test of interest). By looking at the results as a 2 × 2 table (Fig 3.2), there are four subgroups: true positives (disease present and index test positive), true negatives (disease absent and index test negative), false negatives (disease present but index test negative), and false positives (disease absent but index test positive). Sensitivity is then defined as the probability of a positive index test given the knowledge that someone actually has the disease. Specificity is the probability of a

		Gold standard		Totals
		Disease present	Disease absent	
Index test result	Positive	a True positives	b False positives	a + b
	Negative	c False negatives	d True negatives	c + d
	Totals	a + b	c + d	a+b+c+d

$$\text{Sensitivity} = \frac{a}{a + c} \qquad \text{Specificity} = \frac{d}{b + d}$$

$$\text{Pre-test probability (prevalence)} = \frac{a + c}{a + b + c + d}$$

$$\text{Positive predictive value} = \text{post-test probability } (+) = \frac{a}{a + b}$$

$$\text{Post-test probability } (-) = \frac{c}{c + d}$$

$$\text{Negative predictive value} = 1 - \text{post-test probability } (-) = \frac{d}{c + d}$$

Converting between probability and odds

$$\text{Odds} = \frac{\text{probability}}{1 - (\text{probability})} \qquad \text{Probability} = \frac{\text{odds}}{1 + (\text{odds})}$$

Likelihood ratios, and odds-likelihood ratio calculation of post-test probability

$$\text{Likelihood ratio} = \frac{\text{probability of a result given disease}}{\text{probability of the same result given no disease}}$$

$$\text{Likelihood ratio } (+) = \frac{\text{sensitivity}}{1 - (\text{specificity})} \qquad \text{Likelihood ratio } (-) = \frac{1 - (\text{sensitivity})}{\text{specificity}}$$

$$\text{Pre-test odds} = \frac{\text{prevalence}}{1 - (\text{prevalence})} = \frac{\text{pre-test probability}}{1 - (\text{pre-test probability})}$$

$$\text{Post-test odds} = (\text{pre-test odds}) \times (\text{likelihood ratio})$$

$$\text{Post-test probability} = \frac{\text{post-test odds}}{\text{post-test odds} + 1}$$

$$\text{Treatment threshold} = \frac{R/B}{1 + R/B}, \text{ where R is net risk (all types of harm) and B is benefits}$$

FIGURE 3.2 Formulas for diagnostic test use and calculating post-test probability.

negative index test given the knowledge that someone does not have the disease. These criteria indicate how often the index test is correct if you start out knowing about presence or absence of disease, but unfortunately this is not the clinically important information. You need the opposite: what you are looking for, because you do not already have the knowledge about your patient's presence or absence of disease, is the probability that disease is present given either a positive or negative test result—the **post-test probability.**

ii. **Likelihood ratio** is defined as

$$\frac{\text{probability of a particular result given presence of disease}}{\text{probability of the same result given absence of disease}}$$

(1) For a test that can only have a positive or negative result, there are therefore two likelihood ratios: likelihood ratio positive and likelihood ratio negative (see Fig. 3.2). The better the test is, the higher the likelihood ratio positive (infinity would represent a perfect test) and the lower the likelihood ratio negative (0 would represent a perfect test). Using likelihood ratios provides a second, often easier, way to calculate post-test probability.

(2) Considering the D-dimer test, in one study[5] the measure of accuracy was sensitivity = 0.93, specificity = 0.25. From this, the likelihood ratio positive of 1.24, and likelihood negative of 0.28 can be calculated.

b. Pre-test probability

i. As noted above, one common way to establish your patient's pre-test probability of disease is to find a study that looks at prevalence of that disease in patients similar to yours. If such a study has not been done, you may need to rely on an expert opinion. However, there are many **prediction rule** studies in the literature that allow you to determine a score for your patient based on clinical characteristics and to translate that score into a probability. Using one published rule for a PE (Le Gal et al[6]), a pre-test probability for a PE of 0.72 for this patient could be calculated.

c. Calculating Post-Test Probability

    i. Two ways to calculate this number are the "tree method," which uses sensitivity/specificity, and the odds-likelihood ratio method.

d. Using the Tree Diagram (Fig 3.3)

    i. Assume you begin with a large round number of patients (e.g., 10,000) exactly like yours. You perform the gold standard test for each member of this group, the pulmonary angiogram, so that you could know for certain whether each had had a PE. The pre-test probability of 0.72 would mean that 7200 would have disease, and 2800 would not.

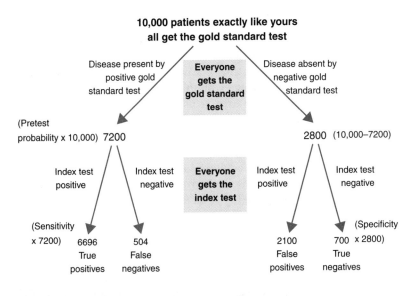

FIGURE 3.3 The tree method of calculating post-test probability.

ii. Assume all 10,000 patients also had a D-dimer test. Sensitivity is 0.93; using the definition of sensitivity above means that 93% of the 7200 with a PE (6696) would have a positive test, leaving 504 with a PE having a negative test. Similarly, using the specificity of 0.25 and its definition, 25% of the 2800 without a PE (700) would have a negative test, leaving 2100 without a PE having a positive test.

iii. What is the **post-test probability** of a PE *given a positive result?* This is the number of patients with a PE, out of all of the patients with a positive test, or 6696/(6696 + 2100) = 0.76. What is the **post-test probability** of a PE *given a negative result?* This is the number of patients *who still have a PE*, out of all of the patients with a negative test, or 504/(504 + 700) = 0.42. You now know what you should conclude about the patient's updated likelihood of a PE if you decide to go ahead and do the D-dimer test. But should you do the test in the first place? You need to return to the threshold model with this new information. However, there is an alternative way to get to the post-test probability that in some cases is easier: the odds-likelihood ratio method.

e. **Using Odds-Likelihood Ratio**

i. Although uncertainty is usually expressed as a probability, it can easily be converted to **odds,** which is defined as the probability of an event occurring divided by the probability of the same event not occurring. The formulas for converting back and forth between probability and odds are simple and are given in Figure 3.2.

ii. The main reason to do this is that it gives you a very easy way to calculate post-test probability. The formula is *post-test odds = pre-test odds × likelihood ratio*, using likelihood ratio positive or negative, depending on the particular test result.

iii. Using the example of possible PE and D-dimer, convert pre-test probability to pre-test odds:

pre-test odds = 0.72/(1 - 0.72) = 2.6

If the D-dimer test is positive:

post-test odds = 2.6 × 1.24 = 3.2

To convert odds back to post-test probability:

probability = 3.2/(1 + 3.2) = 0.76

This is the same answer obtained by using the tree method. Similarly, if the D-dimer test is negative:

post-test odds = 2.6 × 0.28 = 0.73

Converting odds back to post-test probability:

probability = 0.73/(1 + 0.73) = 0.42

This is, again, the same answer obtained with the tree method. Not only is the arithmetic somewhat easier with this odds-likelihood ratio method, but it also becomes very easy to substitute different pre-test odds to see the effect of applying the same test to different patients or to substitute different likelihood ratios to see the impact of choosing different tests.

3. Applying this to the threshold model

a. After calculating the possible post-test probabilities, positive and negative, what is done about doing the D-dimer test? The probabilities are placed on the continuum, along with the pre-test probability of 0.72 and the treatment threshold of 0.17 (Fig. 3.1H). In this case, even a negative D-dimer result would be well above the treatment threshold, even if you were not sure precisely what that threshold value should be. Given this, your conclusion should be that the D-dimer test would not be useful to do for the patient because it would not change any action you would take. You would in fact need a more accurate test or combination of tests, one that would move you further to the left along the continuum, to accomplish that.

b. In general, how far you move left along the continuum is determined by the sensitivity of a test (or likelihood ratio negative), so you need one with a higher sensitivity (or lower likelihood ratio negative); conversely, how far you move right along the continuum is determined by the specificity (or likelihood ratio positive).

4. Receiver operating characteristic (ROC) curve

  a. Rather than consider sensitivity and specificity using a single cutoff of positive versus negative for the index test, much more information is gained by examining an **ROC curve.** The cutoff level is varied, and the resulting sensitivity and speci-ficity at each level are plotted against each other; it reveals the inherent tradeoff between the two. Its value is in allowing you the flexibility to choose where you want to set the cutoff for your own patients and to know the resulting sensitivity and specificity. It also allows you to compare two or more differ-ent diagnostic tests for the same disease, because the best test has the largest area under the curve.

  b. An example of an ROC curve for D-dimer is shown in Figure 3.4.[5] Traditionally the sensitivity is plotted on the y axis from 0 to 1 and the specificity on the x axis from 1 to 0. The sensitivity and specificity that have been used so far

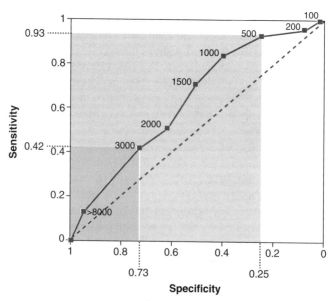

FIGURE 3.4 ROC curve for D-dimer, varying cutoff.

correspond to setting a cutoff of 500 ng/dL for positive, but you can now see what happens if you decide that a different cutoff is more relevant for your own decision making. For example, if you set a cutoff of 3000, you have improved your specificity to 0.73, but you have traded that off for a lower sensitivity of 0.42.

C. Is there an *association*? (risk, prognosis, treatment, and prevention)

1. The other epidemiologic questions that occur with patients are related to possible associations between some type of *exposure* and some type of *outcome*, although what is considered exposure and what is considered outcome changes depending on the particular question. Various common measures of association to express how strongly the two are related come from clinical studies.

2. **Risk**

   a. Does the presence of one factor increase (or decrease) the likelihood of getting a particular disease or having a particular event? This is the question of **risk**. In Problem 1, you want to know if either smoking or using OCPs is a **risk factor** for having a PE.

   b. For risk, *exposure* usually means having a risk factor among a group of people who are initially free of the disease (nonexposure is absence of the risk factor), and *outcome* is the development of the disease or occurrence of the event of interest. Look to see if there is a difference in the proportion getting the outcome, depending on exposure or nonexposure. Exposure might be an environmental toxin, a family history, or a behavior. Sometimes you look at a "protective risk"; for example, you might be interested in whether exposure to bicycle helmet use actually *decreases* the likelihood of the bad outcome of head trauma.

   c. The two most common study designs to look for a risk association are the **cohort study** and the **case-control study**.

      i. A **cohort study** starts with a group of people who are free of the outcome, some of whom have the exposure, and others do not; they are then followed forward to see how many develop the outcome and how many do not. This information is placed in a 2 × 2 table (Fig. 3.5) The following measures of association can be calculated:

Cohort studies or RCTs:

		Outcome			
		Present O^+	Absent O^-	Totals	
Exposure	Yes (cohort 1) E^+	a	b	a + b	Incidence (exposed) = $I_E^+ = \dfrac{a}{a+b}$
	No (cohort 2) E^-	c	d	c+d	Incidence (non-exposed) = $I_E^- = \dfrac{c}{c+d}$
	Totals	a + c	b + d		

Absolute risk = Incidence

$$\text{Relative risk (RR)} = \frac{\text{Incidence (exposed)}}{\text{Incidence (non-exposed)}} = \frac{\dfrac{a}{a+b}}{\dfrac{c}{c+d}}$$

Absolute risk difference (AR) = $(I_E^+) - (I_E^-)$

$$\text{Number needed to treat or harm} = \frac{1}{\text{Attributable risk}}$$

Case-control studies:

		Outcome		
		Present (case) O^+	Absent (control) O^-	Totals
Exposure	Yes E^+	a	b	a + b
	No E^-	c	d	c + d
	Totals	a + c	b + d	

Incidence **cannot be measured**.

Therefore, relative risk **cannot be measured**.

$$\text{It is estimated by the Odds Ratio (OR)} = \frac{\dfrac{a}{c}}{\dfrac{b}{d}} = \frac{a \times d}{c \times b}$$

FIGURE 3.5 Formulas for interpreting studies of risk, prognosis, treatment, and prevention.

(1) **Incidence (absolute risk):** This is the number of new cases in a population, divided by the number of people initially free of disease and potentially able to get it, over a specified time interval. There is an incidence for the cohort of people who were exposed ($I_E{}^+$), and another incidence for those not exposed ($I_E{}^-$).

(2) **Relative risk (RR):** This is the ratio of the incidence in those exposed *divided* by the incidence in those not exposed; it represents the strength of the association. An RR of 1 means no association, an RR >1 means a direct association, and an RR <1 means an inverse association. A risk factor that is linked to a bad outcome (e.g., number dying) will have an RR >1, and a risk factor that is protective against a bad outcome will have an RR <1. (Sometimes studies give their outcomes as good ones, e.g., using number surviving instead of number dying, in which case the interpretation of RR is the opposite). Whereas RR may be important in looking for risk associations, it may distort the real risk for your own particular patient who has a risk factor: if the baseline risk of a disease in a population is very low, then you may find a very high RR despite only a small actual risk for the individual patient.

(3) **Absolute risk difference (AR):** This is the *difference* in the incidence between those exposed and those not exposed and represents the individual increased risk that a person has by virtue of being exposed. This is the number that is most relevant to decision making with individual patients, but it often is not given within a study, so you must be able to calculate it yourself.

(4) **Number needed to harm (NNH):** This is 1/AR and gives information that is analogous to AR but in a way that may be more intuitive for both the patient and the physician. A low NNH means that only a few people need to be exposed for one person to have a bad outcome, compared with a nonexposed person, and therefore means that an individual has a high risk of the

outcome. Alternately, a high NNH means that many people need to be exposed for one person to have the bad outcome, and the individual therefore is at low risk for the outcome. What constitutes a low NNH or a high NNH? There is no single answer because it depends on the outcome and its consequences, along with the nature of reducing risk. For an outcome that is relatively minor (transient pain that resolves completely) or for which modifying the risk factor would be expensive or would itself induce harm, one would need a very low NNH to be concerned about it. However, for an outcome that is devastating (death, disabling myocardial infarction, or stroke) and a risk factor that can be modified without itself causing harm, you would then consider a much higher NNH, one that is worth intervening.

i. As an example, consider a cohort study that looked at the risk of PE in women who were taking oral contraceptives.[7] Among approximately 2186 women currently using OCPs who were followed for 10 years, there were 5 new cases of PE; among approximately 82,924 women who never used OCPs there were 76 new cases. After putting this information in a 2 × 2 table (Fig 3.6), an RR of 2.5, an AR of 0.0014, and an NNH of 714 can be calculated. An interpretation of this would be that there is a direct association between OCP use and a PE (RR >1), but the magnitude of risk for an individual user is not high. This is because the AR means that a user has only a 0.0014 increased risk over 10 years of having a PE, compared with a nonuser; the NNH means that for every 729 users, only 1 will have a PE over 10 years who would not otherwise have had one if she did not use an OCP. This is not a very high risk.

ii. An alternative to the cohort study design is the **case-control study,** in which a group of participants who have already had the outcome is entered ("cases"), along with another group that is comparable with the exception that the group has *not* had the outcome ("controls"). The groups, having been defined on the basis of outcome, can

		Outcome		
		PE	No PE	Totals
Exposure	OCP users	5	2,181	2,186
	OCP non-users	76	82,848	82,924
	Totals	81	85,029	92,110

$$I_E^+ = \frac{5}{2,186} = 0.00229/10 \text{ years} \qquad I_E^- = \frac{76}{82,924} = 0.00092/10 \text{ years}$$

$$\text{Relative risk (RR)} = \frac{0.00229}{0.00092} = 2.5$$

$$\text{Absolute risk difference (AR)} = 0.00229 - 0.00092 = 0.0014/10 \text{ years}$$

$$\text{Number needed to harm (NNH)} = \frac{1}{0.0014} = 714/10 \text{ years}$$

FIGURE 3.6 Example of measuring risk in a cohort study.

then be observed backward to see how many in each group had been exposed in the past. Place this information in another 2 × 2 table (see Fig. 3.5). The advantages of this over the cohort study are that it is generally less expensive, faster (particularly important in the setting of a toxin or infectious epidemic), and may be the only reasonable way to deal with rare diseases (as there may be too few outcomes to be able to have a successful cohort study). The main disadvantage is that it is potentially prone to many more biases in design and execution and must be read very carefully for assessing validity. The other disadvantage is that, because it involves participants who already have or do not have the outcome incidence of outcome cannot be measured; therefore, RR, AR, or NNH cannot be measured. There is only one measure of association:

iii. This is the **odds ratio (OR).** This is the ratio of the odds of exposure among the cases divided by the odds of exposure among the controls. If the study is valid, and if the disease is relatively rare (prevalence <0.01 in the unexposed population), it is a close approximation of the relative risk. Unfortunately, like the RR it does not allow one to know what the actual increased risk is for the individual patient, so it limits the practical information considerably. (If you know the risk of disease in the baseline population of patients similar to yours, you can infer the AR and NNH, but this may be very inaccurate.)

(1) As an example, one case-control study also looked at association between PE and OCP use.[8] The researchers found 26 cases of PE and 111 comparable controls without a PE. Among the cases, 17 were contraceptive users; among the controls, 25 were contraceptive users. Placing this information in a 2 × 2 table (Fig. 3.7), you can calculate an odds ratio of 6.5. The interpretation is that there is a direct association between OCP use and a PE.

3. Prognosis

a. A **prognosis** attempts to **predict** the future for someone who already has a disease. In Problem 1, you want to know what this patient can expect in the future if she currently has a PE.

b. For prognosis studies, *exposure* means having a disease (nonexposure means not having the disease), and *outcome*

		Outcome		
		Cases PE	Controls No PE	Totals
Exposure	OCP users	17	25	42
	OCP non-users	9	86	95
	Totals	26	111	137

$$\text{Odds Ratio (OR)} = \frac{\dfrac{17}{9}}{\dfrac{25}{86}} = \frac{17 \times 86}{9 \times 25} = 6.5$$

FIGURE 3.7 Example of measuring risk in a case-control study.

means a later complication related to the disease. Prognosis studies are sometimes called **natural history** studies, although this can be misleading because patients are often getting some treatment for the disease. Although there are some similarities between risk and prognosis, the main difference is that with "risk" the patients are exposed at a time they are disease-free, and with "prognosis" the exposure starts by having the disease. These terms also generally reflect different medical concerns. With risk, you are most often interested in seeing if there is something that can be modified with the goal of preventing a disease in the future. With prognosis, there is rarely something that can be modified, and you are more interested in knowing what to expect, with the goal being able to inform the patient and be alert for specific problems. In addition, outcomes tend to be relatively infrequent in risk studies and relatively frequent in prognosis studies.

c. Because prognosis considers future problems in someone starting out with an exposure, these are always grouped into **cohort studies**. The same measures of association as with risk are often used: incidence, RR, AR, and NNH, comparing people with a disease to those without a disease. Other measures that are commonly used are survival (Kaplan-Meier) curves and mortality rates (such as 5-year survival).

d. Also consider **prognostic factors**, specific characteristics of patients with a disease that make it more or less likely that they will have an outcome of interest. In that case, exposure is defined as having a disease *and* having a prognostic factor, and nonexposure is having the disease but *not* having the prognostic factor.

e. One PE study[9] followed 2454 patients with acute PE and found that the mortality rate at 3 months was 15.3%. The investigators discovered there were several prognostic factors that increased the likelihood of dying during this time: age >70 years (RR = 1.6), presence of cancer (RR = 2.3), congestive heart failure (RR = 2.4), chronic obstructive pulmonary disease (RR = 1.8), hypotension (RR = 2.9), and tachypnea (RR = 2.0).

4. Treatment

a. Treatment considers if making an intervention will change what happens to a patient. Although treatment includes giving drugs or performing surgery, it is important to think of it more broadly as any type of intervention. This can include actions as diverse as:

i. Counseling about smoking cessation (an individual intervention).

ii. Fluoridating water to prevent dental caries (a societal intervention).

iii. Raising taxes on cigarettes (a societal intervention).

b. For treatment, *exposure* generally means receiving an intervention (nonexposure being no intervention), with *outcome* being occurrence of a disease or other event of interest. In some studies there may be multiple categories of exposure representing alternative treatments rather than a nonexposure group. Either way, the proportion getting the outcome in each group is compared to see if there is a difference.

c. Treatment questions are studied using a **randomized controlled study design.** This is similar to a cohort study, except that the participants do not choose whether they are exposed; this is done by the researcher, using some chance method. Having been assigned to one exposure group or another, the patients are then followed, and the number in each group getting the outcome is recorded. The advantage of this over cohort studies is that, ideally, the randomization process should make each exposure group identical as far as likelihood of developing the outcome, *except for the possible effect of the exposure itself.* This does not always happen, but when it does it eliminates biases that can be present in cohort studies.

d. As with cohort studies, the numbers measured are placed in a 2 × 2 table (see Fig 3.5), and the following measures of association are calculated.

i. **Incidence.** This is the same as in cohort studies.

ii. **RR.** This is the same as in cohort studies. Sometimes a study will report the **relative risk reduction (RRR).** This is 1 - RR and indicates by what percentage the likelihood of a bad outcome is reduced in the exposed group compared with the nonexposed group. As with cohort studies, RRR gives a measure of the strength of association but does not give the relevant information to apply to individual patient benefit.

iii. **AR.** This is the same as in cohort studies and is sometimes referred to as the **absolute risk reduction (ARR).** This indicates the actual amount of benefit a person will get because of the treatment itself and is therefore the number that is important in applying a study's information to an individual patient. As with cohort studies, this number frequently is not given so you have to be able to calculate it yourself.

iv. **Number needed to treat (NNT).** This is 1/AR and gives information analogous to AR, but like NNH it may be more intuitive to use. A low NNT means that only a few people need to be treated for one person to have a good outcome, compared with a nonexposed person, and therefore means that an individual has a high likelihood of benefiting from treatment. A high NNH means that many people need to be treated unnecessarily for one person to get benefit, and the individual therefore is at low likelihood for being helped. As with NNH, there is no single number for NNT that is acceptable for all diseases and all treatments. For a benefit that is relatively minor or for which the treatment would be expensive or could itself induce harm, a very low NNT would be required to consider a treatment worthwhile. However, for preventing an outcome that is devastating and a treatment that itself is not harmful or expensive, a much higher NNT is needed to not consider the treatment.

e. With respect to Problem 1, consider the best way to treat a PE. A study[10] compared 6 weeks of oral anticoagulant therapy with 6 months of the same therapy: 107 participants with a first-time PE were enrolled, with 56 randomized to receive treatment for 6 weeks and 51 randomized to 6 months. Follow-up was for the next 2 years, with the outcome measure being recurrent PE. In the 6-week group there were 15 episodes of recurrent PE, and in the 6-month group there were 7 episodes of recurrent PE. Putting this information into a 2 × 2 table (Fig. 3.8), the measures of association can be calculated: RR = 1.93, ARR = 0.13, and NNT = 7.7. In addition, there was no difference in anticoagulation side effects between the groups. Because the outcome measured in this treatment study was a "bad" one, an interpretation of this would be:

  i. There is a harmful relationship between short-term anti-coagulation and prevention of recurrent PE, compared with the longer treatment (RR >1).

 ii. Using the long-term anticoagulation provides a fairly high likelihood of benefiting the individual patient (the AR means that there is a 13% lower chance of a PE in the next 2 years if long-term treatment is used as com-pared with short-term treatment).

iii. The NNT means that around eight people need to be treated with long-term anticoagulation unnecessarily in

		Outcome		Totals
		Recurrent PE	No recurrent PE	
Exposure	6 weeks of anticoagulant	15	41	56
	6 months of anticoagulant	7	44	51
	Totals	22	85	107

$$I_E^+ = \frac{15}{56} = 0.27/2 \text{ years} \qquad I_E^- = \frac{7}{51} = 0.14/2 \text{ years}$$

$$\text{Relative risk (RR)} = \frac{0.27}{0.14} = 1.93$$

Absolute risk difference (AR) = 0.27 − 0.14 = 0.13/2 years

$$\text{Number needed to treat (NNT)} = \frac{1}{0.13} = 7.7/2 \text{ years}$$

FIGURE 3.8 Example of measuring benefit in a treatment study.

order to prevent a PE in one patient as compared with short-term anticoagulation. If you believe this study is valid, a reasonable conclusion is that long-term treatment is the better approach.

5. **Prevention and screening**

   a. Both of these should be considered subcategories of treatment because they constitute intervening in a person's life with the goal of having better health in the future. Look for randomized controlled trials as evidence that a purported prevention maneuver or screening test is worthwhile. Cohort studies are particularly prone to bias with prevention and screening and should never in themselves be considered definitive proof of benefit.

   b. Because study design is the same as for treatment, use the same measures of association (RR, AR, and NNT) in deciding whether to advocate these interventions.

   c. Screening tests, because they are recommended to be widely used across an asymptomatic population, have other criteria that must be met (Fletcher and Fletcher,[1] Chapter 9):

      i. The disease should represent a substantial burden at the public health level.

      ii. The disease should have a prevalent asymptomatic **critical point** (a point in the course of the disease where there is evidence that intervening earlier will result in a better outcome than intervening later).

      iii. This critical point must be recognizable by some test.

      iv. A good screening test should be available: it must have reasonable sensitivity, specificity, and predictive value; it must have low risk and low cost; and it must be acceptable to both the screener and person screened.

      v. Curative potential should be substantially better in early compared with advanced stages of disease.

      vi. Treatment of screen-detected patients should improve outcome as measured by cause-specific mortality rate, functionality, and quality of life.

      vii. Patients in whom an early diagnosis is achieved will comply with your subsequent recommendations and treatment regimens.

IV. Decision Making in Uncertainty: Decision Analysis

A. When we face decisions that have tradeoffs, it may be obvious whether the benefits of one option outweigh the drawbacks. However, in medicine the complexity of decisions may make it impossible to use intuition as the sole guide to the best choice. This may be due to the intricate ramifications of any one decision, to the various ways that different patients may value different outcomes, or to a combination of both. In these difficult situations, **decision analysis** may be a helpful tool to inform (but not substitute for) decision making (Sox et al,[4] Chapter 6).

B. As an example of how this technique could be used, consider whether to treat the patient in Problem 1 with long-term anticoagulation. The main potential benefit is preventing a future PE that could be fatal. However, this has to be balanced against the bleeding risks associated with anticoagulation use, which could result in a major but nonfatal stroke, among other complications. What makes the decision even more difficult is that, even after testing, it may not be certain that the patient actually has a PE, so there is risk of causing a stroke in someone who potentially would not benefit from the treatment. How do we put all of this together?

C. A simplified version of a decision analysis for addressing this is shown in Figure 3.9. The first step is to diagram the problem in a **decision tree,** a graphic device that shows the decisions or choices that have to be made, the chance events that can ensue, the probabilities of each chance event, and the eventual outcomes. Decision points are shown with boxes, and chance events (not under the control of the decision maker) are shown with circles. At the end of each branch is the ultimate outcome of traveling down that pathway.

D. After creating the tree, you need to find information on the probability of each chance event and then assign a value to each outcome. By straightforward arithmetic, it is then possible to determine which decision option is, on average, most likely to result in the best outcome (Sox et al,[4] Chapter 6).

E. An important piece of this approach is that it allows you to take into account an individual patient's values for different health outcomes and to measure the patient's preferences for health states. This allows you to use the generic decision tree information (the chance events and probabilities) and then individualize the

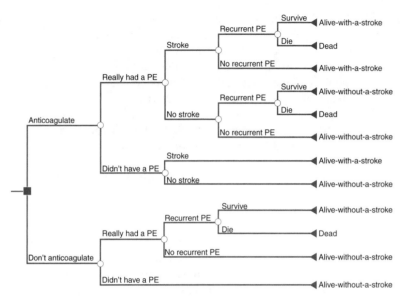

FIGURE 3.9 Simplified decision tree for a PE.

tree to the particular values and personality of your patient. Techniques for this are described in standard textbooks (e.g., Sox et al,[4] Chapters 7 and 8). The answer units are **utilities** (a measure of quality of life) and **quality-adjusted life expectancy** (which takes the actual life expectancy in a given health state and adjusts it downward, based on how bad that health state is for your particular patient).

V. Costs and Cost-Effectiveness

A. If there were no limits on the resources used to deliver health care, the relative costs of different tests and treatments would not need to be considered. For example, on a societal level, there are limits to the amount of money the U.S. government has available to fund Medicare. On a hospital level, there are limits to the number of intensive care unit (ICU) beds available at any given moment. Both of these factors can result in someone needing to make a choice in what care to cover or who should be given an ICU bed. It is in a situation of limited resources that considering **cost-effectiveness** is of value.

B. "Cost-effectiveness" is a term that is frequently used incorrectly.[11] A strategy or approach to a medical problem cannot be described as cost-effective in isolation; cost-effectiveness always requires comparing two or more treatment options (even if one of the options is "do nothing" as there are still costs that result from doing nothing that need to be considered).

C. Other erroneous uses are equating "cost-effective" solely with the most effective approach or with the least costly approach.

D. A strategy can be described properly as "cost-effective" in two situations:

    1. It is *both* more effective *and* less costly than the alternative. This option should always be chosen, but this situation is unusual because in medicine it tends to cost more to get more effectiveness.

    2. It is *more effective* but also *more costly*. However, the increased cost is low enough to make it worthwhile to get that increased effectiveness. This is the more common situation, but it creates a problem because it is not obvious how much is reasonable to spend to get a unit of effectiveness. For this reason, **cost-effectiveness analyses** often do not give an answer as to what is the best strategy but merely inform the decision maker of the relative costs; the ultimate decisions of what to fund have to be based on other issues, which commonly include social equity, ethics, and politics.

E. For this reason, in most cases cost-effectiveness analysis results do not give a direct answer as to what to do with a patient, and in fact there may be a tension between what is in society's best interest and what is in your own patient's best interest. Nevertheless, physicians have a responsibility to society as well as to individual patients; they cannot ignore issues of cost.

F. The proper measure of cost-effectiveness analysis is **marginal** (or **incremental**) **cost-effectiveness**, which is the *increased* amount that must be paid to obtain one unit of effectiveness as compared with the next cheapest strategy. This gives the correct picture of what benefits are provided as resources are diverted to increasingly expensive options. This is in contrast to **average cost-effectiveness** (the cost of a particular strategy divided by its effectiveness), which will often be misleadingly low and does not give any comparative information.

G. Costing needs to consider both the immediate cost of a particular treatment or test and the downstream costs that are incurred because of a particular choice. Costs should be comprehensive, including drug or test costs, physician fees, hospital fees, and any other resources that can be used ("opportunity costs"). Effectiveness units can be anything that is clinically meaningful, but the most common one is **quality-adjusted life expectancy.** The advantage of using the same unit of effectiveness in most cost-effectiveness analyses is that it allows direct comparisons of very disparate options (e.g., childhood immunizations versus screening treadmill tests in middle-aged men).

H. As an example, consider Problem 2, the question of whether to advocate screening mammography for women in their 40s as compared with women in their 50s. A study[12] addressed this by comparing three options: no screening, annually screening women age 50–69 years, and annually screening women age 40–69 years. The results are shown in Figure 3.10.

1. The **marginal cost-effectiveness** means that $45,700 must be spent for each *additional* year of life gained by screening women ages 50–69 years as compared with no screening. Furthermore, an *additional* $159,000 must be spent for each *additional* year of life then gained by screening women ages 40–69 years as compared with screening women ages 50–69 years.

Strategy	Cost ($ millions)	Effectiveness (Total life-years)	Marginal cost (additional $ millions)	Marginal effectiveness (additional years of life)	Average CE ($/year of life)	Marginal CE (additional $/additional year of life gained)
	A	B	C	D	A/B	C/D
No screening	27.03 _A1_	241,950 _B1_	—	—	$112	
50-69 annual	42.08 _A2_	242,279 _B2_	15.05 _(A2-A1)_	329 _(B2-B1)_	$174	$45,700
40-69 annual	52.27 _A3_	242,343 _B3_	10.19 _(A3-A2)_	64 _(B3-B2)_	$216	$159,000

FIGURE 3.10 Example of CE analysis (in a hypothetical population of 10,000 women).

Although the **average cost-effectiveness** looks trivially different among the different strategies, once the marginal cost-effectiveness is examined, you see that in fact almost all of the effectiveness in expanding the screening age down to 40 years is still coming from screening the women who are older than 50 years.

2. What is the right choice? Although there is not a single "reasonable" marginal cost-effectiveness, many people set an upper limit between $50,000 and $100,000 per additional year of life gained. Given that, one interpretation of these results would be that screening women 50–69 years is definitely worth the increased cost, but as there are limited dollars in the United States that can be used for screening as well as all other health care, it is too expensive to divert the money to screening women 40–49 years; instead those resources could be used more efficiently elsewhere (e.g., trying to get more women in their 50s to get screened.)

 MENTOR TIPS

- The core idea of clinical epidemiology is that issues such as diagnosis and treatment outcome are uncertain for individual patients, are therefore expressed as probabilities, and are best estimated by referring to past experience with groups of similarpatients.
- Information from (ideally large) studies is taken and possibly applied one-on-one with each individual patient.
- Most tests in medicine are not perfect; those that are tend to be invasive, expensive, or autopsies (usually not the ideal diagnostic approach). The accuracy of an imperfect test is measured in two ways: sensitivity/specificity and likelihood ratios.
- With questions of treatment, will making an intervention change what happens to a patient? Although treatment certainly includes giving drugs or performing surgery, it is important to think of it more broadly as any type of intervention.
- In prevention and screening, randomized controlled trials are the best evidence that a purported prevention maneuver or screening test is worthwhile. Cohort studies are particularly prone to bias with prevention and screening and should never in themselves be considered definitive proof of benefit.
- When there are decisions that have tradeoffs, it may be obvious whether the benefits of one option outweigh the

drawbacks. However, in medicine the complexity of decisions may make it impossible to use intuition as the sole guide to the best choice. In these difficult situations, decision analysis may be a helpful tool to inform (but not substitute for) decision making.

- A strategy or approach to a medical problem cannot be described as "cost-effective" in isolation; cost-effectiveness always requires comparing two or more treatment options (even if one of the options is "do nothing").
- Marginal (or incremental) cost-effectiveness (which is the increased amount that must be paid to obtain one unit of effectiveness as compared with the next cheapest strategy) is usually more important than average cost-effectiveness.
- Definitions of cost need to consider the immediate cost of a particular treatment or test as well as the downstream costs that are incurred because of the particular choice and the opportunity costs (the other activities could have been done with the money).

References

1. Fletcher RH, Fletcher SW. Clinical epidemiology: The essentials, 3th ed. Lippincott Williams & Wilkins, 2005.
   This is an extremely clear and practical introductory textbook on the principles of clinical epidemiology and their direct use in patient care. Its great strength is its clinical (rather than research) focus and organization, with excellent use of medical examples. All clinicians would benefit from reading this, and it could be considered a core piece of a personal medical library.
2. Guyatt G, Drummond R (eds). Evidence-based medicine working group, users' guides to the medical literature: A manual for evidence-based clinical practice. AMA Press, 2002.
   This is a reference that presents formal but practical methods for finding and evaluating medical literature critically.
3. Guyatt G, Drummond R (eds). Evidence-based medicine working group, users' guides to the medical literature: Essentials of evidence-based clinical practice. AMA Press, 2002.
   A concise pocket-sized version of the preceding textbook.
4. Sox HC, Blatt MA, Higgins MC, et al. Medical decision making. American College of Physicians, 2007.

This is a very straightforward introduction to decision analysis and cost-effectiveness analysis and the ways to quantify individual patient preferences for health states and incorporate those preferences into medical decisions.

5. Goldhaber SZ, Simons GR, Elliott CG, et al. Quantitative plasma D-dimer levels among patients undergoing pulmonary angiography for suspected pulmonary embolism. Journal of the American Medical Association 270:2819–2822, 1993.

6. Le Gal G, Righini M, Roy PM, et al. Prediction of pulmonary embolism in the emergency department: The revised Geneva score. Annals of Internal Medicine 144:165–171, 2006.

7. Grodstein F, Stampfer MJ, Goldhaber SZ, et al. Prospective study of exogenous hormones and risk of pulmonary embolism in women. Lancet 348:983–987, 1996.

8. Parkin L, Skegg DC, Wilson M, et al. Oral contraceptives and fatal pulmonary embolism. Lancet 355:2133–2134, 2000.

9. Goldhaber SZ, Visani L, De Rosa M. Acute pulmonary embolism: Clinical outcomes in the International Cooperative Pulmonary Embolism Registry (ICOPER). Lancet 353:1386–1389, 1999.

10. Schulman S, Rhedin AS, Lindmarker P, et al. A comparison of six weeks with six months of oral anticoagulant therapy after a first episode of venous thromboembolism. New England Journal of Medicine 332:1661–1665, 1995.

11. Doubilet P, Weinstein MC, McNeil BJ. Use and misuse of the term "cost effective" in medicine. New England Journal of Medicine 314:253–256, 1986.
This term has become a catchword in recent years, but at the expense of major misunderstanding about its meaning, interpretation, and proper application. This article very clearly points out the correct and incorrect ways to use the term.

12. Salzmann P, Kerlikowski K, Phillips K. Cost-effectiveness of extending screening mammography guidelines to include women 40 to 49 years of age. Annals of Internal Medicine 127:955–965, 1997.

See the testbank CD for more self-test questions.

Prevention and Screening

Gary J. Martin, MD

I. Epidemiology

A. The general principles that apply to screening are listed in Box 4.1. Frequency and severity of the disease and a long latency period where the disease can be found (or risk factors treated effectively) are key principles.

BOX 4.1

Principles of Screening

- Find disease early while curable (long latency)
- Focus on common problems, major burden of illness
- Consider cost/benefit issues
- Does it make a difference, or did you just find out about it?

B. Table 4.1 lists the lifetime cumulative risk of a number of conditions for which screening is done. This helps put into perspective what the potential yield is and why, as the number gets smaller, false positives become a significant counterbalancing factor for benefit.

TABLE 4.1

Lifetime Cumulative Risks

Pathology	Lifetime Cumulative Risk
Breast cancer for women	10%
Colon cancer	6%
Cervical cancer*	2%
Domestic violence for women	Up to 15%
Hip fracture for white women	16%

*Assuming an unscreened population

C. While thinking critically about tests, remember that:

> Tobacco use, diet and activity, and alcohol use represent the majority of factors for preventable deaths and close to half of all deaths. That is why general counseling is an important preventive measure in addition to screening tests. In fact, probably the single greatest accomplishment a physician can achieve for patients is to help them quit smoking.

D. Box 4.2 lists some of the benefits of screening and prevention. This can help physicians prioritize and make decisions on what to include in their efforts. Some examples of these different measures follow.

  1. Number needed to screen: using a DEXA machine to screen for osteoporosis and then treating patients, one would have to screen 731 women age 65 to 69 years in order to prevent one hip fracture.

  2. The related number of **absolute impact** can be exemplified by looking at breast cancer screening. A meta-analysis of all of the Swedish mammography trials for breast cancer noted that approximately **1.2 fewer women per thousand** would die from breast cancer with screening for women age 40 to 70 years if they were screened over a 12-year period.

  3. Although a different population is involved, it is interesting to compare the preceding number to the approximately **three lives per thousand** saved from colon cancer death in a population of 50- to 75-year-olds screened with annual fecal occult blood testing (8.8/1000 versus 5.9/1000). Based on this, colon cancer screening may actually save more women's lives than mammography. The relative impact

---

BOX 4.2

Methods of Measuring Health Benefits

- Number of patients needed to screen in order to prevent one event
- Absolute and relative impact on morbidity and mortality
- Cost per year of life saved
- Increase in average life expectancy for a population

often sounds more impressive, but both figures are important. The relative impact for occult blood testing from the same data can be stated as a 30% reduction in colon cancer deaths.

4. Cost per year of life data have been estimated for many screening and prevention strategies. Typically, strategies that cost less than $30,000–$50,000/year of life saved are considered "cost-effective." One example at this threshold of approximately $30,000/year of life saved is alendronate use for a 65-year-old woman with osteoporosis.

E. Table 4.2 lists the increases in life expectancy for a population for a number of screening procedures.

F. There are two important concepts to keep in mind while looking at this list:

1. The first is that the average time increase actually applies to no one. In reality, the majority of people screened will not derive any benefit, or possibly a slight negative, from false positives. There will be a small subset of patients who benefit a great deal from being screened. These numbers average out to the reported value. One example is cervical cancer patients. Pap smears cannot benefit the 98% of women who will never get cancer of the cervix, but for the 2% who would develop

TABLE 4.2	Estimated Average Increase in Life Expectancy for a Population
Test or Intervention	**Increase**
Mammography:	
Women 40–50 years old	0–5 days
Women 50–70 years old	1 month
Pap smears 18–65 years old	2–3 months
Screening treadmill for asymptomatic men 50 years old	8 days
Prostate-specific antigen (PSA) and digital rectal examination for men over 50 years old	Up to 2 weeks
Getting a 35-year-old smoker to quit	3–5 years
Beginning regular exercise for 40-year-old men (30 minutes 3 times a week)	9 months to 2 years

cervical cancer, Pap smears may lead to preventing invasive cervical cancer and add as much as 25 years onto those individuals' lives.

2. The second is that although the average numbers appear modest, they are averaged over the entire population so that the number of patient months is a fairly large number. Some physicians have recommended that the gain of a month for a preventive strategy aimed at the general population represents an important intervention.

II. Diseases for Which to Screen in Most Adults

A. The U.S. Preventive Services Task Force (USPSTF) has attempted to balance all these issues rigorously. Table 4.3 lists the majority of its recommendations. However, there are additional procedures to consider for individuals at higher risk for a given disease than

TABLE 4.3	Clinical Preventive Services Recommended by the USPSTF for Normal-Risk Adults
Screening	
Blood pressure, height, and weight	• Periodically, 18 years and older
Cholesterol	• Men, every 5 years, 35 years and older • Women, every 5 years, 45 years and older
Diabetes	• Periodically, adults with hypertension or hyperlipidemia
Pap smear	• Women, every 1–3 years, within 3 years of onset of sexual activity, or 21–65 years old
Chlamydia	• 18–25 years old
Mammography	• Every 1–2 years, 40 years and older
Colorectal cancer	• Periodically, 50 years and older (fecal occult blood annually, and/or sigmoidoscopy every 5 years, or colonoscopy every 10 years) depending on family history
Osteoporosis	• Women, routinely ≥65 years old or ≥60 years old at increased risk for fractures
Abdominal aortic aneurysm	• Once in men who have ever smoked 65–75 years old using ultrasound
Alcohol use	• Periodically, 18 years and older
Vision, hearing	• Periodically, 65 years and older

TABLE 4.3

Clinical Preventive Services Recommended by the USPSTF for Normal-Risk Adults (Continued)

Immunization (www.cdc.gov/nip/recs/adult-schedule.htm)

HPV	• Females <26 years old: three doses
Tetanus-diphtheria (Td)	• Every 10 years, 18 years and older (substitute one Tdap)
Varicella (VZV)	• Susceptibles only—Two doses, 18 years and older
Measles, mumps, rubella (MMR)	• One dose, 18-50 years old if not given series as child or born before 1957
	• Women of childbearing age: **caution**
Pneumococcal	• One dose, 65 years and older
Influenza	• Yearly, 50 years and older
Meningococcal, hepatitis A and B	• Can be considered based on risk

Chemoprevention

Aspirin	Discuss aspirin to prevent cardiovascular (CV) events: CV risk needs to be enough to justify it
	• Men, periodically, 40 years and older
	• Women, periodically, 50 years and older (especially >65 years)
Breast cancer chemoprevention	Discuss breast cancer chemoprevention with women at high risk

Counseling

Calcium intake	• Women, periodically, 18 years and older
Folic acid	• Women of childbearing age, 18–50 years old
Tobacco cessation, drug and alcohol use, STDs and HIV, nutrition, physical activity, sun exposure, oral health, injury prevention (loaded handgun, seat belts, bicycle helmet), and polypharmacy	• Periodically, 18 years and older; upper age limits should be individualized for each patient

In elderly patients, some measures become the priority. For example: vision, hearing, dental evaluations, immunizations (pneumococcal, influenza), fall prevention, hot water heater at less than 120 degrees, and avoidance of polypharmacy.

Adapted from U.S. Preventive Services Task Force: Guide to Clinical Prevention Services, 2nd and 3rd ed. (www.ahrq.gov/clinic/uspstfix.htm).

the general population. In general, family history and social history can identify these patients and are illustrated in the USPSTF report, which is available at www.ahrq.gov/clinic/uspstfix.htm.

B. Regarding age:

> Screening for many conditions begins at age 50 years; however, for those with a significant family history, starting 10 years earlier than when the youngest family member developed a condition is also prudent.

1. For example, if the patient's mother had colon cancer diagnosed at age 55 years, start screening as early as 45 years for the patient.

2. This 10-year advance is also reasonable for breast and prostate cancer screening (although prostate cancer screening with PSA is not mandated by the USPSTF).

C. Some interventions that the USPSTF believes are of uncertain value because of lack of data are recommended by other groups. Some examples are screening the general population for diabetes (with fasting blood sugars), domestic violence, HIV, and depression.

D. The Agency for Healthcare Research and Quality and the Centers for Disease Control and Prevention (CDC) have numerous flow sheets as part of their Put Prevention Into Practice program (www.ahcpr.gov/clinic/ppipix.htm).

E. There are fewer data about when to "sunset" some of these services.

1. Certain cancers, such as cancer of the cervix, become less common in older populations; age 65 years has been offered for consideration as a stopping point, assuming the previous recent Pap smears have been negative.

2. For breast, colon, and prostate cancer, an age of approximately 75 years may be a reasonable time to reevaluate the need for some of these procedures. Because of comorbidities and the fact that so many screening procedures' benefits set in approximately 10 years after screening, a useful approach is estimating the patient's life expectancy.

3. For some older patients with advanced comorbidities, such as severe chronic obstructive pulmonary disease (COPD), congestive heart failure, or immobility, the benefits of some

screening procedures are likely to be close to zero, and other priorities emerge if the patient's life expectancy is less than 10 years. This type of shift in focus needs to be conveyed tactfully, so the patient does not receive the wrong message. The fact that greater attention will be paid to functional capacity, activities of daily living, and optimizing their comorbidities can be explained to both patients and families.

III. Cancer

A. Screening for lung cancer and other cancers as well as coronary artery disease (CAD) with computed tomography/magnetic resonance imaging (CT/MRI) scanning has been commercialized.

  1. There is no proven benefit to lung cancer screening, and nonrandomized comparison group studies offer mixed results.

  2. A 50,000-patient National Institutes of Health (NIH)-funded randomized controlled study has started, using CT scanning for lung cancer screening. Use for abdominal cancers has not been proved.

  3. Screening for CAD with CT is very controversial and unproven but is also the subject of an ongoing 10-year Multiethnic Study of Atherosclerosis (MESA) trial funded by the NIH. Screening for CAD may be worthwhile in higher- (intermediate) risk patients with hypercholesterolemia.

B. Most authorities agree that screening for cancer of the cervix is valuable. For low-risk women, the frequency may be as seldom as every 3 years because increasing the frequency adds little benefit. However, in women at higher risk (for example, a history of multiple sexually transmitted illnesses [STIs], multiple sexual partners, dysplasia), more frequent testing is advisable.

  1. Using a cytobrush to collect cells in the cervical os markedly increases the yield of some practitioners' abilities to collect endocervical cells.

  2. The use of the liquid-based tests as part of the cervical cancer screening collection technique has become a first-line approach in many parts of the country, although its primary benefit is for women who have borderline cytology.

  3. Both the American Cancer Society (ACS) and USPSTF still recommend the traditional collection as acceptable. The USPSTF believes more data are needed before routinely using the liquid-based technologies.

C. There is a lifetime cumulative risk of approximately 10% of developing breast cancer. Pooled data from Scandinavian studies demonstrate a reduction in breast cancer deaths of approximately 1.2 women/1000 screened over a 12-year period. Approximately 5.1/1000 women who are not screened will die of breast cancer over a 12-year period versus 3.9/1000 women who are screened with mammography.

1. Mammography between the ages of 40 and 50 has always been controversial, but in the United States it has become Igenerally accepted. Although the absolute benefit in this age group is quite small and the number of false positives that lead to unnecessary biopsies is relatively large, the USPSTF has recommended that women in this age group continue to have mammography.

   a. Mammography is particularly difficult in this group because breast cancer is less common (only about 1%–1.5% of women will get breast cancer between 40 and 50 years of age), the density of premenopausal breast tissue makes the interpretation of mammography more difficult, and it may be a faster-growing tumor in this premenopausal age group when it does occur and spread earlier.

   b. Although an overall frequency between 1 and 2 years is recommended, it probably makes some sense to use the shorter interval for women between 40 and 50 years of age if one is going to screen this age group. A carefully done breast examination has been a component in some studies and probably adds value.

   c. In recent years, breast cancer deaths have been declining, presumably correlated with the marked decline in hormone replacement therapy since the Women's Health Initiative study results became available.

D. A person's lifetime cumulative risk for colon cancer is approximately 6%. The percentage is a bit lower for those without a family history and higher for those with first-degree relatives who had colon cancer at younger ages.

1. There are three accepted screening techniques for colon cancer.

   a. Fecal occult blood testing annually has led to a 15%–30% reduction in colon cancer deaths in controlled studies.

   b. Flexible sigmoidoscopy is thought to reduce colon cancer deaths by approximately 60%.

   c. Although the benefit of flexible sigmoidoscopy may last for up to 10 years, most experts would recommend a screening sigmoidoscopy every 5 years.

  2. Although colonoscopy has not had as much data regarding a mortality benefit, it is generally believed that it offers at least the potential benefit of flexible sigmoidoscopy. Colonoscopy does, however, have additional costs and risks. No head-to-head comparisons between these techniques have been performed in the same population, but the most important point is that some type of colon cancer screening be offered to patients.

> Colonoscopy is estimated to reduce colon cancer by as much as 80% by removing adenomatous polyps before they progress to colon cancer and by early detection of cancers at a curable stage.

  3. Screening generally starts at age 50 years; however, for those patients with a significant family history, starting 10 years earlier from when the youngest family member developed colon cancer is also prudent (e.g., if the patient's mother had colon cancer diagnosed at age 55, one would start as early as 45 for the patient).

  4. Either endoscopic technique may offer more benefit than fecal occult blood testing, and the choice between them can also be based on the patient's preferences and family history.

  5. Relative to flexible sigmoidoscopy, colonoscopy is more complete but is much more expensive and has a modestly increased risk.

  6. "Virtual" colonoscopy with imaging techniques is evolving, but it misses mucosal lesions and smaller polyps and cannot deal with polyps even if they are seen. It may have a role in the future.

E. The lifetime cumulative risk of prostate cancer in men in the United States is approximately 15%, with three fourths of those being diagnosed after age 65 years.

  1. The likelihood of a man in the United States dying from prostate cancer is only about 3%, so it should be clear that many men diagnosed with prostate cancer would die from other causes, particularly older men. It is also well known that at autopsy, an even higher percentage of men have occult prostate cancer that did not lead to any morbidity during their lifetime.

2. Many experts, including the USPSTF, recommend an individualized discussion between physicians and their patients
about prostate cancer screening as the risk-benefit ratio is
complicated, and therefore personal preferences weigh
highly.

3. Although the early detection of prostate cancer seems desirable,
the risks include false-positive results, unnecessary anxiety,
biopsies, and even potential complications from treating some
early cancers that may never have affected a patient's health
or well-being. These include:
   a. Erectile dysfunction.
   b. Urinary incontinence.
   c. Bowel dysfunction from surgery and radiation treatment.

4. An ongoing National Cancer Institute randomized clinical
trial expected to end later this decade may help clarify the net
benefits of prostate cancer screening. Until then the current data
are considered inconclusive.

IV. Immunizations, Chemoprevention, and Counseling

A. Childhood immunizations are covered in Chapter 26.

B. Table 4.3 lists key immunizations, chemoprevention, and counseling issues for adults. As mentioned earlier, the counseling can be
just as important as any screening test, and smoking cessation is
probably the single biggest event a clinician can help a patient
accomplish.

MENTOR TIPS DIGEST

- Tobacco use, diet and activity, and alcohol use represent the
  majority of factors for preventable deaths and close to half of
  all deaths. That is why general counseling is an important
  preventive measure in addition to screening tests. In fact,
  probably the single greatest support a physician can provide
  for patients is to help them quit smoking.

- Screening for many conditions begins at age 50 years;
  however, for those with a significant family history, starting
  10 years earlier than when the youngest family member developed a condition is also prudent.

- Colonoscopy is estimated to reduce colon cancer by as much
  as 80% by removing adenomatous polyps before they
  progress to colon cancer in addition to early detection.

Resources

Albertson R. A 72-year-old man with localized prostate cancer. Journal of the American Medical Association 274:69–74, 1995.
Ask yourself if patient is likely to live another 10 years.

CDC recommendations and guidelines: Adult immunization schedule (2007). www.cdc.gov/nip/recs/adult-schedule.htm

Clinical Preventive Services for Normal-Risk Adults Recommended by the U.S. Preventive Services Task Force. Put prevention into practice. January 2003. Agency for Healthcare Research and Quality, Rockville, Md. www.ahrq.gov/ppip/adulttm.htm

Elmore JE, Barton MB, Moceri VM, et al. Ten-year risk of false positive screening mammograms and clinical breast examinations. New England Journal of Medicine 338:1089–1096, 1998.
Of women screened with mammography, 24% had at least one false-positive result.

Harris R, Leininger L. Clinical strategies for breast cancer screening: Weighing and using the evidence. Annals of Internal Medicine 122:539–547, 1995.
Good overview of mammography data and risks. Two to four fewer 50-year-old women out of 1000 will die from breast cancer with 10 years of screening.

Olsen O, Gotzsche PC: Cochrane review on screening for breast cancer with mammography. Lancet 358:1340, 2001.
Calls into question the quality of earlier studies of mammography benefit.

U.S. Preventive Services Task Force: Screening for breast cancer: Recommendations and rationale. Annals of Internal Medicine 137:344, 2002.
Start at age 40 years.

U.S. Preventive Services Task Force. Screening for colorectal cancer: Recommendations and rationale. Annals of Internal Medicine 137:129–131, 2002.

U.S. Preventive Services Task Force. Screening for prostate cancer: A recommendation from the U.S. Preventive Services Task Force. Annals of Internal Medicine 2002 137:148, 2002.
Still an individualized decision.

Winawer SJ, Zauber AG, Ho MN, et al. Prevention of colorectal cancer by colonoscopic polypectomy. The National Polyp Study Workgroup. New England Journal of Medicine 329:1977–1981, 1993.
Compared with nonrandomized reference groups, this approach reduced colon cancer incidence by 76%–90%.

Writing Group for the Women's Health Initiative Investigators. Risks and benefits of estrogen plus progestin in healthy postmenopausal women. Journal of the American Medical Association 288:321, 2002.
Risks somewhat outweighed benefits.

Chapter Self-Test Questions

Circle the correct answer. After you have responded to the questions, check your answers in Appendix A.

1. Applying the general principles for screening, which one of the following diseases is most suitable for screening?

    a. Small cell lung cancer

    b. Ovarian cancer

    c. Pancreatic cancer

    d. Rectal cancer

2. Which one of these interventions would have the greatest population impact to decrease preventable deaths?

    a. Encourage aerobic exercise 30 minutes 3 times a week.

    b. Facilitate smoking cessation.

    c. Obtain mammography for women age 50–65 years.

    d. Perform flexible sigmoidoscopy for men age 50–75 years.

3. Screening and treatment in women for which of the following malignancies would yield the greatest impact on longevity?

    a. Ovaries

    b. Colon

    c. Breast

    d. Cervical

See the testbank CD for more self-test questions.

CHAPTER

PREOPERATIVE EVALUATION

Michael Kornfeld, MD, and Kevin O'Leary, MD

I. Overview

A. The purposes of the preoperative evaluation:

1. To assess the patient's risk for surgery
2. To take measures to reduce this risk

B. Communicating the assessment and plan to the surgeon and patient is critical. The more specific and concise the recommendations, the more likely the recommendations will be followed.

C. Anesthesia is generally safe, with an overall mortality rate of <0.3%. The choice of anesthetic is best left to the anesthesiologist. It is important for the medical consultant to have a basic understanding of anesthetic techniques.

1. General anesthesia is drug-induced reversible absence of sensation and consciousness. This is usually done using inhaled anesthetics delivered through an endotracheal tube. Neuromuscular blocking agents are often used.

2. Neuroaxial anesthesia includes spinal and epidural anesthesia.

   a. Spinal anesthesia is accomplished by injecting local anesthetics and/or opioids into the subarachnoid space using a needle or catheter.

   d. Epidural anesthesia is accomplished by injecting local anesthetics and/or opioids into the epidural space.

   i. Both carry a very small risk of epidural hematoma; therefore, the effect of antiplatelet agents and antithrombotic agents needs to have worn off by the time of insertion of the needle.

59

II. Preoperative Testing

A. The general principle for all preoperative testing is that it should be done only if the results will alter clinical management.

B. Preoperative laboratory tests should be ordered for patients who would otherwise require testing, regardless of the plans for surgery. Additional factors to consider include the following.

  1. Complete blood count (CBC) may be useful as a baseline for patients expected to have a large amount of perioperative bleeding.

  2. Prothrombin time (PT) and partial thromboplastin time (PTT) are not indicated unless the patient is on anticoagulants or has a history suggestive of a bleeding disorder.

  3. Low-risk patients going for low-risk surgeries can safely proceed to surgery with no laboratory testing.

  4. If laboratory testing *is* indicated and tests have been done within the past 6 months, there is no need to repeat testing, as long as no change in the patient's clinical status has occurred.

C. Men over 40 and women over 50 years of age who are scheduled for intermediate- to high-risk surgery should have a preoperative electrocardiogram (ECG).

D. Chest x-ray (CXR) indications include symptoms or examination findings suggestive of heart or lung disease.

III. Preoperative Cardiac Assessment and Perioperative Management

A. Perioperative cardiac complications occur in 1.4% of patients 50 years of age and older. Although the incidence of cardiac complication is not very high, the mortality rate of cardiac complications is 15%–50%.

  1. Risk assessment—the Revised Cardiac Risk Index (RCRI) provides a practical method to estimate a patient's risk for cardiac complications related to surgery (Table 5.1). By adding up the number of Risk Factors in the Index, one can estimate the risk for perioperative cardiac events.

  2. Need for noninvasive testing—beyond estimating a patient's risk using the RCRI, noninvasive cardiac testing may further clarify the risk for select patients.

    a. Options for noninvasive cardiac testing include:
      i. Exercise ECG.

TABLE 5.1

Revised Cardiac Risk Index	
Risk Factor	Points
High-risk surgery*	1
Established coronary artery disease	1
Congestive heart failure	1
Cerebrovascular accident or transient ischemic attack	1
Diabetes mellitus (insulin requiring)	1
Chronic renal insufficiency (cr >2.0)	1

*Defined as intraperitoneal, intrathoracic, and suprainguinal vascular procedures.

Rates of complications in patients with 0, 1, 2, ≥3 points were 0.5%, 0.9%–1.3%, 4%–7%, and 9%–11%.

From Lee TH, Marcantonio ER, Mangione CM, et al: Derivation and prospective validation of a simple index for prediction of cardiac risk of major noncardiac surgery. Circulation 1999;100(10):1043–1049.

    ii. Exercise or dobutamine stress echocardiography.

    iii. Exercise or pharmacologically induced stress myocardial perfusion imaging.

  b. The American College of Cardiology/American Heart Association (ACC/AHA) Task Force has published evidence-based guidelines on preoperative cardiac risk assessment and management. These guidelines provide a stepwise approach to help the physician decide which patients may benefit from noninvasive cardiac testing (Fig. 5.1)

    i. Assess the urgency of surgery. If the patient needs to go to surgery emergently, there is no time for risk assessment. The medical consultant's role in this situation is to determine whether measures can be taken to reduce the risk for complications intraoperatively and postoperatively.

    ii. Determine if the patient has significant active cardiac conditions, such as unstable or severe angina, recent myocardial infarction (MI), decompensated or new-onset heart failure, high-grade arrhythmia, or severe valvular disease. If any one of these conditions is present, it should be evaluated and treated preoperatively.

    iii. Surgical procedures may be classified according to the rate of perioperative complications (Table 5.2). Cardiac

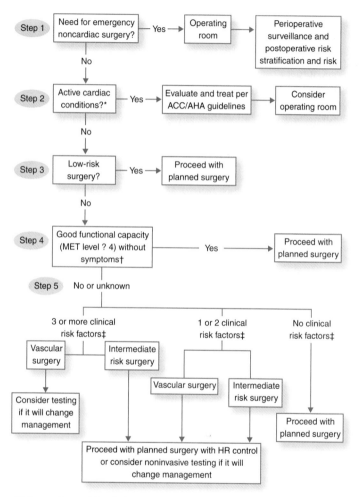

*Active cardiac conditions include unstable or severe angina, recent MI, decompensated
or new-onset heart failure, high-grade arrhythmia, or severe valvular disease.
†See Table 5.3 for estimated MET equivalent.
‡See Table 5.1 for clinical risk predictors.

FIGURE 5.1 Cardiac evaluation and care algorithm for noncardiac surgery
based on active clinical conditions, known cardiovascular disease, or cardiac
risk factors. *(Based in part on recommendations from Eagle KA, Berger PB,
Calkins H, et al: ACC/AHA guideline update for perioperative cardiovascular
evaluation for noncardiac surgery—executive summary: A report of the American
College of Cardiology/American Heart Association Task Force on Practice Guidelines [Committee to Update the 1996 Guidelines on Perioperative Cardiovascular
Evaluation for Noncardiac Surgery]. J Am Coll Cardiol 2002;39[3]:542–553.)*

TABLE 5.2	Cardiac Risk Stratification for Noncardiac Surgical Procedures
Risk Stratification	**Procedure Examples**
Vascular (reported cardiac risk often more than 5%)	Aortic and other major vascular surgery
	Peripheral vascular surgery
Intermediate (reported cardiac risk generally 1%–5%)	Intraperitoneal and intrathoracic surgery
	Carotid endarterectomy
	Head and neck surgery
	Orthopedic surgery
	Prostate surgery
Low (reported cardiac risk generally less than 1%)	Endoscopic procedures
	Superficial procedures
	Cataract surgery
	Breast surgery
	Ambulatory surgery

testing rarely changes management of patients going for low-risk procedures. It is appropriate in these cases to proceed with planned surgery without further cardiac testing.

iv. Management of patients going for vascular or intermediate-/ high-risk nonvascular surgery depends on assessment of their functional capacity. Functional capacity is measured in metabolic equivalents (METs), with <4 METs considered poor functional capacity (Table 5.3). Patients who are not symptomatic and have good functional capacity can generally proceed to planned surgery without further cardiac testing.

v. If functional capacity is poor or cannot be assessed, the decision to perform additional preoperative testing depends on presence of RCRI risk factors. If none of these risk factors is present, patients can generally proceed to planned surgery without further testing. If one or more risk factor is present, additional testing may be considered (see Fig. 5.1).

c. Keep in mind that testing should be ordered only if the results will change the physician's management. In the case of an abnormal noninvasive test result, the physician may

TABLE 5.3	Estimated Energy Requirements for Various Activities	
1 MET	**4 METs**	
Can you take care of yourself? ↓ Eat, dress, or use the ↓ toilet? ↓ Walk indoors around ↓ the house? ↓ Walk a block or two on level ground at 2–3 miles per hour?	Climb a flight of stairs or walk up a hill? ↓ Walk on level ground at ↓ 4 mph? ↓ Run a short distance? ↓ ↓ Do heavy work around the house like scrubbing floors or lifting or moving heavy furniture? Participate in activities such as golf, bowling, dancing, doubles tennis?	
4 METs	**Greater than 10 METs**	
Do light work around the house like dusting or washing dishes?	Participate in strenuous sports like swimming, singles tennis, football, basketball, or skiing?	

From Eagle KA, Berger PB, Calkins H, et al: ACC/AHA guideline update for perioperative cardiovascular evaluation for noncardiac surgery—executive summary: A report of the American College of Cardiology/American Heart Association Task Force on Practice Guidelines (Committee to Update the 1996 Guidelines on Perioperative Cardiovascular Evaluation for Noncardiac Surgery). J Am Coll Cardiol 2002;39(3):542–553.

consider revascularization, adjustment of medications, and/or postoperative surveillance for myocardial damage.

3. Determining the need for revascularization—revascularization can be accomplished with percutaneous coronary angioplasty (PTCA, with or without stent placement) or with coronary artery bypass surgery (CABG).

   a. Issues with PTCA—the majority of patients undergoing PTCA have stents placed in an effort to reduce the risk for restenosis.

      i. Studies show that patients who undergo surgery soon after stent placement may be at high risk for complications. Patients must be on two antiplatelet agents for 4–6 weeks after bare metal stent placement to allow the lumen to become endothelialized.

(1) If antiplatelet agents are stopped too early, the patient is at risk for in-stent thrombosis.

(2) If antiplatelet agents are continued perioperatively, the patient is at risk for bleeding.

ii. Drug-eluting stents have been used to further reduce risk for restenosis.

(1) Drug-eluting stents require a longer period of dual antiplatelet therapy, necessitating a longer delay before surgery can be safely performed.

b. Assessing the potential benefit of revascularization—the Coronary Artery Revascularization Prophylaxis (CARP) study evaluated whether PTCA with stent or CABG prior to major vascular surgery in high-risk patients reduced the risk of cardiac complications.

i. Revascularization prior to surgery did not reduce the risk for perioperative cardiac complications.

ii. Certain patients were excluded from the study, including patients with:

(1) Low ejection fraction.

(2) Severe aortic stenosis.

(3) Left main coronary artery disease.

4. Medication to reduce risk—studies have evaluated the potential benefit of beta blockers, alpha-2 agonists, calcium channel blockers, statins, and nitrates in reducing the risk for perioperative cardiac events.

a. Beta blockers—studies have shown reduced ischemia and mortality for high-risk patients who are treated with beta blockers perioperatively. Indications for beta blockers include:

i. Patients who are already being treated with beta blockers.

ii. Patients with abnormal results on noninvasive cardiac testing who are going for vascular surgery.

iii. Patents with known coronary artery disease who are going for vascular surgery.

iv. Patients with one or more cardiac risk factors going for vascular or intermediate-/high-risk nonvascular surgery, as defined in Table 5.2.

(1) The strength of evidence in support of the use of perioperative beta blockers varies with indication.

        (2) When possible, beta blockers should be adjusted to achieve a resting heart rate of 50–60, as long as the blood pressure tolerates.

    b. Alpha-2 agonists—clonidine has been shown to reduce perioperative cardiac events. Clonidine is most useful for patients who cannot tolerate beta-blocker treatment.

    c. Calcium channel blockers—there is evidence that these medications reduce ischemia and supraventricular tachycardia, although their use in perioperative setting is not well established.

    d. Statins—there are observational data that suggest that statins may have a protective effect in term of reducing perioperative cardiac complications.

    e. Nitrates—oral and intravenous nitrates have not been shown to decrease the risk of perioperative cardiac complications and may induce hypotension.

5. Surveillance—the majority of postoperative myocardial ischemia and infarction cases occur in the absence of typical symptoms. Unfortunately, the optimal strategy to detect perioperative ischemia remains to be determined.

    a. Postoperative ECG—for patients with known or suspected coronary artery disease who are undergoing high- or intermediate-risk procedures, the most cost-effective strategy is to obtain a 12-lead ECG immediately after surgery and on the first 2 postoperative days.

    b. Computerized ST segment monitoring—this should be considered for patients with coronary artery disease or patients undergoing vascular surgery.

    c. Cardiac markers—cardiac troponin I is useful to rule out myocardial infarction should symptoms, ECG changes, or ST monitoring suggest myocardial ischemia.

IV. Preoperative Pulmonary Evaluation, Risk Assessment, and Risk Reduction Strategies for Patients Undergoing Noncardiothoracic Surgery

A. Overview

    1. Postoperative pulmonary complications (PPCs) are common and contribute significantly to mortality and morbidity of surgical patients.

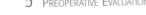

    2. PPCs predict long-term mortality.

    3. Validated patient-related and procedure-related risk factors predict PPCs.

    4. The goal of preoperative pulmonary evaluation is to identify risk factors, optimize preoperative conditions, and to anticipate postoperative interventions that may reduce risk.

B. Scope of significant pulmonary complications

    1. PPCs that are known to contribute to mortality and morbidity or prolong hospital stay include the following:

      a. Atelectasis

      b. Bronchospasm

      c. Exacerbation of chronic obstructive pulmonary disease (COPD)

      d. Pneumonia

      e. Respiratory failure with prolonged mechanical ventilation

C. Interview, physical examination, and laboratory assessment

    1. Focus of the interview

      a. Assess baseline lung disease, such as asthma, COPD, obstructive sleep apnea (OSA), and recent lung infections.

      b. Assess baseline cardiac disease, congestive heart failure (CHF) in particular.

      c. Assess baseline neuromuscular disease.

      d. Assess baseline functional status.

      e. Assess nutritional status, and identify patients with recent weight loss.

      f. Identify patients with unexplained shortness of breath or cough.

      g. Identify patients with significant alcohol use.

    2. Focus of the physical examination

      a. Assess nutritional status

      b. Baseline lung examination important for identifying patients who may need further preoperative evaluation

    3. Laboratory assessment

      a. Preoperative spirometry may be helpful in patients with active asthma, recent COPD exacerbation, or unexplained cough or shortness of breath.

      b. Preoperative arterial blood gas (ABG) is not indicated in most patients. Patients with abnormal baseline ABG are at higher risk for PPCs, but these patients can be identified as high-risk based on findings in history and/or physical examination.

    c. Chest x-ray (CXR) should be considered for:

        i. Patients over the age of 50 years scheduled for intermediate- to high-risk surgery.

        ii. Patients with a history of heart or lung disease scheduled for intermediate- to high-risk surgery.

D. Patient-related risk factors

  1. Age is an important risk factor, even after adjustment for comorbid conditions

  2. Albumin <3.5 g/dL significant independent risk factor for PPCs

  3. American Society of Anesthesiologists (ASA) class >2 (Table 5.4) identifies patients at increased (at least twofold) risk for PPCs

  4. Asthma

    a. Mild or moderate asthma is not a significant risk factor for PPCs.

    b. Risk factors for bronchospasm include recent asthma symptoms, recent treatment for active asthma, and a history of tracheal intubation.

    c. A short course of perioperative steroids does not increase the rate of PPCs in patients with asthma.

    d. For elective surgery, patients with asthma should be optimized to achieve at least 80% of personal best FEV_1 and no wheezing on lung auscultation

  5. COPD

    a. Clinical practice suggests that COPD is a risk factor for PPCs, but the magnitude of this risk is not well established.

    b. No "threshold" spirometric value has been established that should preclude surgery. Experience with lung reduction

TABLE 5.4	**The ASA Physical Status Classification**
Class 1	Healthy patient; no medical problems
Class 2	Mild systemic disease
Class 3	Severe systemic disease but not incapacitating
Class 4	Severe systemic disease that is a constant threat to life
Class 5	Moribund; not expected to live 24 hours irrespective of operation

surgery suggests that even patients with severe COPD may be appropriate candidates for surgery in selected cases.

6. CHF is an established risk factor for PPCs
7. Functional status
   a. Functional dependence defined as inability to perform activities of daily living
   b. Functional dependence is significant risk factor for PPCs
8. Obesity not an independent risk factor for PPCs
9. OSA may increase risk of PPCs
10. Smoking
    a. Cessation of smoking 2 months before surgery may decrease risk of PPCs.
    b. Cessation of smoking within 2 weeks of surgery may increase risk of PPCs.

E. Procedure-related risk factors
1. High-risk surgeries
   a. Abdominal aortic aneurysm repair
   b. Thoracic surgery
   c. Neurosurgery
   d. Upper abdominal surgery
   e. Neck surgery
   f. Vascular surgery
   g. Emergency surgery
2. Duration of surgery (over 3 hours) is independent risk factor

F. Strategies to reduce postoperative pulmonary complications
1. Optimization of baseline cardiopulmonary disease
2. Lung expansion maneuvers, including incentive spirometry and chest physical therapy, reduce risk for PPCs; chest physical therapy involves one or more of the following: deep breathing exercises, percussion and vibration, suctioning and mobilization
3. Postoperative pain control important to promote deep breathing
4. Nasogastric decompression should be used in patients post abdominal surgery who develop symptomatic abdominal distention, nausea, vomiting
5. No conclusive evidence that regional anesthesia superior to general anesthesia in terms of reducing PPCs

V. Preoperative Evaluation of Patients on Antithrombotic or Anticoagulant Therapy

A. Overview

1. Optimal perioperative management of antithrombotic or anticoagulant therapy depends on the original indication for therapy, comorbid conditions, and anticipated bleeding risk associated with the planned procedure.
2. Risk of postoperative bleeding has to be balanced against the risk of postoperative thrombosis.
3. Perioperative strategy must be designed in close consultation with the surgeon.

B. Common antithrombotic medications

1. Aspirin—mechanism of action is irreversible inhibition of platelet function
2. Clopidogrel and ticlopidine—work by inhibiting adenosine diphosphate (ADP)–dependent platelet aggregation
3. Warfarin—mechanism of action is inhibition of vitamin K–dependent clotting factors

C. Patient-specific considerations

1. Age is risk factor for venous thromboembolism
2. Prior history of bleeding raises risk for subsequent bleeding
3. Comorbid conditions
   a. Many cancers raise the risk of thrombosis.
   b. Chronic liver and kidney disease may raise the risk for hemorrhage.
4. Concurrent use of warfarin and antiplatelet agents increase risk for bleeding
5. Common indications for antiplatelet therapy
   a. Cardiac stents
   b. Stroke prevention
   c. Coronary artery disease
6. Common indications for warfarin
   a. Primary or secondary prevention of venous thromboembolism (VTE)
   b. Atrial fibrillation with or without structural heart disease
   c. Mechanical heart valve(s)
   d. Ventricular aneurysm
   e. Hypercoagulable state
   f. Inferior vena cava filter

D. Procedure-specific considerations

    1. Most dental procedures do not require discontinuation of anticoagulation.

    2. Neurosurgical procedures and other procedures that involve tissues where even minimal bleeding may result in significant morbidity and mortality require discontinuation of antiplatelet medications and warfarin.

E. Common perioperative strategies

    1. Low bleeding–risk procedures: warfarin may be continued (International Normalized Ratio [INR] should be adjusted to low end of therapeutic range); antiplatelet agents should be continued

    2. High bleeding–risk procedures

        a. Low thrombotic risk

            i. Discontinue warfarin 3–5 days before the procedure

            ii. Restart warfarin immediately post procedure if allowable from surgical standpoint

            iii. Consider IV heparin 24–48 hours after procedure if allowable from surgical standpoint and INR subtherapeutic

        b. High thrombotic risk

            i. Discontinue warfarin 3–5 days before procedure

            ii. Initiate IV heparin or subcutaneous (SQ) low molecular weight heparin (LMWH) when INR becomes subtherapeutic

            iii. Proceed with surgery when INR <1.5

            iv. Discontinue heparin 6 hours prior to procedure or LMWH 24 hours prior to procedure

            v. Start IV heparin as soon after procedure as is safe from surgical standpoint

            vi. Restart warfarin the night of procedure unless contraindicated from surgical standpoint

VI. Preoperative Evaluation and Management of Endocrine Disorders

A. Preoperative patient with diabetes mellitus

    1. Goals of preoperative assessment

        a. Identify the type and duration of diabetes.

        b. Assess adequacy of glycemic control.

        c. Identify any complications of diabetes.

        d. Evaluate cardiac and renal function.

        e. Establish strategy for perioperative glycemic control.

   2. Perioperative monitoring
      a. Patients on insulin or oral diabetic medications should have blood glucose checked before surgery, every 1–2 hours during surgery, and every 6 hours post surgery.
      b. Patients whose diabetes is controlled with diet should have their blood glucose checked preoperatively.
   3. Perioperative management of diabetic medications
      a. Oral diabetic medications should be held on day of surgery and restarted once patients resume diet
      b. Patients on insulin therapy
         i. Short-acting insulin should be held the morning of surgery and restarted once patients resume diet.
         ii. Patients should be given half to two thirds of their long-acting insulin on the day of surgery.
         iii. Many patients will require IV insulin drips during major surgery.
B. Stress dose corticosteroids
   1. Who is at risk for perioperative adrenal insufficiency?
      a. Patients with history of adrenal insufficiency, either primary or secondary
      b. Patients who have received prolonged courses of systemic corticosteroids in the year preceding surgery at risk for secondary adrenal insufficiency
         i. Patients who have received 20 mg of prednisone or an equivalent dose of another corticosteroid medication for 3 weeks or longer.
         ii. Patient who have received multiple short courses of corticosteroids in the past year.
      c. Patients with severe hyperthyroidism undergoing emergent surgery
   2. ACTH stimulation test may be helpful for assessment of hypothalamic-pituitary-adrenal axis in patients with suspected adrenal suppression
   3. Perioperative stress corticosteroid regimens for patients at risk for perioperative adrenal insufficiency
      a. Major surgery—give 100 mg IV hydrocortisone prior to surgery, then 50 mg hydrocortisone every 8 hours for 48–72 hours, then resume usual dose of steroids
      b. Minor procedure—give usual dose of steroids, no additional supplementation

C. Preoperative patient with thyroid disease
   1. Surgery in patients with hypothyroidism
      a. Mild to moderate hypothyroidism does not increase perioperative risk.
      b. Patients with severe hypothyroidism or myxedema coma should be treated prior to surgery.
   2. Surgery in patients with hyperthyroidism
      a. Mild hyperthyroidism—patients should be started on a beta blocker and proceed to surgery
      b. Severe hyperthyroidism
         i. Patients can be started on antithyroid agents and prepared for surgery in 3–8 weeks.
         ii. Patients who are hyperthyroid at the time of surgery are at risk for atrial fibrillation, adrenal insufficiency, and thyroid storm.
         iii. Thyrotoxic patients undergoing urgent surgery should be treated with antithyroid medications, beta blockers, and stress dose steroids and receive very close hemodynamic monitoring.

MENTOR TIPS

- Communicating the assessment and plan to the surgeon and patient is critical. The more specific and concise the recommendations, the more likely the recommendations will be followed.
- Anesthesia is generally safe, with an overall mortality rate of <0.3%.
- In general, preoperative testing should only be done if the results might alter clinical management.
- Men over 40 and women over 50 years of age who are planned for intermediate- to high-risk surgery should have a preoperative ECG.
- A thorough history and exam is essential in preoperative risk assessment. Special attention should be made to identifying active symptoms and underlying risk factors for cardiac disease.
- Surgeries that carry a high risk for perioperative cardiac complications include emergent surgeries, aortic and peripheral

vascular surgeries, and prolonged surgeries with large fluid shifts and/or blood loss.

- Revascularization prior to noncardiac surgery has not been shown to reduce the risk for perioperative cardiac complications.
- Beta blockers have been shown to reduce ischemia and mortality in high-risk patients.
- Cessation of smoking 2 months prior to surgery decreases the risk for postoperative pulmonary complications. However, cessation of smoking within 2 weeks of surgery may paradoxically increase risk.
- Lung expansion maneuvers reduce the risk for postoperative pulmonary complications.
- Optimal perioperative management of antithrombotic or anti-coagulant therapy depends on the original indication for therapy, comorbid conditions, and anticipated bleeding risk associated with planned procedure.
- Patients who have received prolonged courses of systemic corticosteroids in the year preceding surgery are at risk for secondary adrenal insufficiency.
- Mild hypothyroidism does not confer an increased risk for perioperative complications. Similarly, mild hyperthyroidism does not confer an increased risk for perioperative complications.

Resources

Arozullah AM, Conde MV, Lawrence VA. Preoperative evaluation for postoperative pulmonary complications. Medical Clinics of North America 87:154–173, 2003.

Cohn SL. The role of the medical consultant. Medical Clinics of North America 87:1–6, 2003.

Fleisher LA, Beckman JA, Brown KA, et al. ACC/AHA 2007 guidelines on perioperative cardiovascular evaluation and care for noncardiac surgery: Executive summary. Journal of the American College of Cardiology 50:1707–1732, 2007.

Fleisher LA, Beckman JA, Brown KA, et al. ACC/AHA 2006 guideline update on perioperative cardiovascular evaluation for noncardiac surgery: Focused update on perioperative beta-blocker therapy. Circulation 113:2662–2674, 2006.

Kaboli P, Henderson MC, White RH. DVT prophylaxis and anticoagulation in the surgical patient. Medical Clinics of North America 87:77–110, 2003.

Lee TH, Marcantonio ER, Mangione CM, et al. Derivation and prospective validation of a simple index for prediction of cardiac risk of major noncardiac surgery. Circulation 100:1043–1049, 1999.

McFalls EO, Ward HB, Moritz TE, et al. Coronary-artery revascularization before elective major vascular surgery. New England Journal of Medicine 351:2795–2804, 2004.

Schiff RL, Welsh GA. Perioperative evaluation and management of the patient with endocrine dysfunction. Medical Clinics of North America 87:175–192, 2003.

Smetana GW. Preoperative pulmonary evaluation. New England Journal of Medicine 340:937–944, 1999.

Smetana GW, Lawrence VA, Cornell JE. Preoperative pulmonary risk stratification for noncardiothoracic surgery: Systematic review for American College of Physicians. Annals of Internal Medicine 144:581–595, 2006.

Smetana GW, MacPherson DS. The case against routing preoperative testing. Medical Clinics of North America 87:7–40, 2003.

Chapter Self-Test Questions

Circle the correct answer. After you have responded to the questions, check your answers in Appendix A.

1. A 65-year-old man with history of kidney transplant, atrial fibrillation treated with warfarin, and stroke needs to undergo kidney biopsy to evaluate worsening renal function. What is the optimal perioperative strategy with respect to management of his anticoagulation?

   a. Continue warfarin throughout the operative interval.

   b. Discontinue warfarin 3–5 days before the procedure, and restart immediately after the procedure.

   c. Discontinue warfarin 3–5 days before the procedure; when INR <2 start heparin infusion until 4–6 hours before the procedure. Resume heparin infusion several hours after the procedure, and resume warfarin the night of the procedure.

   d. Discontinue warfarin 3–5 days before the procedure; when INR <2 start subcutaneous heparin 5000 units every 12 hours. Resume warfarin the night of the procedure.

2. Which of the following statements accurately describes the rationale for preoperative evaluation?

   a. Clear the patient for surgery.

   b. Order and evaluate routine preoperative tests.

   c. Recommend the safest type of anesthesia.

   d. Take measures to reduce perioperative risk.

3. A 65-year-old male with a history of hypertension will undergo cataract surgery. He has no additional past medical or surgical history or symptoms. The physical examination result is normal. His only medication is hydrochlorothiazide 25 mg daily. What preoperative test should he have?

   a. No testing

   b. Electrocardiogram

   c. Exercise cardiac stress test

   d. Exercise cardiac stress test with perfusion imaging

See the testbank CD for more self-test questions.

PART two

DIAGNOSIS AND MANAGEMENT OF COMMON OUTPATIENT SYMPTOMS

6

HEADACHE

Gary J. Martin, MD, and James J. Foody, MD

I. Background

A. Headache is one of the most common complaints a primary care clinician will encounter

B. Features

1. Only intracranial structures with sensation are meninges and circle of Willis and a few centimeters of its branches

2. Primary headache results from neurogenic mistakes in processing pain information

3. Term "vascular headaches" is a misnomer: blood vessels are not the cause of headaches, although vascular response is a component of some primary headaches
4. Episodic primary headache runs across continuum of clinical presentations from typical migraine with aura to common everyday headache that people self-treat with over-the-counter analgesics
5. Secondary headache is result of anatomical pathology

 Primary headaches arise from brain dysfunction.

C. Headache classification
   1. Primary headache
      a. Migraine
      b. "Tension-type"
      c. Chronic daily
      d. Cluster
   2. Secondary headache
      a. Increased intracranial pressure
      b. Intracerebral hemorrhage
      c. Trauma
      d. Tumor
      e. Post concussion
D. Clinical manifestation of primary headache
   1. Migraine
      a. Aura precedes a headache in fewer than 20% of all migraineurs. Aura is a neurologic disturbance of the cerebral cortex due to spreading electrochemical depression followed by cortical oligemia. Aura, especially visual aura, may precede headache onset by as much as an hour and typically lasts about 20 minutes.
      b. Migraine pain has any or all of following characteristics: throbbing; unilateral; accompanied by nausea with or without vomiting; gastroparesis; light, smell, or sound hypersensitivity; severity that is moderate or worse and lasts 4–72 hours.

c.Migraine syndrome is ~4 times more common in women. Many women have variation of frequency and severity that correlates with menses (catameneal migraine).

d. Migraine exhibits a strong familial pattern.

e. Most people with migraine will exhibit one or more of the following: tendency for motion sickness, pain on chilling of roof of mouth ("freezer brain"), ice pick–like head pains lasting for seconds, or personal history of colic in infancy.

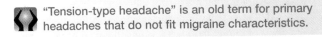 Migraine is a primary headache characterized by moderate to severe unilateral throbbing pain lasting 4–72 hours, often accompanied by nausea and vomiting.

2. "Tension-type"

    a. Hypothetical pathologic mechanism is same as migraine

        i. Studies demonstrate there is no muscle tension in "tension-type" headache.

        ii. Stress or tension as headache inducer is not different from migraine.

    b. Distinguished by lesser severity and absence of patterns typical for migraine

    c. ~90% of people have some headaches during lifetime

    d. Most of these headaches never require medical attention because acetaminophen or nonsteroidal anti-inflammatory drug (NSAID) analgesics relieve pain

"Tension-type headache" is an old term for primary headaches that do not fit migraine characteristics.

3. Chronic daily headache

    a. Occurs with background of frequent primary headache treated with analgesic

    b. Headache rebounds after treatment until rebound headache and primary headache overlap

    c. Recurrent episodic primary headache can transform into headache that is present on most days

> Frequent use of medicine that aborts primary headache can cause chronic daily headache.

4. Cluster
   a. Manifested by severe, boring type of pain perceived behind one eye; is always unilateral
   b. Male-to-female prevalence 10:1
   c. Clustering of headaches multiple times daily for a few to several days, followed by weeks to months of no episodes
   d. Initial headache of a cluster episode almost always begins during sleep at night
   e. Each episode of headache lasts 20–30 minutes, often repeated several times a night

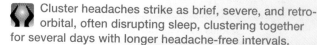

> Cluster headaches strike as brief, severe, and retro-orbital, often disrupting sleep, clustering together for several days with longer headache-free intervals.

5. Diagnostic guidelines
   a. "Sinus" headache is almost always a primary headache syndrome. Head pain from sinusitis is usually easy to distinguish.
   b. No one seeks medical care without first trying self-medication with over-the-counter drugs.
   c. History of chronic episodic headache and normal neurologic examination is sufficient for diagnosis. Primary headache is not a "diagnosis of exclusion."
   d. Patients with cluster headache often have a peculiar history of hitting their head against the wall because pain is so severe.
E. Clinical manifestations of secondary headache
   1. History of *new* onset headache in adult or *change* in pattern of chronic primary headache should alert to possibility of pain caused by something else.
   2. Neurologic examination is *normal* in primary headache. Abnormal neurologic examination results suggest secondary headache caused by another disorder. Neurologic abnormalities in setting of headache always need thorough evaluation.

3. Cluster headache can be an exception to the rule about normal physical examination. During a headache, it is possible to demonstrate ipsilateral Horner syndrome.
4. Head computed tomography (CT) scan without infusion is 100% sensitive for clinically significant intracerebral hemorrhage.
5. Subarachnoid hemorrhage, meningitis, and meningeal malignancy require examination of cerebrospinal fluid (CSF). Imaging is seldom, if ever, diagnostic.

> Change in pattern of headache is an important alert for secondary headache. Head CT scan and/or CSF examination would be necessary.

II. Approach to the Patient

A. History

1. Inquire about age at onset. Primary headache syndromes start in childhood or adolescence. However, patients may not recognize any pattern until adulthood.
2. Ask patient to describe typical headache duration. If headaches are episodic, attempt to identify typical intervals between headaches.
3. Ask what measures have been used to treat headaches and what response to treatment has been.
4. Listen for triggers

> Identify common lifestyle triggers, including sleep deprivation, occasional excessive sleep, caffeine, caffeine withdrawal, alcohol, fasting, life stresses, or any relationship to menstrual cycle.

5. A headache that exists on awakening in the morning means nothing. The notion that such a headache suggests brain tumor is wrong.
6. Ask about family history, symptoms of motion sickness, cold-induced head pain, and ice pick–like head pains. Positive responses may bolster the diagnosis of primary headache.
   a. Note that many patients may deny family history of migraine but report that mothers used to get sinus headaches.
   b. Parents need to provide history of colic.

B. Physical examination

    1. Primary headache syndromes do not cause physical examination abnormalities

    2. Palpation of entire head and auscultation for intracranial bruit rarely yield abnormality yet may be only early clue for secondary headache

    3. Mandatory elements

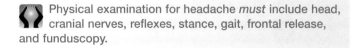 Physical examination for headache *must* include head, cranial nerves, reflexes, stance, gait, frontal release, and funduscopy.

C. Laboratory evaluation

    1. Consider complete blood count and glucose.

    2. If intracranial hemorrhage is a possibility, head CT scan without contrast is an emergency procedure.

    3. If subarachnoid hemorrhage or meningitis is a possibility, CSF examination is an emergency procedure. Many would choose an imaging procedure first to exclude increased intracranial pressure.

    4. Magnetic resonance imaging (MRI) is more sensitive for small tumors, encephalitis, some unusual infections, stroke, and demyelinating disease but not as an emergency procedure.

D. Remember to consider reason that patients with primary headache seek medical attention; they often worry about brain tumor; careful history and competent physical examination are adequate to rule out brain tumor

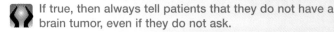 If true, then always tell patients that they do not have a brain tumor, even if they do not ask.

    1. Failure to thus reassure often results in treatment failure.

III. Treatment

A. Headache treatment is not simple; lifestyle interventions are effective and safe; drugs may be necessary to abort a headache episode or prevent headache recurrences; no distinct line in the spectrum of headache delineating which should require more specific drug treatment

1. Transformation to chronic daily headache is a limiting factor with drugs that relieve episodic headaches. Transformation is unlikely if fewer than 10 doses are required in a month; transformation is common when abortive drugs are generally used three or more times a week. Any abortive drug, even acetaminophen, can result in transformation to chronic daily headache. Compound medicines that contain caffeine or barbiturate are more prone to cause transformation.

 Transformation of episodic headaches to chronic daily headache is unlikely if abortive drug use does not exceed 10 doses per month.

B. Lifestyle
   1. Regularize sleeping hours; oversleeping is as likely to trigger headache as sleep deprivation.
   2. Avoid fasting; eat something for breakfast.
   3. Standardize caffeine intake.
      a. Most people tolerate two to three cups of coffee or equivalent in a day.
      b. Some may need to avoid caffeine totally.
      c. Include caffeinated soft drinks in estimating total daily intake.
   4. Regulate alcohol.
      a. Red wines may be especially provocative.
      b. Alcohol can interfere with sleep maintenance, leading to headache.
   5. Observe for any consistent trigger.
   6. Contrary to popular belief, chocolate does not induce migraine.
C. Abortive (Table 6.1)
   1. Acetaminophen
      a. Least side effects, but almost everyone has tried it prior to medical consultation
   2. Aspirin or NSAID
      a. Aspirin maximal dose 650 mg
      b. NSAIDs have higher maximal equivalent dose
         i. Ibuprofen 200 mg = naproxen 220 mg = aspirin 650 mg
         ii. No comparative evidence demonstrating superiority of any NSAID
         iii. COX-2 inhibitors not superior to standard NSAIDs

TABLE 6.1	
Drug Classes to Stop Primary Headache	
Drug Class	**Route(s) of Administration**
Acetaminophen	Oral
Aspirin	Oral
NSAID	Oral
Triptans	Oral
	Intranasal
	Transbuccal
	Subcutaneous
Dihydroergotamine (DHE)	Intranasal
	Intramuscular
	Intravenous
Narcotics	Intranasal
	Parenteral
	Oral

3. Triptans

 Triptans have the greatest efficacy. Early treatment is best. They differ primarily in route of administration.

    a. Gastroparesis is often a part of migraine, so oral drug availability may be impaired, but oral drugs may have a longer duration of effectiveness.
    b. The subcutaneous route is fastest.
    c. Intranasal spray is absorbed as quickly as injected.
    d. The sublingual route is almost as quickly absorbed as injected.
    e. Oral tablets have variable absorption but greatest patient acceptance.
4. Ergot derivatives
    a. DHE
        i. Most effective early at headache onset; effectiveness diminishes quickly with headache duration
        ii. Intranasal spray for outpatients
        iii. Intravenous bolus or infusion for inpatients
    b. Constituent of many unregulated "homeopathic" and "natural" compounds

5. Narcotics

   a. Using potentially addictive agent for lifelong disorder is troublesome; migraine-specific drugs (i.e., triptans and DHE) as potent or more effective than narcotic analgesics

   b. Oral narcotics

      i. Poor pharmacologic availability due to delayed absorption

      ii. Slow onset of action can lead to excessive dosing

      iii. Caution with potentially addictive agent for a chronic condition

      iv. Lipophilic preparations, such as oxycodone and meperidine, have extremely high abuse potential

   c. Parenteral narcotics

      i. Quick pharmacologic availability

      ii. Occasionally used in emergency room setting

   d. Intranasal narcotics

      i. Butorphanol available as intranasal spray

      ii. Mixed agonist-antagonist activity theoretically less prone to addiction

      iii. Use in pregnancy not unusual; no studies exist demonstrating relative safety

   e. Anti-nausea drugs

      i. Drugs that prevent or relieve nausea have no direct effect on primary headache but may be useful as adjunct treatment (e.g., metoclopramide, promethazine)

D. Preventive (Table 6.2)

TABLE 6.2	Drugs to Prevent Primary Headache
Drug	**Dosing Suggestion**
Divalproex	125–2500 mg/day
Amitriptyline/nortriptyline	10–50 mg at bedtime
Topiramate	
Beta blockers	
Verapamil	40–320 mg/day
Cyproheptadine	4–16 mg/day

1. Frequent use of any drug that aborts primary headache will lead to transformation to chronic daily headache. When patients require abortive treatment more than two to three times a week, they can prevent headaches by taking daily preventive medication. Several drug classes are effective. Clinical trials, in particular comparative trials, have been small.
2. Lack of efficacy of one drug class does not predict failure of drugs from other classes. Switching drugs within a class might improve side effects, but drugs within a class likely have the same beneficial effects.
3. Preventive benefits may not be apparent for 2–6 weeks.
4. There are no clinical trials for use in pregnancy. Almost all preventive drugs are potent CNS serotonin antagonists, suggesting possible fetal intrauterine developmental risk.
5. Divalproex
   a. Comparative results suggest modestly greater effectiveness than other agents.
   b. The initial dose is small, 125 mg once or twice a day.
   c. The dose is gradually increased until successful or until reaching maximal anticonvulsant dose.
   d. Ill-defined malaise and fatigue are not uncommon side effects.
   e. Hepatotoxicity occurs in children and adolescents. Hepatotoxicity occurs rarely, if at all, in adults.
   f. Clinical effectiveness is 60%–80%.
6. Tricyclic drugs
   a. Amitriptyline and nortriptyline most commonly used
   b. Effective dose much lower than dose necessary for antidepressant properties; 10–50 mg is usual range
   c. Little or no antidepressant effect at this dose
   d. Sedating side effect can be advantageous if sleep disorder contributes to triggering headaches
   e. Mild weight gain common and problematic.
   f. Dry mouth common limiting side effect
   g. Clinical effectiveness approximates that of divalproex

Low-dose tricyclic drugs are useful in preventing primary headache. Their sedating side effect can be useful if sleeping is a problem.

7. Beta-adrenergic blockers
  a. First agent to demonstrate preventive effectiveness
  b. Dose range identical to that for treating hypertension
  c. Clinical effectiveness ~40%
8. Topiramate
  a. Dose range identical to anticonvulsant dosage
  b. Lacks substantial comparative trials
  c. Hypothetical mechanism of action differs from that of divalproex
  d. Mild weight gain common
  e. Subjective adverse effects common
9. Calcium channel blockers
  a. Verapamil 40–320 mg daily
  b. Bradycardia, constipation, and hypotension frequent side effects
  c. Mild weight gain common
  d. Clinical effectiveness 20%–40%
10. Antihistamine serotonin antagonist
  a. Cyproheptadine 4–16 mg daily
  b. Extensive experience in childhood migraine makes it drug of choice for children and adolescents
  c. Sedation often prominent at initiation but typically improves with continued use
  d. Weight gain very common and problematic
  e. Dry mouth very common and problematic
11. SSRI antidepressants
  a. It is questionable if SSRI agents are effective in headache prevention.
  b. Depression is a frequent co-morbid condition with primary headache syndromes. Untreated depression can aggravate underlying headache.
E. Nonspecific treatment
  1. Therapies such as stress reduction techniques, biofeedback, massage therapies, stretching exercises, and relaxation training all may be useful adjuncts for selected patients. There are no clinical trials demonstrating effectiveness.
  2. Vitamin and nutritional supplement therapy lacks evidence-based support.

3. Many over-the-counter nutritional supplements and homeopathic remedies contain compounds that interact with pharmaceutical treatment.

 MENTOR TIPS DIGEST

- Primary headaches arise from brain dysfunction.
- Migraine is a primary headache characterized by moderate to severe unilateral throbbing pain lasting 4–72 hours, often accompanied by nausea and vomiting.
- "Tension-type headache" is an old term for primary headaches that do not fit migraine characteristics.
- Frequent use of medicine that aborts primary headache can cause chronic daily headache.
- Cluster headaches strike as brief, severe, and retro-orbital, often disrupting sleep, clustering together for several days with longer headache-free intervals.
- Change in pattern of headache is an important alert for secondary headache. Head CT scan and/or CSF examination would be necessary.
- Identify common lifestyle triggers, including sleep deprivation; occasional excessive sleep; caffeine; caffeine withdrawal; alcohol; fasting; life stresses; or any relationship to menstrual cycle.
- Physical examination for headache *must* include head, cranial nerves, reflexes, stance, gait, frontal release, and funduscopy.
- If true, then always tell patients that they do not have a brain tumor, even if they do not ask.
- Transformation of episodic headaches to chronic daily headache is unlikely if abortive drug use does not exceed 10 doses per month.
- Triptans have the greatest efficacy. Early treatment is best. They differ primarily in route of administration.
- Low-dose tricyclic drugs are useful in preventing primary headache. Their sedating side effect can be useful if sleeping is a problem.

Resources

Dodick D, Freitag F. Evidence-based understanding of medication-overuse headache: Clinical implications. Headache 46:S202–S211, 2006.

This article discusses the problem of medication-overuse headache from a variety of perspectives, based on the best available evidence.

Lipton RB, Bigal ME. Migraine prevalence, disease burden, and the need for preventive therapy. Neurology 68: 343–349, 2007.
Objectives: to reassess the prevalence of migraine in the United States; to assess patterns of migraine treatment in the population; and to contrast current patterns of preventive treatment use with recommendations for use from an expert headache panel

Rothrock, JF. Let's put "mixed headache" to rest. Headache 47: 94–97, 2007.

Chapter Self-Test Questions

Circle the correct answer. After you have responded to the questions, check your answers in Appendix A.

1. Primary headache differs from secondary headache in that:

    a. Primary headache describes the first headache of a person's life.

    b. Primary headache describes neurogenic headache.

    c. Aura precedes secondary headache.

    d. Triptans are the drugs of choice for secondary headache.

2. The following statement about headache is true:

    a. Most persons with headache will sometime seek medical attention for their headache.

    b. Almost all people will experience headache.

    c. Women are four times more likely than men to have headaches.

    d. Prevention is a critical factor in treating most headaches.

3. The aura of migraine headache typically demonstrates:

    a. A sharp jabbing pain that can feel as if an ice pick is jammed in the head.

    b. Sudden onset of visual scotoma (circumscribed vision loss) often relieved by using triptan drugs

c. Gradual onset of vision distortion that becomes progressively greater over 20 minutes.

d. Cerebral ischemia due to constriction of middle or posterior cerebral artery.

 See the testbank CD for more self-test questions.

COMMON SLEEP DISORDERS

Helen Gartner Martin, MD

I. Introduction

A. Sleep disturbances are very common problems in primary care.

B. Sleep disturbances can affect quality of life and be significant medical problems.

C. Questions to ask patients to evaluate their sleep include:

1. How is your sleep at night?

2. Are you too sleepy during the day?

3. Does anything unusual happen during your sleep?

D. Some of the most common sleep disorders are insomnia, obstructive sleep apnea (OSA), and restless leg syndrome/periodic leg movements of sleep.

II. Insomnia

A. Definition/epidemiology

1. Insomnia is defined as difficulty with sleep initiation, duration, or consolidation or quality, despite adequate time and opportunity for sleep.

2. There should be an associated complaint of some daytime impairment (e.g., lack of energy, difficulty concentrating, irritability).

 30%–40% of adults experience insomnia within any given year.

 10%–15% of adults have chronic insomnia, defined as persisting for at least several weeks.

B. Classification
  1. Acute insomnia
     a. Insomnia occurring in association with identifiable stressor
     b. Should resolve within several days to weeks as stressor resolves
C. Chronic insomnia—lasting more than several weeks
  1. Psychophysiologic insomnia
     a. The patient "learns" sleep-preventing associations, commonly after an acute stressor, and develops excessive anxiety concerning sleep
  2. Paradoxical insomnia
     a. Also called sleep state misperception
     b. Characterized by marked overestimate of lack of sleep as well as overestimate of daytime impairment
  3. Insomnia associated with psychiatric disorder
     a. Insomnia commonly associated with depression, bipolar disorder, anxiety
  4. Insomnia associated with drug or substance abuse
     a. Insomnia commonly associated with caffeine, amphetamines, other central nervous system (CNS) stimulants
     b. Insomnia may be unintended side effect of some prescription medications (e.g., antidepressants, antihypertensives, antiepileptics, theophylline)
     c. Acute and chronic alcohol abuse as well as abrupt withdrawal from alcohol may disrupt sleep
  5. Insomnia due to a medical condition
     a. Chronic pain
     b. Respiratory disorders, e.g., asthma
     c. Gastroesophageal reflux disorder
     d. Medical conditions associated with nocturia
     e. Neurologic disorders
     f. Menopause
  6. Insomnia not otherwise classified
D. Evaluation of patient with insomnia
  1. History

 A complete sleep history is the most important tool in evaluating insomnia.

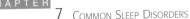

    a. History should be tailored based on whether insomnia is acute or chronic.

      i. Acute insomnia

        (1) Has there been a recent stressful life event?

        (2) Has there been a recent change in sleeping environment?

        (3) Are there any acute medical or surgical issues?

        (4) Has the patient started taking any new medications or stopped any chronic medications?

        (5) Has the patient experienced any recent time changes (e.g., shift work or jet lag?)

      ii. Chronic insomnia

        (1) Has the patient had a long history of difficulty sleeping?

        (2) What are the duration and frequency of the problem?

        (3) What are usual bedtime and waking times for weekdays and weekends?

        (4) What are the patient's sleep-related habits? Does the patient read or watch television in bed? If not able to sleep, does the patient remain in bed or leave the bedroom?

        (5) Does the patient have a medical or psychiatric problem which might be interfering with sleep?

        (6) Does the patient use caffeine, alcohol, or tobacco? When, and how much?

        (7) Does the patient snore or have leg movements during sleep? These questions are frequently better answered by a bed partner.

        (8) Is the patient's sleep disrupted by bed partner (including pets)?

        (9) Has the patient traveled?

        (10) What are the patient's work hours?

        (11) What are the daytime consequences of the patient's insomnia?

  2. Physical examination

    a. Looking for signs of thyroid disorders (tremor, goiter, lid lag) or congestive heart failure (CHF) (edema, rales, jugular venous distention [JVD], S_3) is reasonable.

3. Sleep diary

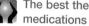 Recording daily sleep diary for 1–2 weeks can help determine extent of problem and may uncover poor sleep habits. Information includes wake and sleep times, nocturnal awakenings, time spent awake during the night, and quality of sleep as determined by patient and bed partner.

4. Polysomnography
  a. Occasionally, a formal sleep study may be indicated if a problem such as sleep apnea or nocturnal leg movements is suspected as a cause of sleep disruption.
  b. If a sleep study is performed, the comparison of the recorded information with the patient's perception of the night's sleep may help physician better evaluate patient's complaints.

E. Treatment
  1. Review of sleep hygiene measures is appropriate in most cases.
  2. Acute insomnia
    a. Alter, if possible, any precipitating factor (e.g., stop medication causing problem, treat nocturnal pain adequately).
    b. Treatment with hypnotics may be valuable for current symptoms and help avoid the development of "learned" or conditioned insomnia.
  3. Chronic insomnia
    a. Treat any sleep-disturbing issues, such as apnea and leg movements.
    b. Optimize any medical conditions disturbing sleep.
    c. It is very important to establish reasonable goals and expectations at the beginning of treatment.

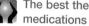 The best therapy for chronic insomnia involves both medications and cognitive behavioral therapy.

    d. Medications:
      i. The use of medications for chronic insomnia is controversial, as most hypnotics have been approved for short-term use only. However, more recently, at least one hypnotic has been approved for long-term use.

(1) Benzodiazepine (BDZ) receptor agonists
  (A) Almost all drugs approved for treatment of insomnia in the United States are BDZ receptor agonists or similar agents because of overall safety and (at least short-term) efficacy
  (B) Include estazolam, eszopiclone, flurazepam, temazepam, triazolam, zaleplon, and zolpidem
  (C) All generally well-tolerated but recommended for short-term use
  (D) Eszopiclone has been studied over 6 months, and it retains efficacy; eszopiclone and the extended-release form of zolpidem are the only medications not limited to short-term treatment of insomnia; effects longer than 6–12 months have not been documented
  (E) Potential side effects include tolerance; these medications are frequently prescribed on an intermittent basis to avoid tolerance, but this approach has not been systematically studied
  (F) Another side effect is complex sleep related behaviors; in March 2007 U.S. Food and Drug Administration (FDA) requested labeling to include stronger warnings
(2) Melatonin receptor agonists
  (A) Ramelteon approved for treatment of insomnia.
  (B) Data supporting efficacy still evolving
(3) Antidepressants
  (A) Although not specifically indicated for treatment of insomnia, trazodone, amitriptyline, and mirtazapine identified as three of top four drugs prescribed to treat insomnia in 2002
  (B) Little systematic evidence that these drugs are effective
(4) Other
  (A) Over-the-counter medications frequently contain antihistamines. These drugs may promote drowsiness but generally do not improve the quality of sleep and have the disadvantage of long half-lives and may result in morning "hangover" effects.

(B) Melatonin is a normal product of the pineal gland, but it has had limited efficacy in most patients with insomnia.

(C) Valerian is a commonly used herbal supplement, but few data support efficacy in promoting sleep.

e. Cognitive behavioral therapy:

 Cognitive behavioral therapy is as effective as medication in long-term treatment of insomnia.

i. Components of treatment include combinations of several of the following:

(1) Stimulus control therapy—a set of instructions designed to promote the association of the bed and bedroom with sleep and to help establish a consistent sleep schedule

(2) Sleep restriction therapy—method designed to limit the time in bed to time spent actually sleeping. As sleep becomes more consolidated, time in bed is gradually increased.

(3) Relaxation training—training to reduce tension and intrusive thoughts interfering with sleep onset

(4) Cognitive therapy—psychological training aimed at changing perceptions of insomnia and its effect on daytime function

(5) Sleep hygiene education—general guidelines for optimizing conditions for sleep, including:

(A) Maintaining regular sleep-wake schedule

(B) Establishing a relaxing pre-sleep ritual

(C) Going to bed only when sleepy

(D) Using bed for sleep and sex only

(E) Avoiding naps, especially past early afternoon

(6) Avoid stimulants (e.g., caffeine and nicotine) and alcohol before bedtime

(7) Maintain comfortable sleep environment (comfortable temperature; dark, quiet room)

(8) Avoid heavy exercise or stimulating activity (including computer work) in late afternoon

(9) Exercise regularly in the morning or afternoon

(10) Do not eat heavy meals close to bedtime

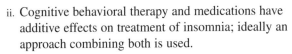

  ii. Cognitive behavioral therapy and medications have
      additive effects on treatment of insomnia; ideally an
      approach combining both is used.

III. Obstructive Sleep Apnea (OSA)

A. Definition

  1. An obstructive apnea is defined as an obstruction to airflow
       during sleep for at least 10 seconds with continued respiratory
       effort.

  2. An obstructive hypopnea is an incomplete apnea with some air-
       flow maintained and should be associated with either an arousal
       or a decrease in oxygen saturation.

  3. Apneas and hypopneas are grouped together in the Apnea/
       Hypopnea Index (AHI), the number of apneas and hypopneas
       per hour.

  4. OSA syndrome defined as:

   a. Five or more respiratory events/hour associated with
         either:

     i. Excessive daytime sleepiness or

     ii. Symptoms of (two or more):

       (1) Choking or gasping episodes during sleep

       (2) Recurrent awakenings

       (3) Unrefreshing sleep

       (4) Daytime fatigue

       (5) Impaired concentration

  5. Severity of OSA defined by frequency of respiratory events:

   a. Mild: AHI between 5 and 15

   b. Moderate: AHI between 15 and 30

   c. Severe: AHI >30

B. Prevalence of OSA

  1. Defined as AHI >5, with symptoms of daytime sleepiness, ages
       30–60 years

 Prevalence of OSA: 4% in men; 2% in women.

C. Signs and symptoms of OSA

  1. Nocturnal symptoms

   a. Loud snoring

   b. Witnessed apneas (often interrupt snoring)

    c. Gasping and/or choking episodes that arouse patient from sleep

    d. Restless sleep ("tossing and turning")

    e. Nocturia

  2. Daytime symptoms

    a. Excessive daytime sleepiness (EDS)

    b. Sense that sleep was nonrestorative

    c. Personality changes, problems with concentration or memory

    d. Dry throat and mouth on awakening

    e. Impotence

D. Pathophysiology of OSA

 OSA involves abnormal balance between forces maintaining airway patency and forces promoting airway collapse.

  1. Promoting airway patency

    a. Pharyngeal dilator muscles

    b. Increased lung volume

  2. Promoting airway collapse

    a. Negative pressure in airway on inspiration

    b. Extraluminal positive pressure

      i. Small anatomic airway

      ii. Excess fat deposition in neck or airway

      iii. Excess tissue (e.g., large tongue, uvula, or tonsils) in airway

      iv. Small or posteriorly placed mandible

E. Pertinent physical examination for OSA

  1. Examine face for retro- or micrognathia

  2. Examine nose for deviated septum, obstruction, or narrowing of nares

  3. Examine upper airway for evidence of obstruction: small oropharynx, excessive tissue in pharynx, enlarged tonsils, large uvula, large tongue

  4. Measure neck (size >17 inches increased risk of OSA)

  5. Cardiovascular and respiratory examination

F. Diagnosis of OSA

 Standard is overnight study monitored in laboratory.

1. Study includes recordings of:
   a. Sleep stages
   b. Heart rate and rhythm
   c. Airflow and respiratory effort
   d. Oxygen saturation
   e. Leg movements
2. A variety of portable devices are available, often for home use, that can record some of the standard data (e.g., oxygen saturation, respiratory effort)
   a. Not well standardized
   b. Can be useful for screening large populations
G. Consequences of OSA

 OSA has far-reaching consequences across many domains of health and safety.

1. Impairment of cognitive function and performance
   a. Patients with OSA have more auto accidents
2. Cardiovascular (CV) function
   a. Increased incidence of hypertension
   b. Increased risk of CV events (e.g., myocardial infarction and stroke)
3. Metabolic dysfunction
   a. Increased glucose intolerance
   b. Increased insulin resistance
H. Treatment of OSA
   1. Conservative measures
      a. Avoid use of alcohol and central nervous system depressants close to time of sleep
      b. Avoid sleep in the supine position
      c. Lose weight (if patient overweight or obese)
   2. Medications
      a. Little role in treatment of OSA
      b. Small studies have shown mild improvement in AHI with protriptyline and mirtazapine
      c. Oxygen, especially transtracheal oxygen, may improve apneas slightly; oxygen can also prolong apneas; patients must have sleep study on oxygen before it is prescribed

3. Surgical options may improve apnea in appropriately selected candidates; surgical options include:

   a. Nasal surgery (repair of deviated septum, etc).

   b. Uvulopalatopharyngoplasty (removal of excess tissue from posterior pharynx).

   c. Mandibular advancement for retrognathia.

   d. Radiofrequency ablation for reduction in size of tongue and other tissue.

   e. Tracheotomy: ultimate (but drastic) treatment of OSA as it bypasses the upper airway obstruction entirely.

4. Mechanical devices

   a. Mandibular advancement devices are worn at night to move mandible forward; may be helpful in appropriate patient with mild apnea

   b. Continuous positive airway pressure (CPAP)

 CPAP is the standard of care for OSA.

   i. CPAP is effective in almost all patients, although not all patients choose to use CPAP.

   ii. Treatment consists of a bedside device (CPAP unit) that compresses room air. The compressed air is fed into the patient's airway via a mask (commonly a mask that covers only the nose) that maintains airway patency with the positive pressure of the compressed air.

   iii. CPAP has been documented to reverse the CV effects of OSA. Various types of CPAP and many masks are available to increase patient comfort and compliance.

IV. Restless Leg Syndrome (RLS)/Periodic Leg Movements of Sleep (PLMD)

A. Introduction

   1. Restless legs syndrome (RLS) and periodic leg movement disorder (PLMD) are closely related syndromes, with significant clinical overlap.

RLS is an intense urge to move the legs and is an *awake* phenomenon. PLMD is a series of repetitive involuntary movements occurring *during sleep*.

2. Approximately 80% of RLS patients also have PLMD.

3. RLS is not as common in association with PLMD.

4. Research studies of treatment often combine the two phenomena.

B. Prevalence

    1. The prevalence of RLS is estimated to be approximately 10%–15%. It can be severe during pregnancy.

    2. PLMD is rare earlier than age 30 years but increases dramatically after age 50 years. The estimated prevalence is estimated to be 45% in the elderly.

C. Diagnosis

    1. RLS

 RLS is a clinical diagnosis requiring four criteria:

    a. There is an urge to move the legs, usually accompanied by paresthesias or dysesthesias.

    b. Symptoms of RLS begin or worsen during periods of rest or inactivity.

    c. Symptoms are relieved or significantly improved by movement.

    d. Symptoms are worse in the evening or at night.

    2. PLMD

 PLMD is a diagnosis made by sleep study.

    a. A sequence of four or more leg movements, each with duration of 0.5–5 seconds, and separated by intervals of 5–90 seconds

    b. Periodic leg movement index (PLMI), number of leg movements/hour, should exceed 15

    c. Movements may be asymptomatic or may disturb sleep

    d. Although movements typically involve legs, they may also involve arms and, occasionally, trunk

D. Evaluation of patients with RLS and PLMD

    1. Physical examination

        a. Frequently normal results

        b. Look for evidence of peripheral neuropathy, which can be associated with RLS/PLMD

2. Laboratory tests
   a. Serum ferritin (low levels may worsen symptoms)
   b. Renal function (can have RLS/PLMD in association with severe renal insufficiency)
   c. Diagnostic test for pregnancy (if indicated)
E. Pathophysiology of RLS/PLMD
   1. Not clearly established
   2. Significant inherited component
   3. Likely involves dopaminergic system
F. Treatment
   1. Substances to avoid include nicotine, alcohol, and caffeine
   2. Medications that can worsen symptoms include some antidepressants, many antihistamines, most anti-nausea drugs, many antipsychotics
   3. Anecdotal evidence for hot baths, leg massage, counterstimulation, heat or ice packs, regular exercise, supplemental calcium, folate, vitamin E, vitamin C, magnesium
   4. Iron supplementation: serum ferritin levels of <50 mcg/L (normal 20–300) associated with increased symptoms and supplementation can improve symptoms
   5. Four types of medications used for treatment

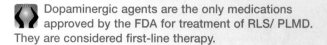
Dopaminergic agents are the only medications approved by the FDA for treatment of RLS/ PLMD. They are considered first-line therapy.

   a. Dopaminergic agents—pramipexole (0.125–0.5 mg qhs) and ropinirole (0.25–2.0 mg qhs)
      i. Problems with these medications include rebound (symptoms worsen at end of dosing period), augmentation (symptoms develop earlier in the day or become more severe), and tolerance (decreased effectiveness with time).
      ii. Pathologic gambling or other compulsive behaviors have rarely been reported with these medications).

b. Anticonvulsants
   i. Gabapentin (100–1200 mg qhs) best studied
   ii. May produce drowsiness (sometimes beneficial)
c. Benzodiazepines—e.g., clonazepam (0.5–2.0 mg qhs)
   i. Some of the first drugs used to treat RLS/PLMD
   ii. Generally less effective than dopaminergic agents and gabapentin
d. Opioids—e.g., oxycodone (5–15 mg) and propoxyphene (100–200 mg)
   i. Can probably generalize effects to most narcotics
6. General principles of use of medications in treating RLS/PLMD
a. Start with one of the dopaminergic agents, unless there is pain or insomnia; then consider starting with gabapentin.
b. Use medications at lowest effective dose, and increase dose slowly.
c. Combinations of medications may be needed.
d. Medications may need to be administered in divided doses (dinner and bedtime) to control early evening symptoms of RLS.
e. Optimal treatment is often determined empirically.

MENTOR TIPS DIGEST

- 30%–40% of adults experience insomnia within any given year.
- 10%–15% of adults have chronic insomnia, defined as persisting for at least several weeks.
- A complete sleep history is the most important tool in evaluating insomnia.
- Recording in a daily sleep diary for 1–2 weeks can help determine extent of a problem and may uncover poor sleep habits. Information includes wake and sleep times, nocturnal awakenings, time spent awake during the night, and quality of sleep as determined by patient and bed partner.
- The best therapy for chronic insomnia involves both medications and cognitive behavioral therapy.
- Cognitive behavioral therapy is as effective as medication in long-term treatment of insomnia.
- Prevalence of OSA: 4% in men; 2% in women.

- OSA involves abnormal balance between forces maintaining airway patency and forces promoting airway collapse.
- For diagnosis of OSA, the standard is overnight study monitored in laboratory.
- OSA has far-reaching consequences across many domains of health and safety (from auto accidents to cardiovascular events and many others).
- CPAP is the standard of care for OSA.
- RLS is an intense urge to move the legs and is an *awake* phenomenon. PLMD is a series of repetitive involuntary movements occurring *during sleep.*
- RLS is a clinical diagnosis requiring four criteria (discussed in text).
- PLMD is a diagnosis made by sleep study.
- Dopaminergic agents are the only medications approved by the FDA for treatment of RLS/PLMD. They are considered first-line therapy.

Resources

Insomnia

Edinger JD, Sampson WS. A primary care "friendly" cognitive behavioral insomnia therapy. Sleep 26:177–182, 2003
  This study demonstrates efficacy of cognitive behavioral therapy and also describes how it is performed.

National Institutes of Health state of the science conference statement on manifestations and management of chronic insomnia in adults, June 13–15, 2005. Sleep 28:1049–1057, 2005.
  Overview of the scope of the problem, with many classic references.

Schenck CH, Mahowald MW, Sack RL. Assessment and management of insomnia. Journal of the American Medical Association. 289:2475–2479, 2003.
  A more clinical approach to managing insomnia.

Obstructive Sleep Apnea

Drager LF, Bortolotto LA, Figueiredo AC, et al. Effects of continuous positive airway pressure on early signs of atherosclerosis in obstructive sleep apnea. American Journal of Respiratory and Critical Care Medicine 176:706–712, 2007.
  Documents efficacy of CPAP in reversing adverse CV effects of OSA.

Yaggi HK, Concato J, Kernan WN, et al. Obstructive sleep apnea as a risk factor for stroke and death. New England Journal of Medicine 353:2034–2041, 2005.
One of the articles documenting OSA as a risk factor for increased CV mortality.

Young T, Palta M, Dempsey J, et al. The occurrence of sleep-disordered breathing among middle-aged adults. New England Journal of Medicine 328:1230–1235, 1993.
One of the classic studies measuring prevalence of OSA in employed adults.

RLS/PLMD

Bogan RK, Fry JM, Schmidt MH, et al. Ropinirole in the treatment of patients with restless legs syndrome: A U.S.-based randomized, double-blind, placebo-controlled clinical trial. Mayo Clinic Proceedings 81:17–27, 2006.
One of the classic articles demonstrating efficacy of treatment with dopaminergic agents.

Phillips B, Young T, Finn L, et al. Epidemiology of restless legs symptoms in adults. Archives of Internal Medicine 160:2137–2141, 2000.
A study measuring prevalence of restless leg syndrome in adults; documents increasing prevalence with increasing age.

Trenkwalder C, Paulus W, Walters AS. The restless legs syndrome. Lancet 4:465–475, 2005
A recent, thorough review with specific recommendations for treatment.

Chapter Self-Test Questions

Circle the correct answer. After you have responded to the questions, check your answers in Appendix A.

1. How common is chronic insomnia among American adults?

    a. <1%

    b. 15%–20%

    c. 50%–70%

    d. >90%

2. A 47-year-old woman presents to you because she has difficulty falling asleep. She typically will lie in bed awake for hours. There have been nights during which she did not sleep at all. She has trouble concentrating at work. Her difficulty sleeping began 1 week ago when her husband told her he wanted a divorce. Which of these choices is most appropriate for your response?

   a. She should immediately begin to take lorazepam 0.5–1 mg every 4–6 hours to relieve anxiety.

   b. She should have a polysomnogram (overnight sleep study).

   c. She should begin to drink 1–2 glasses of wine before bedtime.

   d. You can reassure her that her insomnia is very likely to remit spontaneously, and zolpidem can be used short-term along with counseling if necessary.

3. A 56-year-old man complains of insomnia with daytime difficulty maintaining attention since hospital discharge 6 weeks ago. His hospital stay was due to angina, treated with coronary angioplasty and stent. His discharge medicines, all newly prescribed, include clopidogrel, aspirin, atorvastatin, fluoxetine, and lisinopril. Which of his medicines is most likely to cause sleep disturbance?

   a. Clopidogrel

   b. Atorvastatin

   c. Fluoxetine

   d. Lisinopril

See the testbank CD for more self-test questions.

8 CHAPTER

DIZZINESS

John E. Butter, MD

I. Background
   A. Dizziness is a common disorder that can be challenging for patients to describe and physicians to evaluate.
   B. Complexity and vagueness of symptoms arise from interaction of multiple systems that maintain a person's proper perception of relationship to the environment.
   C. Disturbances in the cardiovascular, visual, vestibular, and proprioceptive pathways can produce dizziness. Dizziness may be related to multiple causative factors in nearly half of all patients.
   D. Patients' descriptions are frequently vague due to difficulty communicating what disturbs them.

II. Epidemiology
   A. Dizziness common in all age groups but more common in elderly and women
   B. Over 7 million office visits for dizziness in the United States each year
   C. 15%–30% of patients experience dizziness severe enough to seek medical attention at some time in their lives
   D. Most patients present to primary care physicians

III. Approach to the Patient
   A. History is the most crucial part of the evaluation.
   B. A common mistake is for the physician to say too much. Avoid "putting words in patients' mouths" or offering them a list of descriptors from which to choose.

   When eliciting the history from patients who are dizzy, allow them to describe the sensation in their own words before offering multiple choices.

C. Facilitative questions or comments include "Tell me what you mean by dizzy," or "I'm not sure I understand what you mean when you say you are dizzy; please tell me more."

IV. Classification of Type of Dizziness

> Categorize the diagnosis into one (or more) of four categories: vertigo, presyncope, disequilibrium, or vague lightheadedness.

A. Each category has its own differential diagnosis and treatment.
B. Typical statements include the following:
  1. "I feel like the room is spinning" (vertigo).
  2. "I feel like I'm going to pass out" (presyncope).
  3. "I feel like I'm off balance, like I'm going to fall down" (disequilibrium).
  4. "I just feel dizzy, like I'm woozy" (vague lightheadedness).
C. The evaluation can proceed when the dizziness has been placed in one (or more) of these categories.

V. Vertigo

A. A rotatory sensation is hallmark
B. Caused by disturbance in the vestibular system, which normally functions to provide an awareness of the body's position in space.
C. Key questions are:
  1. How long do the symptoms last?
  2. Does a change in head position provoke symptoms?
  3. Is there hearing loss?
  4. Are there other neurologic symptoms such as dysphagia, diplopia, dysarthria, hemiparesis, or ataxia?
D. Differential diagnosis
  1. Benign positional vertigo
  2. Vestibular neuronitis
  3. Labyrinthitis
  4. Ménière disease
  5. Central nervous system (CNS) disorders
E. Benign positional vertigo (BPV)
  1. Classic history: "When I turned over in bed, I felt like the room was spinning for a few minutes."
  2. Symptoms resolve spontaneously after a few minutes.
  3. Hearing is not affected.

4. The cause may include accumulation of organic debris in the posterior circular canal.

5. Clinical test:

> BPV can be confirmed by reproduction of symptoms with the Dix-Hallpike maneuver, also known as the Bárány test (Fig. 8.1).

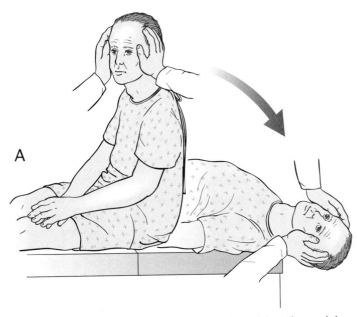

FIGURE 8.1 Dix-Hallpike maneuver *(A)*. With the patient sitting, the neck is extended and turned to one side. The patient is then placed supine rapidly so that the head hangs over the edge of the bed. The patient is kept in this position and observed for nystagmus for 30 seconds. Nystagmus usually appears with a latency of a few seconds and lasts less than 30 seconds. It has a typical trajectory, beating upward and torsionally, with the upper poles of the eyes beating toward the ground. After it stops and the patient sits up, the nystagmus will recur but in the opposite direction. Therefore, the patient is returned to upright and again observed for nystagmus for 30 seconds. If nystagmus is not provoked, the maneuver is repeated with the head turned to the other side *(B)*. If nystagmus is provoked, the patient should have the maneuver repeated to the same (provoked) side; with each repetition, the intensity and duration of nystagmus will diminish. *(Modified from Foster CA, Baloh RW: Episodic vertigo. In Rakel [ed]: Conn's Current Therapy, 47th ed. WB Saunders, Philadelphia, 1995, p. 873.)*

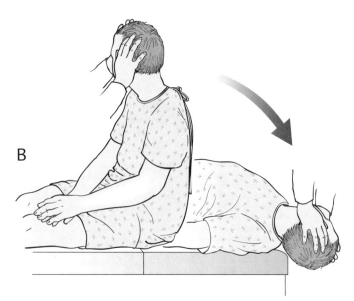

B

FIGURE 8.1 *Continued*

    a. To perform this test, have the patient sit on the examination table, then move the patient's head down over the end of the examination table to about 30 degrees below the horizontal plane, and then turn the head toward one side. Frequently, the patient will say "It's coming on now—I feel dizzy." If there is no response after about 30 seconds, return the patient to the sitting position, and repeat the maneuver, but this time turn the head in the opposite direction so the other ear is dependent.

    b. Classic positive response on the Dix-Hallpike maneuver (Bárány test) is:

        i. Vertigo, which occurs after a latency of a few seconds.

        ii. Nystagmus.

        iii. Fatigability—the symptoms are less severe if the maneuver is repeated.

  F. Vestibular neuronitis

    1. Classic history: "The room has been spinning for days, and I'm nauseous and have been vomiting."

    2. Symptoms last much longer than those of BPV—generally a few days, then resolve spontaneously.

3. Residual unsteadiness may last for weeks after the attack.

4. Hearing is not affected.

5. Spontaneous nystagmus may be present.

G. Labyrinthitis

1. Classic history: "The room is spinning, my hearing is diminished, and I hear ringing in my ears."

2. Labyrinthitis, unlike BPV or vestibular neuritis, causes diminished hearing.

3. Symptoms typically follow a viral upper respiratory tract infection.

4. Symptoms last a few weeks, then resolve without recurrence.

H. Ménière disease

1. Classic history: "My ears feel full, I can't hear so well, there's ringing in my ears, and I feel dizzy."

2. There is a triad of hearing loss, vertigo, and tinnitus, frequently accompanied by aural fullness.

3. Hearing loss is frequently low-frequency and fluctuates.

4. The typical patient is a 30–60-year-old male.

5. Cause of Ménière disease is abnormal collection of endolymphatic fluid in the inner ear.

I. Other causes of peripheral vestibular disturbances include ototoxic drugs such as loop diuretics, aspirin, quinine, caffeine, alcohol, aminoglycosides, and cisplatinum.

J. CNS:

 CNS causes of vertigo are manifested by additional neurologic symptoms, not dizziness alone.

1. Clues to a CNS cause of vertigo include more gradual onset and less intense symptoms.

2. The lower brainstem or cerebellum is frequently involved, producing symptoms such as diplopia, dysarthria, paresthesias, and changes in sensory or motor function.

3. Cerebellar dysfunction may be difficult to separate from a peripheral vestibular disorder. Difficulty with rapidly alternating movements and finger-nose-finger testing supports a cerebellar cause. In contrast, patients with a peripheral cause of vertigo are able to complete finger-nose-finger testing

accurately because visual fixation partly compensates for the vestibular defect.

4. Causes of CNS vertigo include neoplastic, vascular, and demyelinating disorders. Neoplasms such as acoustic neuromas grow slowly and often cause imbalance, tinnitus, and hearing loss. Multiple sclerosis may cause vertigo. Stroke or transient ischemic attack (TIA) may cause dizziness but in conjunction with other neurologic symptoms. One of the most common brainstem syndromes is Wallenberg syndrome, caused by infarction of the lateral medulla by occlusion of the posterior inferior cerebellar artery (PICA). Wallenberg syndrome produces a characteristic clinical picture of vertigo, ataxia, diplopia, dysphagia, Horner syndrome, ipsilateral facial numbness, and contralateral decreased pain and temperature sensation.

K. Nystagmus from peripheral causes usually evokes horizontal beating. Vertical nystagmus (up and down beating) is suggestive of central causes of vertigo. Table 8.1 compares and contrasts central versus peripheral causes.

VI. Presyncope

A. Classic history: "I feel faint, like I'm going to black out."

B. Presyncope is the impending loss of consciousness caused by decreased blood flow to the brain.

TABLE 8.1

Central Versus Peripheral Vertigo		
	Central	Peripheral
Duration	Long	Brief
Intensity	Moderate	Severe
Nausea and/or vomiting	Mild	Moderate to severe
Neurologic symptoms	Common	Rare
Hearing loss	Rare	May be present
Affected by head position	Not usually	Frequently

C. Differential diagnosis includes vasovagal hypotension and cardio-vascular disease and disorders that produce orthostatic hypotension.

D. Vasovagal reaction (neurocardiogenic presyncope)
1. Most common cause of presyncope and syncope in young adults
2. Episodes often precipitated by stressful or painful stimuli that lead to drop in heart rate and peripheral resistance.
3. Vasovagal syncope often accompanied by prodrome of diaphoresis, pallor, and nausea
4. Tilt table test, which demonstrates an exaggerated fall in blood pressure and pulse on assuming an upright posture, may be helpful in diagnosing vasovagal syncope

E. Orthostatic hypotension may be the result of dehydration, hemorrhage, diarrhea, vomiting, or excessive diuresis. Drugs are a common cause and include antihypertensives, anticonvulsants, antipsychotics, and antiparkinson medications.

F. Peripheral neuropathy, such as that caused by diabetes or alcohol, can contribute to orthostatic hypotension.

G. Cardiovascular disease
1. The mechanism of cardiovascular causes is valvular disease or arrhythmias.
2. Valvular disease such as aortic stenosis causes presyncope during or shortly after exercise due to the inability of the heart to augment cardiac output combined with exercise-induced vasodilation leading to a fall in blood pressure. Physical examination followed by echocardiography can confirm this diagnosis.
3. Arrhythmias usually have a short or absent prodrome. Advanced age; history of coronary artery disease; depressed ejection fraction; or an electrocardiogram (ECG) showing left-axis deviation, left ventricular hypertrophy (LVH), or left bundle branch block (LBBB), should raise suspicion of arrhythmias.

VII. Disequilibrium
A. Classic history: "I feel unbalanced when I walk—like I might fall."
B. Disequilibrium-type dizziness commonly causes dizziness when walking but not when sitting or supine.
C. Disequilibrium is common in the elderly.
D. Disequilibrium results from a constellation of impaired sensory deficits, including visual impairments, neuropathy, vestibular disorders, and musculoskeletal disturbances.

VIII. Vague Lightheadedness

    A. Classic history: a vague description of dizziness often accompanied by anxiety and/or a positive review of systems.

    B. Dizziness is common in patients with anxiety, panic disorder, depression, or somatization.

    C. Frequent accompanying symptoms include palpitations, headaches, weakness, chest pain, dyspnea, and paresthesias.

    D. A subset of anxiety disorders with dizziness is provoked by hyperventilation.

IX. Treatment

    A. Effective treatment depends on reaching a probable diagnosis.

    B. Treatment for vertigo

        1. Vestibular suppressants such as meclizine do not alter the natural history of the disease but can reduce symptoms.

        2. The canalith respositioning maneuver (Eply maneuver) (Fig. 8.2), which involves turning the patient 360 degrees to reposition the otoliths in the semicircular canals, is one of the most effective treatments for BPV. Patients with BPV can be cured with this maneuver.

        3. Methylprednisolone has been shown to induce a more rapid and complete recovery in patients with vestibular neuritis.

        4. Salt restriction and diuretics can be helpful for patients with Ménière disease.

    C. Treatment for presyncope

        1. For orthostatic hypotension, eliminating offending medications or volume depletion can be curative.

        2. Support stockings may be helpful to augment venous return.

        3. Fludrocortisone or midodrine are pharmacologic treatments that may be helpful.

        4. Valvular heart disease such as aortic stenosis requires surgical evaluation.

        5. Arrhythmias may require pharmacologic therapy, ablation, or treatment with an automatic implantable cardiac defibrillator (AICD).

    D. Treatment dysequilibrium

        1. Patients with disequilibrium usually have multiple sensory deficits that are not easily corrected.

        2. Correcting any visual problems such as refractive errors or cataracts may be helpful.

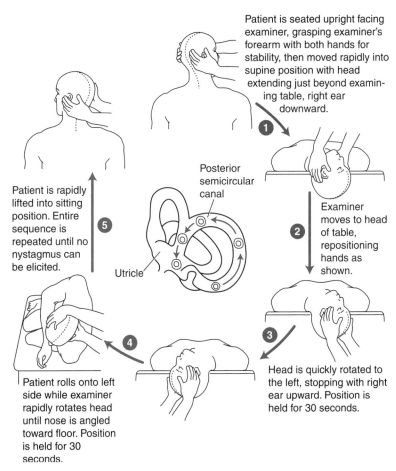

Patient is seated upright facing examiner, grasping examiner's forearm with both hands for stability, then moved rapidly into supine position with head extending just beyond examining table, right ear downward.

1

Posterior semicircular canal

Examiner moves to head of table, repositioning hands as shown.

2

Patient is rapidly lifted into sitting position. Entire sequence is repeated until no nystagmus can be elicited.

5

Utricle

3

Head is quickly rotated to the left, stopping with right ear upward. Position is held for 30 seconds.

4

Patient rolls onto left side while examiner rapidly rotates head until nose is angled toward floor. Position is held for 30 seconds.

FIGURE 8.2 Particle repositioning maneuver. In patients with benign paroxysmal positional vertigo due to canalithiasis, the particle repositioning maneuver encourages the calcium carbonate debris to migrate toward the common crus of the anterior and posterior canals and exit into the utricular cavity. Step 1 is the standard Dix-Hallpike positioning test. *(Modified from Foster CA, Baloh RW: Episodic vertigo. In Rakel [ed]: Conn's Current Therapy, 47th ed. WB Saunders, Philadelphia, 1995, p. 873.)*

3. Physical therapy and devices such as a cane or walker can be helpful.

E. Treatment for vague lightheadedness

  1. For patients with anxiety, panic disorder, or depression, a selective serotonin reuptake inhibitor is effective.

  2. Psychological counseling and cognitive behavioral therapy can be helpful.

F. Vestibular rehabilitation helpful for chronic or multifactorial dizziness of various causes, including BPV, psychological factors, head injury, and multifactorial dizziness common in elderly

---

 MENTOR TIPS DIGEST

- When eliciting the history from patients who are dizzy, allow them to describe the sensation in their own words before offering multiple choices.
- Categorize the diagnosis into one (or more) of four categories: vertigo, presyncope, disequilibrium, or vague lightheadedness.
- BPV can be confirmed by reproduction of symptoms with the Dix-Hallpike maneuver, also known as the Bárány test.
- CNS causes of vertigo are manifested by additional neurologic symptoms, not dizziness alone.

Resources

Eaton DA, Roland PS. Dizziness in the older adult, part 1: Evaluation and general treatment strategies. Geriatrics 58:28–36, 2003.

Hoffman RM, Einstadter D, Kroenke K. Evaluating dizziness. American Journal of Medicine 107:464–478, 1999.

Kroenke K, Hoffman RM. How common are various causes of dizziness? A critical review. Southern Medical Journal 93:160–167, 2000.

Radtke A, Von Brevern M, Tiel-Wilck K, et al. Self-treatment with a modified Eply procedure resolved positional vertigo. Neurology 63:150–152, 2004.

Sloan PD, Coeytaux RR, Beck RS, et al. Dizziness: State of the science. Annals of Internal Medicine 134:Supplement, 823–832, 2001.

Strupp M, Zingler VC, Arbusow V, et al. Methylprednisolone, valacyclovir, or the combination for vestibular neuritis. New England Journal of Medicine 351:354–361, 2004.

Tusa R. Dizziness. Medical Clinics of North America 87: 609–641, 2003.

Warner EA, Wallach PM, Adelman HM, et al. Dizziness in primary care patients. Journal of General Internal Medicine 7:454–63, 1992.

 See the testbank CD for more self-test questions.

CHEST PAIN

CHAPTER 9

Gary J. Martin, MD

I. Pathophysiology

A. Chest pain can be caused by any of the structures within or adjacent to the chest, including the chest wall and upper abdomen. The vascular causes are the most concerning.

II. Epidemiology

A. It is useful to separate acute causes of chest pain from chronic causes. Box 9.1 lists many of the causes of acute chest pain. Box 9.2 lists some of the common causes of episodic or chronic recurrent chest pain.

> In a primary care setting, the most common causes of chest pain are musculoskeletal followed by gastrointestinal and cardiac causes. Less common are psychiatric and pulmonary causes.

BOX 9.1

Common Causes of Acute Chest Pain

- Myocardial infarction
- Aortic dissection
- Pulmonary embolism
- Pericarditis
- Esophageal reflux or spasm
- Pneumonia
- Chest wall disorders (musculoskeletal, zoster, breast disease)
- Psychogenic
- Upper abdominal causes (pancreatitis, peptic ulcer, cholelithiasis)

Common Causes of Episodic or Recurrent Chest Pain

- Esophagitis
- Esophageal spasm
- Biliary colic
- Chest wall pain
- Psychogenic causes including anxiety, depression, and panic attacks
- Stable angina from coronary artery disease (CAD)

III. Signs and Symptoms

A. Classic patterns of chest pain include:

1. *Angina:* central pressure associated with exertion, lasting approximately 1–2 minutes and relieved with rest; myocardial infarction is similar but typically lasts 30 minutes to 2 hours or longer—unusual to last more than 6 hours

> Classic angina is usually a pressure sensation, and patients may even deny pain. Less often it can be described as a burning, ache or, although rarely, a sharp pain.

2. *Pericarditis:* central pain that can be aggravated when lying down and relieved when sitting up; duration can be hours to days

3. *Esophageal pain:* typically described as burning (reflux) or squeezing (spasm) and aggravated by lying down after a meal or triggered by certain foods or alcohol; patient's mouth may also have a bitter taste; duration may be minutes to an hour

4. *Pleuritic chest pains:* by definition are aggravated by taking a deep breath

5. *Chest wall pain:* can also be aggravated by taking a deep breath or by other position changes; can last for minutes or hours

IV. History and Physical

A. History

1. Key points to collect information on include:

   a. Classic cardiac risk factors such as smoking, diabetes, hypertension, hyperlipidemia, and family history

b. Quality, location, duration, radiation, precipitating factors, relieving factors

c. Past medical history of cardiac and gastrointestinal disease and psychiatric disorders

2. Box 9.3 lists criteria for classic angina, atypical chest pain, and nonanginal/nonischemic chest pain

 Your history-taking skills are able to classify patients into these three useful categories.

a. Using these categories for pain, along with the patient's age and gender, a reliable estimate of the likelihood of finding significant CAD can be made. Table 9.1 demonstrates the probabilities based on a large number of patients.

BOX 9.3

Criteria to Classify Chest Discomfort

Criteria

1. Precipitated by exercise
2. Brief duration (2–15 min)
3. Relieved promptly by rest or nitroglycerin
4. Substernal location
5. Radiation from chest to jaw, left arm, or neck
6. Absence of other causes for pain

Classification

I. Typical angina pectoris
   • Criteria 1–3 all positive
   • Any four criteria positive
II. Atypical chest pain
   • Any two criteria positive
   • Only criteria 4–6 positive
III. Nonanginal chest pain
   • Only one criterion positive

From Patterson RE, Horowitz SF: Importance of epidemiology and biostatistics in deciding clinical strategies for using diagnostic tests: A simplified approach using examples from coronary artery disease. JACC 1989; 13:1653–1665.

TABLE 9.1 — Approximate Clinical Probability (%) of Coronary Disease

	Age (yr)	Nonanginal Chest Pain	Atypical Chest Pain	Typical Angina Pectoris
Females	35	.5-1	4	27
	45	5	13	57
	55	12	37	80
	65	20	55	89
Males	35	6	23	71
	45	15	46	88
	55	21	58	91
	65	27	72	93

Adapted from Patterson RE, Horowitz SF. Importance of epidemiology and biostatistics in deciding clinical strategies for using diagnostic tests: A simplified approach using examples from coronary artery disease. JACC 1989;13(7):1653–1665.

B. Physical examination

1. Comparison of blood pressure in each arm can be useful for detecting aortic dissection.

2. Chest auscultation can detect pleural rubs, consolidation suggesting pneumonia, or decreased breath sounds consistent with a pneumothorax.

3. Cardiac examination can detect pericardial rubs, an aortic stenosis murmur, and other evidence of underlying heart disease.

4. Pressure on the chest wall or certain arm or shoulder maneuvers may reproduce the patient's pain, but patients with serious internal conditions including myocardial infarction can say "yes" to chest wall tenderness, so the clinician needs to be careful not to eliminate such possibilities prematurely.

V. Laboratory Tests

A. Even though for most patients chest pain can be diagnosed by history with additional help from the physical examination, a subset of patients benefit from additional tests.

1. An electrocardiogram (ECG) *during* the pain is quite helpful in diagnosing cardiac disease. However, an ECG test result can be quite normal *after* an episode of angina. ST segment changes and T-wave inversions are usually associated with ischemia. ST segment elevation may also be present (and, classically, PR depression) in pericarditis. For prolonged chest pain, troponin levels are quite sensitive for cardiac ischemia.

2. A chest x-ray is another useful test for detecting pneumothorax, pneumonia, pleural effusions, and even a dilated aorta associated with a dissection.

3. More advanced testing could include esophageal manometry, pH monitoring, and stress testing with or without imaging. Transesophageal echo, computed tomography (CT) and magnetic resonance imaging (MRI) can help with acute pain syndromes such as aortic dissection and pulmonary embolism.

VI. Management

A. Acute coronary problems:

1. Initial office treatment includes chewable aspirin and transportation as soon as possible to a monitored setting or a cardiac catherization laboratory for possible thrombolytic therapy or percutaneous coronary intervention. Time is critical because opening the occluded artery within 60–90 minutes gives the best results.

 Unstable angina and acute myocardial infarction (acute coronary syndromes) need immediate attention.

B. For chronic CAD, long-term use of aspirin, beta blockers, and statins are the mainstay of therapy. Angiotensin-converting enzyme (ACE) inhibitors are particularly helpful for the subset of coronary patients with a prior myocardial infarction or left ventricular dysfunction. Control of other risk factors, such as smoking, hypertension, and diabetes, is important.

Control of cholesterol with statins, use of aspirin, and use of beta blockers all have a major impact on recurrent events and mortality in patients with chronic coronary disease.

C. Reflux disease is usually improved with proton pump inhibitors. Some patients can be managed with just diet or over-the-counter H_2 blockers.

D. Chest wall pain usually only requires reassurance, but local physical therapy measures such as cold packs and pain medications would be useful adjuncts.

 MENTOR TIPS DIGEST

- In a primary care setting, the most common causes of chest pain are musculoskeletal followed by gastrointestinal and cardiac causes. Less common are psychiatric and pulmonary causes.
- Classic angina is usually a pressure sensation, and patients may even deny pain. Less often it can be described as a burning, ache or, although rarely, a sharp pain.
- Your history-taking skills are able to classify patients into three useful categories: classic angina, atypical chest pain, and non-anginal/nonischemic chest pain.
- Unstable angina and acute myocardial infarction (acute coronary syndromes) need immediate attention.
- Control of cholesterol with statins, use of aspirin, and use of beta blockers all have a major impact on recurrent events and mortality in patients with chronic coronary disease.

Resources

ACC/AHA 2002 guideline update of the management of patients with chronic stable angina—summary article: A report of the American College of Cardiology/American Heart Association task force on practice guidelines (committee on the management of patients with chronic stable angina). Circulation 107:149–158, 2003.
Use of aspirin, statins, beta blockers, and in some cases ACE_I are key interventions for these patients.

Goldman L. A computer-derived protocol to aid in the diagnosis of emergency room patients with acute chest pain. New England Journal of Medicine 588–596, 1982.
A decision tree for acute chest pain that has been validated.

Klinkman MS, Stevens D, Gorenflo DW. Episodes of care for chest pain: A preliminary report from Michigan Research Network. Journal of Family Practice 38:345, 1994.

Episodes of chest pain totaling 399 were collected and used for analysis from a community-based network. Musculoskeletal chest pain accounted for 20.4% of all diagnoses, followed by reflux esophagitis (13.4%) and costochondritis (13.1%). Stable angina pectoris was the primary diagnosis in only 10.3% of episodes, unstable angina or possible myocardial infarction in 1.5%.

Patterson RE, Horowitz SF. Importance of epidemiology and biostatistics in deciding clinical strategies for using diagnostic tests: A simplified approach using examples from coronary artery disease. JACC 13:1653–1665, 1989.

Useful evidence-based overview of the diagnosis of CAD, using probability to enhance the approach.

Chapter Self-Test Questions

Circle the correct answer. After you have responded to the questions, check your answers in Appendix A.

1. Which is characteristic of typical angina?

  a. Retrosternal pressure chest pain lasting for a few seconds

  b. Retrosternal pressure chest pain lasting for 2–5 minutes associated with exertion

  c. Retrosternal pressure chest pain lasting for a few hours to days, exacerbated by supine posture

  d. Retrosternal burning chest pain lasting for seconds to an hour

2. Which is characteristic of pericarditis?

  a. Retrosternal pressure chest pain lasting for seconds and associated with exertion

  b. Retrosternal pressure chest pain lasting for 2–15 minutes

  c. Retrosternal pressure chest pain lasting for hours to days, exacerbated by supine posture

  d. Retrosternal burning chest pain lasting for seconds to an hour

3. A 47-year-old man comes to the emergency department because of chest pain. He describes a squeezing retrosternal pain that began shortly after he went to bed. He had attended a party that evening and imbibed adult beverages. The pain lasted for over an hour and remitted when paramedics administered sublingual nitroglycerin. What is the most appropriate management at this time?

a. Reassure him that he experienced esophageal reflux and to control alcohol intake.

b. Prescribe a proton pump inhibitor, and arrange for follow-up later in the week.

c. Obtain an ECG.

d. Admit to CCU for observation.

See the testbank CD for more self-test questions.

SINUSITIS, BRONCHITIS, AND PHARYNGITIS

CHAPTER 10

Heather Heiman, MD

I. Sinusitis
A. Pathophysiology
1. Viruses lead to *rhinosinusitis*, also known as the common cold and viral upper respiratory infection.
2. Blockage of the osteomeatal complex from viral rhinosinusitis can lead to acute bacterial sinusitis.

> Clinicians use the term "sinusitis" to imply acute bacterial sinusitis.

3. The microbes causing sinusitis depend on the host.
  a. Immunocompetent hosts
  i. *Streptococcus pneumoniae* and *Haemophilus influenza* are the most common.
  ii. *Moraxella catarrhalis, Streptococcus pyogenes, Staphylococcus aureus,* and anaerobic bacteria are less common.
  b. Patients having diabetes may also get fungal infections such as mucormycosis
4. Chronic sinusitis, which lasts longer than 12 weeks, more commonly involves different bacteria.
  a. Anaerobic bacteria
  b. *S. aureus*
  c. Gram-negative rods

B. Epidemiology

1. Occasional upper respiratory infection (URI) comorbidity

 Sinusitis complicates about 0.5%–2% of URIs.

2. Other risk factors for sinusitis include environmental, anatomic, and genetic conditions:

a. Allergic rhinitis

b. Swimming

c. Anatomic disorders such as nasal polyps

d. Ciliary dysmotility syndromes such as cystic fibrosis

e. Immunodeficiency states such as HIV

3. Uncommon complications:

 About 1/10,000 cases of sinusitis lead to severe complications such as local or central nervous system (CNS) infection.

C. Prevention

1. Hand hygiene has been shown to prevent the spread of viral URIs.

 Antimicrobial agents do not alter the course of the common cold or prevent bacterial sinusitis.

D. History and physical

 History and physical examination in the office focus on differentiating viral rhinosinusitis from bacterial sinusitis.

1. Some symptoms increase the likelihood of a bacterial cause.

a. Maxillary toothache is specific for bacterial sinusitis.

b. History of colored nasal discharge is usually described.

c. Poor response to decongestants is common.

d. The presence of symptoms for more than 7 days is needed to diagnose sinusitis.

 Mental status changes or vision changes are red flags for CNS spread.

2. The physical examination can be helpful but is less so than the history.
   a. Tenderness to sinus palpation is neither sensitive nor specific.
   b. Abnormal sinus transillumination may be helpful: opaque or dull transillumination predicts bacterial source.
      i. Transillumination is done by shining a light source on the sinus in a darkened room and watching the transmission of light through the sinus.
      ii. Transillumination can be done for the frontal and maxillary sinuses.
   c. Purulent secretions in the nares increase the likelihood of bacterial sinusitis.
   d. Periorbital edema is a red flag for orbital cellulitis or osteomyelitis.
E. Differential diagnosis
   1. Radiologic studies do not differentiate bacterial from viral sinusitis, as over 80% of viral rhinosinusitis cases show abnormalities on plain film or computed tomography of the sinuses.
   2. Sinus aspirate by puncture is invasive and not performed routinely.

> Diagnosis of acute sinusitis is made empirically. National guidelines endorsed by the U.S. Centers for Disease Control and Prevention (CDC) recommend reserving the diagnosis of acute bacterial rhinosinusitis for patients with rhinosinusitis symptoms lasting 7 days or more with maxillary pain or tenderness in the face or teeth (especially when unilateral) and purulent nasal secretions.

   3. Sinus symptoms are occasionally caused by noninfectious illness.
      a. Rhinitis medicamentosum (overuse of topical decongestants leading to rebound congestion)
      b. Allergic rhinitis
      c. Idiopathic (vasomotor) rhinitis
      d. Migraine headache
      e. Wegener granulomatosis
E. Management
   1. Antimicrobial therapy
      a. Two thirds of cases of acute bacterial sinusitis will get better on their own.

b. Amoxicillin and penicillin have a small, statistically significant benefit over placebo in terms of cure or improvement of symptoms.

 Newer, non-penicillin antibiotics are not shown to be more effective than amoxicillin.

 Amoxicillin (500 mg three times daily in adults) is first-line therapy for acute sinusitis.

   i. Patients who are allergic to penicillin may be treated with doxycycline or trimethoprim-sulfamethoxazole.

   ii. Patients who used antibiotics in the past month should be treated with broader-spectrum antibiotics such as amoxicillin/clavulanic acid or quinolones.

2. Supportive therapy

   a. Antihistamines and intranasal steroids are effective for patients with a history of allergic rhinitis.

   b. Patients without a history of allergic rhinitis are not known to benefit from antihistamines, intranasal corticosteroids, or decongestants.

3. Referral to an otolaryngologist for consideration of surgical therapy reasonable for patients with more than three episodes of sinusitis per year

II. Acute Bronchitis

A. Pathophysiology

   1. Infection leading to inflammation and desquamation of the bronchial epithelium

   2. Microbiology

 Acute bronchitis is almost always viral.

     a. Viruses involved

       i. Influenza

       ii. Respiratory syncytial virus

       iii. Adenovirus

       iv. Rhinovirus

    v. Coronavirus

    vi. Parainfluenza

  b. Atypical bacteria

 Atypical bacterial causes of acute bronchitis are thought to be far less common than viral.

    i. *Bordatella pertussis* probably accounts for 1% of cases of acute bronchitis.

    ii. *Chlamydia pneumoniae* accounts for 5% of cases.

    iii. *Mycoplasma pneumoniae* accounts for 1% of cases.

  c. Intubated patients or patients with chronic obstructive pulmonary disease may get bronchitis from typical bacteria such as *S. pneumoniae, H. influenza,* or *M. catarrhalis*

B. Epidemiology

  1. Bronchitis affects about 5% of adults each year.

  2. It is most common in winter.

  3. Recurrent episodes of bronchitis are associated with development of adult-onset asthma, but the link is poorly understood.

C. Prevention

  1. Hand hygiene prevents spread of viruses.

  2. Pertussis immunization is given in childhood, and a booster dose is given once in adulthood.

D. History and physical

  1. A cough is almost always the presenting manifestation of bronchitis.

    a. The common cold is associated with a cough, which usually follows sore throat, sneezing, and congestion.

    b. Cough in bronchitis is persistent.

 In bronchitis, cough persists for more than 5 days, usually 10–20 days.

    c. Cough may be productive or nonproductive.

  2. Chest pain may be present and is often pleuritic.

 Dyspnea is typically absent in bronchitis.

3. The vital signs follow.
   a. Fever may not occur
      i. Usually present in patients with influenza and adenovirus
      ii. Most often absent in patients with rhinovirus or coronavirus
   b. Others

 Tachypnea, tachycardia, and hypoxemia should not be present in bronchitis and are concerning for pneumonia, bronchiolitis, or severe asthma.

E. Chest examination

Either normal breath sound or wheezing is heard in bronchitis.

   1. Signs of consolidation (rales, egophony) should not be present.
F. Differential diagnosis
   1. Other possible diagnoses
      a. Asthma may present jointly with bronchitis or be the sole diagnosis.
      b. Bronchiolitis presents with wheezing, tachypnea, and hypoxemia.
      c. Bronchiectasis presents with a chronic cough with dilation of the bronchi on imaging.
      d. Chronic bronchitis occurs in smokers who have cough with sputum on most days for more than 3 months of the year for 2 years running.
      e. Upper respiratory infection typically manifests with cough less than a week.
      f. Pneumonia usually presents with consolidation or vital sign abnormalities, although patients over 75 years may lack these findings.
   2. Laboratory testing in patients with a clinical presentation of bronchitis
      a. Chest x-ray (CXR) for certain indications

CXR is recommended for patients with signs of consolidation on lung examination, or with tachycardia, tachypnea, hypoxemia, or fever >101°F (38.3°C)

      b. Nasopharyngeal swabs can detect pertussis, mycoplasma, and influenza in epidemics

      c. 40% of patients have transient decrement in forced expiratory volume in the first second, but pulmonary function testing is not necessary routinely

   G. Management

      1. Antimicrobial therapy

 Bronchitis is a self-limited illness; antibiotics reduce cough by a fraction of a day but have no benefit for overall quality of life.

      a. Nevertheless, 60% of patients with bronchitis receive antibiotics.

      b. Patients with influenza benefit from initiation of neuraminidase inhibitors within the first 48 hours of symptoms.

      c. Spread of pertussis can be reduced by initiating macrolide therapy during the paroxysmal (cough) phase, although therapy after 14 days of the illness does not reduce symptoms for the individual.

      d. Tetracyclines or macrolides treat *M. pneumoniae* and *C. pneumoniae.*

      2. Supportive therapies

      a. Nonsteroidal anti-inflammatory medications with or without antihistamines reduced cough in some studies.

      b. No consistent benefit has been seen with use of beta agonist.

      c. Trials of mucolytic or antitussive agents, such as guaifenesin and codeine, have had mixed results.

III. Pharyngitis

   A. Pathophysiology

      1. Viral

 Viruses are the most common cause of pharyngitis.

      a. Rhinoviruses are the leading viral cause.

      b. Coronavirus, adenovirus, and herpes simplex virus are also frequent.

c. Less commonly, pharyngitis is caused by parainfluenza, influenza, Epstein-Barr virus (EBV), cytomegalovirus, HIV, coxsackievirus

2. Streptococcus causes almost all bacterial pharyngitis.

> 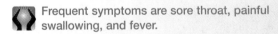 *Streptococcus pyogenes* (group A beta-hemolytic streptococcus) accounts for 15%–30% of pharyngitis episodes in children and 10% in adults.

  a. Groups C and G beta-hemolytic streptococci are common causes as well.
  b. *Arcanobacterium hemolyticum* may cause pharyngitis that mimics a streptococcal infection.
B. Epidemiology
  1. There are 18 million office visits yearly in the United States for pharyngitis.
  2. Winter is the most common time for pharyngitis outbreaks.
  3. *S. pyogenes* often colonizes the oropharynx, especially in school-age children.
C. Prevention
  1. Prevention of strep throat through tonsillectomy in patients with recurrent episodes is controversial.
  2. Influenza vaccination in October through May can prevent influenza pharyngitis.
D. History and physical
  1. Streptococcal pharyngitis
    a. Symptoms

> Frequent symptoms are sore throat, painful swallowing, and fever.

      i. Sometimes patients have headaches, abdominal pain, and chills.
    b. Signs

> Key signs are temperature above 101°F (38.3°C), exudate on the tonsils, and tender cervical adenopathy.

    i. Other signs

      (1) Significant erythema of the throat

      (2) Edema of the uvula

      (3) A white blood cell count of greater than $12,000/mm^3$

c. Be alert for complications of streptococcal pharyngitis

    i. Suppurative complications

      (1) Peritonsillar abscess

> In peritonsillar abscess, the tonsil may be displaced toward the midline, and the voice may sound muffled, classically described as a "hot potato."

      (2) Retropharyngeal abscess, jugular venous thrombophlebitis, otitis media, mastoiditis can complicate strep throat

    ii. Nonsuppurative complications

      (1) Acute rheumatic fever

> Acute rheumatic fever occurs in 3% of patients with untreated streptococcal tonsillitis (one case per million people annually in the United States) and manifests with heart and joint involvement, chorea, subcutaneous nodules, and fever.

      (2) Poststreptococcal glomerulonephritis may occur in children

      (3) Reactive arthritis may occur

2. Viral pharyngitis

  a. Exudative pharyngitis often observed with adenovirus and EBV

  b. Ulcers, vesicles occur with herpes simplex and coxsackievirus

  c. Diphtheria, occurring occasionally in the United States, presents with grayish "pseudomembrane"

  d. Possibilities with HIV

> Acute HIV can manifest with fever and a nonexudative pharyngitis.

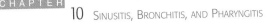

    e. Mild nonexudative pharyngitis occasionally occurs with oral infection with *Neisseria gonorrhea*

    f. Influenza may present with nonexudative pharyngitis, muscle aches, headache, cough

E. Differential diagnosis

  1. It is critical to distinguish between streptococcal infection, which requires antimicrobial therapy to prevent suppurative and nonsuppurative complications, and viral causes of pharyngitis.

    a. Although only 10% of adults with sore throat have a strep infection, 75% of adults receive antibiotics.

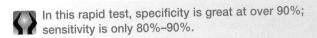
The Centor criteria are a validated clinical prediction rule to help diagnose strep; one point is given for each of the following criteria.

      i. Fever

      ii. Tonsillar exudates

      iii. Tender cervical lymphadenopathy

      iv. Absence of cough

      v. Age sometimes included in modification of the criteria, with age under 14 years giving one point and over 45 years taking away one point

    b. Guidelines for use of Centor criteria, according to the American College of Physicians:

      i. Patients with zero or one Centor criterion do not need further testing, because risk of strep is 10% or less.

      ii. Patients with two Centor criteria should be tested with one of the methods discussed in the following section.

      iii. Patients with three or more Centor criteria can be tested or empirically treated because risk is at least 28%.

  2. Laboratory testing for strep

    a. Rapid strep enzyme immunoassay

In this rapid test, specificity is great at over 90%; sensitivity is only 80%–90%.

      i. Advisory committees consider that the rapid test is not sensitive enough to be used alone in children and adolescents.

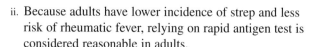
ii. Because adults have lower incidence of strep and less risk of rheumatic fever, relying on rapid antigen test is considered reasonable in adults.

b. Throat culture

 Throat culture is the gold standard and should be done in children if results of rapid testing are negative.

3. Laboratory testing for other causes

a. Heterophile antibody can be checked to evaluate for EBV.

b. Testing for gonorrhea requires culture on Thayer-Martin medium.

c. Rapid testing on an oropharyngeal swab can detect influenza virus.

F. Management

1. Antimicrobial therapies

a. Penicillin cures group A strep, and essentially no resistance has been seen.

   i. 10 days of oral penicillin VK

   ii. Injection of benzathine penicillin

 Treatment within 9 days of onset of symptoms is sufficient to prevent rheumatic fever.

b. Patients with mononucleosis (EBV) who are treated with ampicillin or amoxicillin for presumed strep often get a diffuse, pruritic skin eruption.

2. Supportive therapies

a. OTC pain relievers

 Ibuprofen is more effective than acetaminophen in relieving pain in the throat in children.

b. Warm saltwater gargles, throat lozenges may also help.

MENTOR TIPS DIGEST

Sinusitis

- Clinicians use the term "sinusitis" to imply acute bacterial sinusitis.
- Sinusitis complicates about 0.5%–2% of URIs.
- About 1/10,000 cases of sinusitis lead to severe complications such as local or CNS infection.
- Antimicrobial agents do not alter the course of the common cold or prevent bacterial sinusitis.
- History and physical examination in the office focus on differentiating viral rhinosinusitis from bacterial sinusitis.
- Mental status changes or vision changes are red flags for CNS spread.
- Diagnosis of acute sinusitis is made empirically. National guidelines endorsed by the CDC recommend reserving the diagnosis of acute bacterial rhinosinusitis for patients with rhinosinusitis symptoms lasting 7 days or more with maxillary pain or tenderness in the face or teeth (especially when unilateral) and purulent nasal secretions.
- Newer, non-penicillin antibiotics are not shown to be more effective than amoxicillin.
- Amoxicillin (500 mg three times daily in adults) is first-line therapy for acute sinusitis.

Bronchitis

- Acute bronchitis is almost always viral.
- Atypical bacterial causes of acute bronchitis are thought to be far less common than viral.
- In bronchitis, cough persists for more than 5 days, usually 10–20 days.
- Dyspnea is typically absent in bronchitis.
- Tachypnea, tachycardia, and hypoxemia should not be present in bronchitis and are concerning for pneumonia, bronchiolitis, or severe asthma.
- Either normal breath sound or wheezing is heard in bronchitis.
- CXR is recommended for patients with signs of consolidation on lung examination, or with tachycardia, tachypnea, hypoxemia, or fever >38.3°C.
- Bronchitis is a self-limited illness; antibiotics reduce cough by a fraction of a day but have no benefit for overall quality of life.

Pharyngitis

- Viruses are the most common cause of pharyngitis.
- *Streptococcus pyogenes* (group A beta-hemolytic streptococcus) accounts for 15%–30% of pharyngitis episodes in children and 10% in adults.
- Frequent symptoms in streptococcal pharyngitis are sore throat, painful swallowing, and fever.
- Key signs in streptococcal pharyngitis are temperature above 39.4°C, exudate on the tonsils, and tender cervical adenopathy.
- In peritonsillar abscess, the tonsil may be displaced toward the midline, and the voice may sound muffled, like a "hot potato."
- Acute rheumatic fever occurs in 3% of patients with untreated streptococcal tonsillitis (one case per million people annually in the United States) and manifests with heart and joint involvement, chorea, subcutaneous nodules, and fever.
- Acute HIV can manifest with fever and a nonexudative pharyngitis.
- The Centor criteria are a validated clinical prediction rule to help diagnose strep; one point is given for each criterion (see text).
- In rapid strep enzyme immunoassay, specificity is great at over 90%; sensitivity is only 80%–90%.
- Throat culture of strep is the gold standard and should be done in children if results of rapid testing are negative.
- Penicillin cures group A strep. Treatment within 9 days of onset of symptoms is sufficient to prevent rheumatic fever.
- Ibuprofen is more effective than acetaminophen in relieving pain in the throat in children.

Resources

Bisno A. Acute pharngitis. New England Journal of Medicine 344:205–211, 2001
This is a helpful review article that pays special attention to the differential diagnosis of pharyngitis and the clinical characteristics of the various viral and bacterial etiologies.

Bisno A. Pharyngitis. In Mandell GL, Bennett JE , Dolin R, eds. Principles and practice of infectious diseases, 6th ed. Elsevier, Philadelphia, 2005.

This comprehensive chapter explains the pathophysiology, clinical syndromes, diagnosis, and treatment of all causes of pharyngitis.

Brook I. Acute and chronic bacterial sinusitis. Infectious Disease Clinics of North America 427–448, 2007.
This is a detailed review article about the microbes causing acute and chronic sinusitis.

Ebell MH, et al. The rational clinical examination: Does this patient have strep throat. Journal of the American Medical Association 2912–2918, 2000.
This article is a focused exploration of the sensitivity and specificity of signs and symptoms for diagnosing strep pharyngitis. It explores available clinical prediction rules such as the Centor criteria.

Gonzalez R, et al. Principles of appropriate antibiotic use for treatment of nonspecific upper respiratory infections in adults: Background. Annals of Internal Medicine 134:490–494, 2001.
A clinical practice guideline for treating ambulatory patients with suspected sinusitis.

Gwaltney J. Acute bronchitis. In Mandell GL, Bennett JE , Dolin R, eds. Principles and practice of infectious diseases, 6th ed. Elsevier, Philadelphia, 2005.
Gwaltney explores the pathogenesis and clinical manifestations of the viral and nonviral causes of acute bronchitis.

Gwaltney J. Sinusitis. In Mandell GL,Bennett JE, Dolin R, eds. Principles and practice of infectious diseases, 6th ed. Elsevier, Philadelphia, 2005.
Gwaltney explores sinusitis.

Hahn RG, Knox LM, Forman TA. Evaluation of poststreptococcal illness. American Family Physician 1949–1954, 2005.
This article details the suppurative and nonsuppurative complications of streptococcal pharyngitis.

Piccirillo J. Acute bacterial sinusitis. New England Journal of Medicine 351:902–910, 2004.
Excellent review article.

Snow V, et al. Principles of appropriate antibiotic use for acute pharyngitis in adults. Annals of Internal Medicine 506–517, 2001.
This is a brief clinical guideline focusing on the diagnosis of strep throat and avoidance of unnecessary antibiotic use.

Steinman MA, et al. Changing use of antibiotics in community-based outpatient practice, 1991–1999. Annals of Internal Medicine 525–533, 2003.

Cross-sectional study showing a high incidence of antibiotic prescribing for common viral diagnoses such as acute bronchitis.

Wenzel RP, Fowler AA. Acute bronchitis. New England Journal of Medicine 2006;355:2125–30.

This article offers a practical approach to the common clinical presentation of acute bronchitis.

Williams JW, et al. Antibiotics for acute maxillary sinusitis. The Cochrane Database of Systematic Reviews 2007.

A compilation of the high-quality studies of antibiotics for sinusitis, which in summary show a marginal benefit of antibiotics.

Williams JW, Simel DL. Does this patient have sinusitis: Diagnosing acute sinusitis by history and physical examination. Journal of the American Medical Association 1242–1246, 1993.

An installment in the rational clinical examination series that explores utility of signs and symptoms in distinguishing bacterial sinusitis from the common cold.

Chapter Self-Test Questions

Circle the correct answer. After you have responded to the questions, check your answers in Appendix A.

1. What is the most effective proven technique for preventing the common cold?

   a. Hand washing

   b. Paper face masks covering nose and mouth

   c. Decongestant nasal spray

   d. Prophylactic antibiotic therapy

2. A 32-year-old man presents to you because his wife has a "sinus" infection for which a provider prescribed amoxicillin/clavulanate. He is aware of extensive news coverage of MRSA in the community. He would like a prescription to prevent a sinus infection. Which is the most appropriate response?

a. Prescribe amoxicillin/clavulanate.

b. Prescribe clindamycin.

c. Reassure and explain that sinus infections are not contagious.

d. Reassure and recommend temporary change in home sleeping arrangements.

3. Which is the most common organism causing acute bacterial sinusitis in immunocompetent adults?

a. *Staphylococcus aureus*

b. *Streptococcus pneumoniae*

c. *Legionella pneumoniae*

d. *Escherichia coli*

 See the testbank CD for more self-test questions.

CHAPTER 11

ABDOMINAL PAIN

Mitchell S. King, MD

I. Introduction

A. Common with a variety of presenting symptoms and potential etiologies.

B. Diagnostic possibilities from chronic and benign illnesses, such as irritable bowel syndrome, to acute and life-threatening conditions, such as abdominal aortic aneurysm (AAA).

C. Differential diagnosis includes intra-abdominal conditions; pulmonary, cardiac, musculoskeletal, and dermatologic disease (Table 11.1).

D. Chronic abdominal pain not assumed as benign

TABLE 11.1	Differential Diagnosis of Abdominal Pain by Location
Location	**Differential Diagnosis**
Poorly localized	Abdominal aortic aneurysm (AAA)
	Mesenteric ischemia
	Early obstruction
	Early appendicitis
	Inflammatory bowel disease
	Gastroenteritis
	Pancreatitis
	Peritonitis
	Sickle cell anemia crisis
Epigastric	Gastroesophageal reflux disease
	Peptic ulcer disease
	Gastritis

Differential Diagnosis of Abdominal Pain by Location (Continued)

Location	Differential Diagnosis
	Pancreatitis
	Cholecystitis
	Musculoskeletal
	Cardiac (myocardial infarction/pericarditis)
Right upper quadrant	Cholecystitis
	Other liver disease (hepatitis, cholangitis, abscess)
	Gastritis
	Peptic ulcer disease
	Renal (stones, pyelonephritis)
	Pulmonary (pneumonia, pleural disease, pulmonary embolus)
	Musculoskeletal
	Herpes zoster
	Appendicitis
	Subdiaphragmatic abscess
Left upper quadrant	Peptic ulcer disease
	Gastritis
	Splenic (splenomegaly, infarction, injury)
	Pancreatitis
	AAA
	Cardiac (infarction, pericarditis)
	Pulmonary (pneumonia, pleural disease, pulmonary embolus)
	Musculoskeletal
	Herpes zoster
Right lower quadrant	Appendicitis
	Mesenteric adenitis
	Crohn disease
	Diverticular disease, including Meckel
	Cholecystitis/biliary tract
	Musculoskeletal
	Pancreatitis
	Herpes zoster
	Gynecologic (pelvic inflammatory disease, ectopic pregnancy, endometriosis)
	Renal (stones, infection)

(continued on page 144)

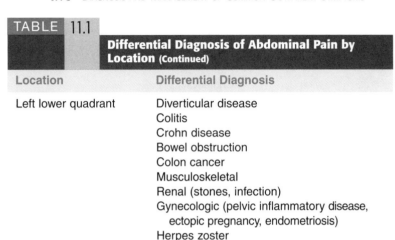

TABLE 11.1	Differential Diagnosis of Abdominal Pain by Location (Continued)
Location	**Differential Diagnosis**
Left lower quadrant	Diverticular disease
	Colitis
	Crohn disease
	Bowel obstruction
	Colon cancer
	Musculoskeletal
	Renal (stones, infection)
	Gynecologic (pelvic inflammatory disease, ectopic pregnancy, endometriosis)
	Herpes zoster

II. Approach to the Patient

A. Initial evaluation of abdominal pain

1. History (Box 11.1): characterizing the pain and assessing risk for the different diseases that can cause abdominal pain are important elements of the history.

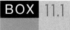

BOX 11.1	Important History Elements to Evaluate in Patients With Abdominal Pain

- Onset of pain
- Location of pain
- Aggravating/alleviating factors
- Associated symptoms
- Fever
- Past medical and surgical history
- Medication use
- Family history
- Smoking history
- Dietary history

a. Onset

> Pain that develops suddenly suggests a vascular etiology (e.g., organ infarction, AAA) or perforation/rupture of an abdominal organ (perforated ulcer, esophageal rupture).

   i. Onset of pain with peptic ulcer disease, diverticulitis, appendicitis, bowel obstruction, biliary or renal colic, and pancreatitis is generally over minutes to hours.

   ii. The exact onset of pain with chronic abdominal pain is often difficult to define.

> In patients with chronic abdominal pain, the presence of "alarm" symptoms such as onset at older than 50 years of age, rectal bleeding, weight loss, or recent change in bowel function raises suspicion for organic disease.

b. Location of pain (see Table 11.1)

   i. Pain radiation patterns: e.g., midepigastric pain of pancreatitis is referred through to the back; pain of biliary colic may be referred to the scapular region

   ii. Evolution of the pain: e.g., pain of appendicitis starts in periumbilical region but as process progresses, pain can localize to right lower quadrant

c. Aggravating/alleviating factors: ingesting food, passing bowel movements, or changing position

   i. *Food* may alleviate the symptoms of ulcer disease but worsen the symptoms associated with bowel obstruction, cholecystitis, pancreatitis, and irritable bowel syndrome.

   ii. *Bowel movements* may bring some relief to patients with irritable bowel syndrome.

   iii. The *reclining position* may aggravate the symptoms of pancreatitis and gastroesophageal reflux disease (GERD).

iv. *Body movement* may aggravate the pain in conditions with peritoneal inflammation, such as appendicitis, diverticulitis, or ruptured viscus. The pain of renal colic occurs independently of the above factors.

  d. Associated symptoms

    i. *Nausea* and *vomiting* are common.

> Pain that precedes emesis suggests a potential surgical condition, whereas emesis that is followed by pain points more toward a nonsurgical condition.

    ii. *Hematemesis,* or "coffee ground" emesis, occurs with upper gastrointestinal (GI) bleeding seen with peptic ulcer disease, gastritis, esophagitis, or esophageal varices.

    iii. *Heme-positive stools* (can occur with either upper or lower GI blood loss) and abdominal pain may be caused by peptic ulcer disease, gastritis, inflammatory bowel disease, infectious colitis, mesenteric ischemia, diverticular disease, or colon cancer.

    iv. *Diarrhea* associated with crampy abdominal pain is present with gastroenteritis, colitis, lactose intolerance, and inflammatory bowel disease.

    v. *Jaundice* in association with abdominal pain suggests liver disease or biliary tract obstruction.

    vi. *Colicky or wavelike discomfort* is consistent with an intestinal obstruction. Vomiting is common, particularly in proximal obstruction. Obstruction that is more distal tends to be less painful and is associated with less vomiting than proximal obstruction.

    vii. *Fatigue and weight loss* may indicate inflammatory bowel disease or a malignancy as the underlying cause for abdominal pain.

    viii. *Extraintestinal manifestations* such as iritis, arthritis, aphthous ulcers, and dermatologic findings of erythema nodosum and pyoderma gangrenosum may occur with inflammatory bowel disease.

    ix. *Referred pain* from a cardiac or pulmonary process should be considered if patients complain of shortness of breath, cough, or chest pain. For patients with stigmata of alcohol abuse, such as spider hemangioma, palmar erythema, or testicular atrophy, pancreatitis should be considered.

x. *Gynecologic conditions* should be considered in female patients. Timing of the pain in relation to the menstrual cycle may point to either endometriosis or mittelschmerz. Finally, vaginal discharge and a history of sexually transmitted disease may indicate the possibility of pelvic inflammatory disease.

 Symptoms that are significantly associated with ovarian cancer are pelvic/abdominal pain, urinary urgency/frequency, increased abdominal size/bloating, and difficulty eating/feeling full when present for <1 year and occurring >12 days per month.

xi. *Fever* is common with infectious enteritis, diverticulitis, appendicitis, cholecystitis, intra-abdominal abscesses (psoas, subdiaphragmatic), and pulmonary, gynecologic, and urinary tract infections.

2. Past medical and surgical history may suggest etiologies:
   a. Gallstones, nephrolithiasis, or diverticular disease may indicate a recurrence.

 Of the adult Western population, 10%–15% will develop gallstones.

   b. Previous abdominal surgery should lead to consideration of bowel obstruction due to adhesions.
   c. Known hypertension or vascular disease is a risk factor for a vascular cause, such as AAA, or mesenteric infarction.
   d. Cholelithiasis and alcohol abuse are the most common conditions associated with pancreatitis.
   e. Prior ectopic pregnancies, a history of a sexually transmitted disease, or pelvic inflammatory disease may suggest a gynecologic etiology.

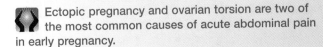 Ectopic pregnancy and ovarian torsion are two of the most common causes of acute abdominal pain in early pregnancy.

   f. Ketoacidosis may present with abdominal pain and should
      be considered in diabetic individuals.
   3. Medication use:
      a. Nonsteroidal anti-inflammatory medications (NSAIDs) may
         cause *Helicobacter pylori*–negative ulcer disease.
      b. Fenofibrate and gemfibrozil are associated with gallstone
         formation.
      c. Azathioprine, 6-mercaptopurine, didanosine, and other
         medications can cause pancreatitis.
   B. Physical examination (Table 11.2)

TABLE 11.2 Diagnostic Clues to Etiologies of Abdominal Pain	
Diagnosis	**Typical Symptoms**
Gastroesophageal reflux disease	Regurgitation, dysphagia
Peptic ulcer disease	Gnawing epigastric pain, nausea, vomiting, bloating
Gastritis	Same as peptic ulcer disease
Nonulcer dyspepsia	Upper abdominal/epigastric pain, bloating, belching, flatulence, nausea
Cholelithiasis	Colicky right upper quadrant pain, worse with meals, radiation to scapular region
Pancreatitis	Severe constant midabdominal pain
Inflammatory bowel disease	Chronic diarrhea, hematochezia, weight loss, anorexia, fever
Irritable bowel syndrome	Chronic abdominal cramps, alternating diarrhea and constipation; *no* weight loss, fever, or hematochezia
Gastroenteritis	Acute illness with nausea, vomiting, diarrhea
Bowel obstruction	Pain followed by absent stool, flatus, nausea, vomiting, abdominal distention
Peritonitis	Severe abdominal pain, worsens with movement, cough; fever
Nephrolithiasis	Flank pain radiating to the groin, intense, writhing to get comfortable, ± hematuria

Diagnostic Clues to Etiologies of Abdominal Pain (Continued)

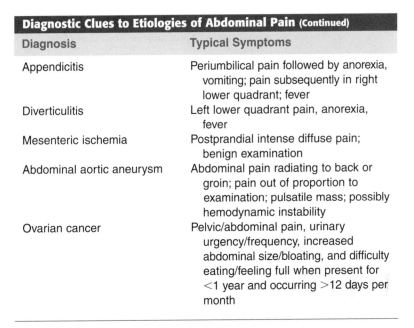

Diagnosis	Typical Symptoms
Appendicitis	Periumbilical pain followed by anorexia, vomiting; pain subsequently in right lower quadrant; fever
Diverticulitis	Left lower quadrant pain, anorexia, fever
Mesenteric ischemia	Postprandial intense diffuse pain; benign examination
Abdominal aortic aneurysm	Abdominal pain radiating to back or groin; pain out of proportion to examination; pulsatile mass; possibly hemodynamic instability
Ovarian cancer	Pelvic/abdominal pain, urinary urgency/frequency, increased abdominal size/bloating, and difficulty eating/feeling full when present for <1 year and occurring >12 days per month

1. Vital signs
   a. Hypotension may signify AAA, rupture of an intra-abdominal organ, significant blood loss, dehydration, or sepsis.
   b. Fever may occur with appendicitis, diverticulitis, pancreatitis, and cholecystitis as well as with pulmonary, gynecologic, or urinary tract infections.
2. General appearance and posture
   a. Patients in severe pain should generally be evaluated in an emergency room setting.

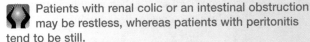 Patients with renal colic or an intestinal obstruction may be restless, whereas patients with peritonitis tend to be still.

   b. A patient with pancreatitis may prefer to sit up and lean forward and may be more uncomfortable in the supine position.

3. Chest

    a. Evaluate for pericardial or pleural rubs and signs of lower lobe consolidation.

4. Abdomen

    a. Inspection

      i. *Abdominal distention* may indicate bowel obstruction (however, it is nonspecific).

      ii. *Scars* from prior surgeries should be noted.

      iii. *Rash* could indicate presence of herpes zoster.

      iv. *Skin discoloration* or *bruising* should be noted and may indicate retroperitoneal bleeding as may occur with hemorrhagic pancreatitis. Jaundice suggests biliary disease or hepatitis.

    b. Auscultation

      i. *Hyperactive bowel sounds* occur with gastroenteritis or bowel obstruction, with high-pitched, tinkling bowel sounds being characteristic of the latter.

      ii. *Hypoactive bowel sounds* may be present with diverticulitis or appendicitis and late bowel obstruction. A silent abdomen often indicates generalized peritonitis.

      iii. *Abdominal bruits* suggest potential vascular pathology.

    c. Palpation

      i. *Begin with light palpation* in areas away from the abdominal pain.

      ii. *Abdominal guarding,* presence of masses, hernias, or organomegaly should be noted during palpation.

      iii. *Rebound tenderness* can be elicited by asking the patient to cough.

      iv. *Localization of the pain* is very helpful in narrowing the differential diagnosis (see Table 11.1). For example, a positive Murphy sign, increased pain on palpation of the right upper quadrant while the patient inspires, suggests cholecystitis.

      v. *Generalized* severe abdominal tenderness indicates diffuse peritoneal inflammation.

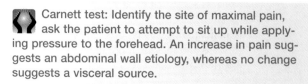 Carnett test: Identify the site of maximal pain, ask the patient to attempt to sit up while applying pressure to the forehead. An increase in pain suggests an abdominal wall etiology, whereas no change suggests a visceral source.

> Significant abdominal pain in the absence of significant physical examination findings may suggest mesenteric ischemia. (However, be circumspect; this finding is also common in somatoform disorder and malingering.)

5. Rectal examination
   a. Evaluate for masses, and check the stool for occult blood.
6. Pelvic examination
   a. Evaluate for pelvic masses, cervical/vaginal discharge, and presence of cervical motion tenderness.
7. Testicular examination
   a. Evaluate for testicular torsion or epididymitis.
C. Diagnostic studies (Table 11.3)

TABLE 11.3	Diagnostic Testing to Evaluate Abdominal Pain
Laboratory test	**Useful for**
Complete blood count	Anemia/hemorrhage, infection
Urinalysis	Renal infection, renal stones, diabetes
Liver panel	Cholecystitis, hepatitis
Amylase	Pancreatitis
Lipase	Pancreatitis
Serum calcium	Pancreatitis
Basic metabolic panel	Nausea/vomiting/diarrhea, dehydration, impaired renal function, diabetes
Lipids	Pancreatitis
Human chorionic gonadotropin	Pregnancy/ectopic pregnancy
Hemoccult testing of stool	Gastrointestinal blood loss (any source)
Stool for leukocytes	Bacterial gastroenteritis, inflammatory bowel disease
Stool culture	Bacterial gastroenteritis
Stool for ova and parasites	Diarrhea/abdominal pain due to parasites
Stool for *Clostridium difficile* toxin	Diarrhea/abdominal pain from pseudomembranous colitis

(continued on page 152)

TABLE 11.3	
Diagnostic Testing to Evaluate Abdominal Pain (Continued)	
Radiologic test	**Useful for**
Plain film	Perforated viscus, bowel obstruction, ± renal stones
Computer tomography scan	Organ infection, infarction or tumor, bowel obstruction, pancreatitis, appendicitis, diverticulitis, hemorrhage, abdominal aortic aneurysm (AAA)
Magnetic resonance scan	Imaging patients for whom the risk of radiation or the potential nephrotoxicity of iodinated contrast is a major concern; evaluating pregnant patients with acute lower abdominal pain believed to have an extrauterine cause such as appendicitis or torsion. MRI with gadolinium should be avoided in patients with end stage renal disease.
Ultrasound	Cholecystitis, pancreatitis, renal infection/obstruction, AAA in women and children: appendicitis, gynecologic disease
Intravenous pyelogram	Renal stones/obstruction, hematuria evaluation
Barium swallow	Esophageal cancer, stricture, diverticula, reflux, ± spasm
Upper gastrointestinal series	Small bowel source of blood loss when other source negative, bowel obstruction, inflammatory bowel disease, small bowel malignancies (rare)
Barium enema	Colon cancer, polyps, colitis, Crohn disease, bowel obstruction
Esophagogastroduodenoscopy	Gastroesophageal reflux disease, esophageal stricture, cancer, peptic ulcer disease, gastritis, gastric cancer
Colonoscopy	Colon cancer, colitis, polyps, inflammatory bowel disease

1. Laboratory studies
   a. *Complete blood count (CBC):* detects the presence of anemia or an elevated white blood cell count suggesting the presence of an acute inflammatory or infectious process; in elderly patients, the differential is extremely important because a shift to immature forms of white blood cells can indicate significant disease in patients with just mildly elevated or normal white blood cell counts
   b. *Urinalysis:* look for pyuria and/or hematuria, thus pointing to urinary tract as potential source for abdominal pain
   c. *Liver function tests* and *amylase/lipase:* when elevated, may signify liver and/or pancreatic disease; when a patient has had recurrent episodes of hepatitis and pancreatitis, this may not be true
   d. *Basic metabolic panel:* can assess hydration, renal function, and electrolytes; an elevated glucose with low serum bicarbonate is consistent with ketoacidosis
   e. *H. pylori* testing (Table 11.4): in patients who are not taking ulcerogenic medications, *H. pylori* accounts for almost 90% of ulcer disease

TABLE 11.4 — Diagnostic Tests for *Helicobacter pylori*

Test	Comments
Rapid urease test	• Most commonly used test • Performed on endoscopically obtained tissue sample • Test is inexpensive but requires endoscopy • Results promptly obtained • Sensitive/very specific
Histologic staining	• Requires endoscopy culture • Often performed in conjunction with rapid urease test • Takes longer to receive results • More expensive than rapid urease test
Serology	• Noninvasive • Inexpensive • Documents exposure but not active disease

(continued on page 154)

TABLE 11.4	
Diagnostic Tests for *Helicobacter pylori* (Continued)	
Test	**Comments**
	• Cannot document eradication
	• Used more in younger patients (age <40 years)
	• High rate of positive tests in asymptomatic elderly limits usefulness
Urea breath tests	• Noninvasive
	• Variable cost but can be inexpensive
	• Sensitive/specific
	• Can document eradication
Stool antigen testing	• Requires stool sample
	• 95% sensitive and specific
	• Can document eradication

   i. *Rapid urease test* analyzes tissue samples obtained during endoscopy for the presence of urease (the presence of urease is consistent with *H. pylori* infection). This test has a sensitivity of approximately 90% and a specificity of 98%. The test itself is inexpensive and quickly performed but requires endoscopy to obtain tissue.

   ii. *Histologic staining* can also detect *H. pylori* and may be performed if the rapid urease test is negative in a patient with ulcers or gastritis. Histologic staining has an excellent sensitivity and specificity; however, it is slower and more expensive than the urease test.

   iii. *Serologic testing* for *H. pylori* has the advantage of being noninvasive, inexpensive, and highly sensitive and specific (>90%). The disadvantages are that serology will remain indefinitely positive, and a positive test does not distinguish between prior or current infection. Patients in their twenties are rarely positive, whereas those in their sixties are positive more than 50% of the time.

> This test is useful in younger populations and for diagnosing *H. pylori* in radiographically diagnosed duodenal ulcers, but it cannot be relied on in older patients with gastric ulcers or for following therapeutic response.

iv. *H. pylori* stool antigen testing requires collecting a stool sample. It can be used to test for cure of the disease and is 95% sensitive and specific.

v. *Urea breath testing* involves having the patient ingest urea labeled with radioactive carbon. If *H. pylorus* is present, urease hydrolyzes the urea, and the patient exhales labeled carbon dioxide. The test is both sensitive and specific but is expensive and not readily available.

2. Radiologic testing

   a. *Plain film* is useful for detecting intestinal obstruction and free air, which suggests a perforated viscus. Plain film has a sensitivity of 30%–60% for detecting free air and is diagnostic for 50%–60% of cases of bowel obstruction. Additional information from plain films is limited.

   b. *Computed tomography* (CT) has become one of the most widely used tests for evaluating undifferentiated acute abdominal pain as well as cases of pancreatitis, appendicitis, and diverticulitis. The CT scan has a sensitivity and specificity of over 90% for appendicitis and diverticulitis.

   c. *Magnetic resonance imaging* (MRI) is a useful modality for patients for whom the risk of radiation or the potential nephrotoxicity of iodinated contrast is a major concern. MRI is also useful in evaluating pregnant patients with acute lower abdominal pain that is believed to have an extrauterine cause, such as appendicitis or torsion.

   d. *Ultrasound* is commonly used to evaluate patients with abdominal pain and suspected gallstones, renal stones, pyelonephritis, appendicitis, or gynecologic disease. Ultrasound is commonly the first radiologic study performed for patients being evaluated for cholecystitis. The ultrasound can detect the presence of gallstones, gallbladder wall edema, and biliary duct obstruction. For renal disease, ultrasound can detect ureteral obstruction and demonstrate parenchymal disease or abscess formation. In women with lower quadrant pain, ultrasound is commonly the test first used because of lower cost and lack of radiation exposure. Ultrasound has a sensitivity of approximately 85% and specificity of approximately 90% for diagnosing appendicitis. Ultrasound can also assess the uterus, fallopian tubes, and ovaries for gynecologic disease in patients with abdominal pain.

    e. *Intravenous pyelogram* can demonstrate urinary tract obstruction and is useful for evaluating patients with hematuria and the renal system for traumatic damage. However, CT scan is usually the initial test for patients with abdominal trauma; it can also detect internal bleeding and kidney or other organ damage.

    f. *Barium studies* can be useful in evaluating the colon (barium enema) and upper GI tract (barium swallow or upper GI with small bowel follow through). This test is useful in detecting anatomical abnormalities and esophageal spasm, and it may detect esophageal reflux. However, barium studies have a lower sensitivity than endoscopy for detecting ulcerations, erosions, polyps, and tumors, and they do not allow tissue diagnosis.

3. Endoscopy

    a. *Esophagogastroduodenoscopy (EGD)* is the diagnostic tool most frequently used in evaluating symptoms of heartburn or dysphagia and in assessing the upper GI tract in patients with GI blood loss. EGD detects esophagitis, erosions, ulcerations, malignancies, webs, diverticula, and strictures, and it can be therapeutically useful in treating ulcer disease and strictures.

    b. *Colonoscopy* is most commonly used in assessing patients with suspected lower intestinal blood loss. In patients with negative CT scans, it is often used to rule out colonic sources of abdominal pain.

III. Management (Tables 11.5, 11.6, and 11.7)

A. "Acute" abdomen

  1. Patients typically present in emergency rooms but may, rarely, present to physician's office

  2. Often present with sudden onset of severe abdominal pain with associated generalized tenderness

  3. Acute abdominal pain presenting with rigid abdomen and hemodynamic instability may be due to perforation, infarction, obstruction of abdominal organ, or ruptured aneurysm

  4. Patients require urgent surgical consultation, stabilization

  5. Clinicians have historically withheld opiate analgesics from patients with acute abdominal pain until after surgical evaluation, based on concern that physical findings may be altered; new evidence shows whereas physical findings may be altered, no significant increase in management errors occurs.

(continued on page 160)

TABLE 11.5 Medical Therapies for Some Common Causes of Abdominal Pain

Cause	Medical Therapies
Gastroesophageal reflux disease	**Behavioral changes** • No food or drink 2 hours before reclining • Lose weight • Avoid overeating, tight clothing, and certain foods (spicy, citrus, mints, alcohol, caffeine) • Elevate head of bed **Medications** • H_2 blockers (cimetidine, famotidine, nizatidine, ranitidine) • Proton pump inhibitors (lansoprazole, omeprazole) • Motility agents (metoclopramide)
Peptic ulcer disease (PUD)	***H. pylori*–positive disease** • 7–14 days of antibiotics: clarithromycin and ampicillin or metronidazole; bismuth subsalicylate, metronidazole, and tetracycline. • 4–8 weeks of H_2 blocker or proton pump inhibitor therapy for duodenal ulcers and 6–12 weeks for gastric ulcers • Follow-up EGD to document eradication of gastric ulcers ***H. pylori*–negative disease** • H_2 blockers or proton pump inhibitor therapy as for *H. pylori*–positive disease • Follow-up EGD as for *H. pylori*–positive disease • Removal of causative agents (e.g., NSAIDs) • Misoprostol can help prevent NSAID-induced ulcers

(continued on page 158)

TABLE 11.5	Medical Therapies for Some Common Causes of Abdominal Pain (Continued)
Cause	**Medical Therapies**
Nonulcer dyspepsia	**Behavioral changes** • Physician reassurance of nonserious nature of the disease • Avoidance of provocative foods and medications **Medications** • H_2 blockers or proton pump inhibitors for PUD and GERD-like symptoms • With dysmotility symptoms, motility agents can be tried • Can try to step down or use intermittent therapy after about 4 weeks of therapeutic success
Pancreatitis	• Intravenous (IV) hydration • Nothing by mouth until pain subsides, pancreatic enzymes decline • Pain relief as appropriate • Monitor for complications: necrosis, abscess, pseudocyst, hypocalcemia, hyperglycemia, hypotension, renal failure, shocks
Cholecystitis	• IV hydration, antibiotics, surgery • For nonsurgical candidates and chronic symptoms, ursodiol may be used
Diverticulitis	• IV hydration • Nothing by mouth until pain subsides • Antibiotic therapy (see Table 11.6) • Monitor for complications: peritonitis, abscess formation, strictures, fistulae • Follow-up colonoscopy to document no other underlying cause for the patient • Symptoms (i.e., colon cancer)

TABLE 11.6   Examples of Antibiotic Coverage for GI Organism

Route and Indication	Examples
Outpatient/oral (for diverticulitis)	Trimethoprim/sulfamethoxazole 160/800 mg bid **or** Ciprofloxacin 500 mg bid **plus** metronidazole 500 mg qid **or** Amoxicillin/clavulanic acid 500 mg tid **or** 875 mg bid
Outpatient/oral (for *H. pylori*)	Omeprazole 40 mg qd **and** clarithromycin 500 mg tid **and** ampicillin 500 mg **or** metronidazole 250 mg qid **or** Ranitidine 150 mg bid **and** bismuth subsalicylate 2 tabs qid **and** metronidazole 250 mg qid **and** tetracycline 500 mg qid
Inpatient/intravenous (for diverticulitis)	Ciprofloxacin 400 mg IV q 12 h **or** Gentamicin 2 mg/kg loading dose **then** 1.7 mg/kg IV q 8 h **or** Cefotaxime 2 g IV q 4–8 h **or** Aztreonam 2 g IV q 8 h **plus** metronidazole 500 mg IV q 6 h **or** Clindamycin 450–900 mg IV q 8 h **plus** ampicillin/sulbactam 3 g IV q 6 h **or** Cefoxitin 2 g IV q8 h **or** Cefotetan 2 g IV q 12 h **or** Ticarcillin/clavulanic acid 3.1 g IV q 6 h **or** Piperacillin/tazobactam 3.375 g IV q 6 h

TABLE 11.7	Indications for Abdominal Pain Referral
Referral Type	**Indications**
Gastroenterology referral	• Dysphagia • Evidence of bleeding • Early satiety • Recurrent vomiting • Weight loss • Atypical symptoms • Diagnostic uncertainty • Refractory to therapy • For possible endoscopic retrograde cholangiopancreatography in patients with pancreatitis or cholecystitis • Suspected colon cancer • Inflammatory bowel disease • Follow-up endoscopy for gastric ulcers and diverticulitis
Surgical referral	• Appendicitis • Diverticulitis • Bowel obstruction/perforation • Abdominal aortic aneurysm • Mesenteric ischemia • Resectable malignancy • Cholecystitis • Nephrolithiasis

B. Surgical conditions
   1. Abdominal aortic aneurysm, mesenteric ischemia, and appendicitis are surgical conditions.
   2. Cholecystitis is generally treated surgically; however, for patients who have chronic disease who are not surgical candidates, ursodiol may be utilized.
   3. Bowel obstruction is initially treated with bowel rest, supportive care, and nasogastric suction. In instances when the obstruction is caused by adhesions, these measures may resolve the obstruction. Surgery is needed for persistent obstruction and for those with mechanical lesions such as colon cancer.

4. Therapy for peritonitis is dictated by the underlying cause. Antibiotic therapy and other supportive measures are important for all patients; for those with peritonitis from an organ perforation (e.g., peptic ulcer, appendicitis, diverticulitis), surgery is indicated.

5. Patients with painful renal stones need intravenous hydration, narcotic pain medications, and often antibiotics until their stones pass. Stones that have not passed within 48–72 hours or that are associated with infection or uncontrollable pain require surgical intervention.

C. Medical conditions

1. Acute pancreatitis

   a. Typically hospitalized

   b. Nothing by mouth to limit stimulation of pancreatic enzyme secretion and provided intravenous hydration and pain medication until symptoms resolve

   c. Monitoring for hypotension, infection, respiration, renal and fluid/electrolyte abnormalities are cornerstones of therapy

2. Chronic pancreatitis

   a. Chronic pain, steatorrhea, and diabetes are complications that may require therapy.

      i. Chronic pain should be treated initially with nonnarcotic pain medication.

      ii. Cautious use of narcotic medications is recommended along with monitoring the patient's use of these medications for potential abuse.

      iii. Consider pancreatic enzymes.

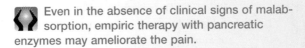 Even in the absence of clinical signs of malabsorption, empiric therapy with pancreatic enzymes may ameliorate the pain.

      iv. Refractory pain may require nerve blocks or surgical intervention.

3. Pancreatic pseudocysts

   a. They are a complication of either acute or chronic pancreatitis.

   b. Pseudocysts may resolve spontaneously.

    c. Pseudocysts present for more than 6 weeks are less likely to resolve spontaneously.

    d. Pseudocysts that are more than 5 cm in size have an increased rate of complication that includes rupture, hemorrhage, or infection.

    e. Ultrasound or CT can be used to monitor the presence and size of pseudocysts.

    f. For patients at increased risk of complications, surgical or gastroenterology consultation should be considered for possible operative or endoscopic surgical drainage.

4. Diverticulitis

    a. Patients with mild diverticulitis can be managed as outpatients with antibiotics active against gram-negative rods and anaerobes (see Table 11.6).

    b. Patients may be placed on a clear liquid diet, with advancement of the diet as tolerated, if clinical improvement is noted within the following 2–3 days.

    c. Antibiotic therapy is continued for 7–14 days.

    d. Outpatient evaluation (CT scan) and follow-up colonoscopy are often recommended.

    e. To prevent further episodes, fiber supplements or high-fiber diets are prescribed.

5. GERD

    a. Spectrum ranges from minimal symptoms and objective findings to severe disease with associated complications such as stricture, bleeding, or Barrett esophagus.

    b. Therapy should be tailored to the patient.

       i. Mild GERD: behavioral or lifestyle modifications (see Table 11.5), along with over-the-counter (OTC) H_2 blockers or antacids.

       ii. For patients with more severe symptoms or patients unresponsive to OTC medications, prescription H_2 blockers, proton pump inhibitors, or motility agents can be prescribed, along with continued reinforcement of lifestyle modifications.

    c. If symptoms are relieved, then maintenance therapy can be initiated.

    d. Symptoms persisting beyond 6 weeks merit referral for endoscopy.

e. Recurrence of GERD is very high because the underlying pathophysiologic process is unchanged when therapy is discontinued.
f. Therapy for moderate to severe esophagitis may require long-term treatment. Nonetheless, attempts to step down therapy should be attempted after 8 weeks of symptom control.
g. Some patients may require only intermittent therapy along with continued lifestyle modifications.

> Severe esophagitis, Barrett esophagus, and stricture are markers of severe reflux and require long-term treatment and follow-up, even in the absence of symptoms, in order to reduce the risk of esophageal carcinoma, bleeding, or disease progression.

6. Peptic ulcer disease and gastritis
   a. Therapy is dependent on the presence of *H. pylori*.
      i. If *H. pylori* is present, then therapy directed against this organism is indicated (see Tables 11.5 and 11.6).
      ii. After completion of the antibiotic regimen, proton pump inhibitors are generally continued for 4–8 weeks for duodenal ulcers and for 6–12 weeks for gastritis or gastric ulcers.

> Patients with gastric ulcer require follow-up EGD to document ulcer healing and to exclude the possibility of malignancy as the underlying cause of the ulcer.

   b. NSAID-related ulcers are generally treated with acid suppression therapy and discontinuing the NSAID.
      i. If NSAIDs must be used, options include switching the patient to a non-acetylated salicylate, such as salsalate (Disalcid), with an enterically coated preparation, using a COX-2 inhibitor, and prescribing the lowest effective dose.
      ii. If NSAIDs must be used in patients with a history of ulcer, misoprostol (Cytotec) can help prevent recurrence.

7. Nonulcer dyspepsia

 Therapy involves avoidance of precipitating foods or medications, reassurance regarding the absence of serious disease, and medications directed at the predominant symptoms.

    a. For patients with ulcer-like or reflux symptoms, acid-suppressing agents can be used.

    b. For patients with dysmotility-related symptoms, e.g., nausea, bloating, or early satiety, motility agents such as metoclopramide can be tried.

    c. If treatment is initially successful, 4 weeks of continuous therapy can be employed, followed by a trial off medication.

    d. Some patients may benefit from intermittent therapy, whereas others may require continuous treatment. In such cases, periodic trials off medication should be attempted to see if medication is still necessary.

IV. Referral or Consultations

    A. Whereas many of the conditions associated with abdominal pain can be managed medically, many require specialty referral for further evaluation or therapy. Indications for gastroenterology and surgical referral are outlined in Table 11.7.

MENTOR TIPS DIGEST

- Pain that develops suddenly suggests a vascular etiology (e.g., organ infarction, AAA) or perforation/rupture of an abdominal organ (perforated ulcer, esophageal rupture).
- In patients with chronic abdominal pain, the presence of "alarm" symptoms such as onset at older than 50 years of age, rectal bleeding, weight loss, or recent change in bowel function raises suspicion for organic disease.
- Pain that precedes emesis suggests a potential surgical condition, whereas emesis that is followed by pain points more toward a nonsurgical condition.
- Symptoms that are significantly associated with ovarian cancer are pelvic/abdominal pain, urinary urgency/frequency, increased abdominal size/bloating, and difficulty eating/feeling full when present for <1 year and occurring >12 days per month.

- Of the adult Western population, 10%–15% will develop gallstones. Ectopic pregnancy and ovarian torsion are two of the most common causes of acute abdominal pain in early pregnancy.
- Patients with renal colic or an intestinal obstruction may be restless, whereas patients with peritonitis tend to be still.
- Carnett test: Identify the site of maximal pain, ask the patient to attempt to sit up while applying pressure to the forehead. An increase in pain suggests an abdominal wall etiology, whereas no change suggests a visceral source.
- Significant abdominal pain in the absence of significant physical examination findings may suggest mesenteric ischemia. (However, be circumspect; this finding is also common in somatoform disorder and malingering.)
- Serologic testing for *H. pylori* is useful in younger populations and for diagnosing *H. pylori* in radiographically diagnosed duodenal ulcers, but it cannot be relied on in older patients with gastric ulcers or for following therapeutic response.
- In chronic pancreatitis, even in the absence of clinical signs of malabsorption, empiric therapy with pancreatic enzymes may ameliorate the pain.
- Severe esophagitis, Barrett esophagus, and stricture are markers of severe reflux and require long-term treatment and follow-up, even in the absence of symptoms, in order to reduce the risk of esophageal carcinoma, bleeding, or disease progression.
- Patients with gastric ulcer require follow-up EGD to document ulcer healing and to exclude the possibility of malignancy as the underlying cause for the ulcer.
- In nonulcer dyspepsia, therapy involves avoidance of precipitating foods or medications, reassurance regarding the absence of serious disease, and medications directed at the predominant symptoms.

Resources

Ables AZ, Simon I, Melton ER. Update on *Helicobacter pylori* treatment. American Family Physician 75: 351–358, 2007.
Reviews the epidemiology of H. pylori *disease along with a discussion of the various tests and treatments available.*

Camilleri M. Management of patients with chronic abdominal pain in clinical practice. Neurogastroenterology and Motility 18:499–506, 2006.

Dickerson LM, King DE. Evaluation and management of nonulcer dyspepsia. American Family Physician 70:107–114, 2004.
Presents an approach to evaluating the patient with dyspepsia along with different treatment options for patients with nonulcer dyspepsia.

Dominguez EP, Sweeney JF, Choi YU. Diagnosis and management of diverticulitis and appendicitis. Gastroenterology Clinics of North America 35:367–391, 2006.
Review of diagnosis and care for diverticulitis and appendicitis.

Flaser MH, Goldberg E. Acute abdominal pain. Medical Clinic of North America 90:481–503, 2006
Presents an approach to assessment of patients with acute abdominal pain.

Goff BA, Mandel LS, Drescher CW, et al. Development of an ovarian cancer symptom index: Possibilities for earlier detection. Cancer 109:221–227, 2007.

Mayerle J, Simon P, Lerch MM. Medical treatment of acute pancreatitis. Gastroenterology Clinics of North America 33:855–869, 2004.
Reviews diagnosis, treatment, and complications for acute pancreatitis.

Smith L. Updated ACG guidelines for diagnosis and treatment of GERD. American Family Physician 71:2376–2381, 2005.

For self-test questions, see the testbank CD.

DIARRHEA

Michael J. Polizzotto, MD, and Martin S. Lipsky, MD

I. Definitions and Overview

A. Diarrhea is one of the most common conditions seen in a primary care setting. Acute diarrhea is defined as the passage of more than three abnormally loose stools per 24 hours during fewer than 2 weeks. Chronic diarrhea is recurrent diarrhea or diarrhea that persists for more than 30 days.

B. Acute diarrhea has the following features.

  1. Acute diarrhea can be divided into two clinical presentations: a watery noninflammatory diarrhea and an inflammatory diarrhea with the presence of either blood or white blood cells in the stool.

  2. Diarrhea can also be classified as mild (no effect on daily activity), moderate (some activity limitations), or severe (patient is confined to bed).

  3. It is important to ask about exposure to individuals with similar symptoms; recent travel; intake of caffeine, alcohol, and sorbitol; and antibiotic or other medication use.

> Antibiotic use within 2 weeks suggests that diarrhea may be from either an alteration of bowel flora or *Clostridium difficile* infection.

  4. Grossly bloody diarrhea indicates mucosal damage and is most commonly seen with an invasive bacterial infection or inflammatory bowel disease.

5. Most acute diarrhea cases are caused by infection.
   a. Viral cases have the following features.

 Viral gastroenteritis accounts for most cases of acute infectious diarrhea.

       i. Typically, stools are watery and accompanied by a low-grade fever, nausea, or vomiting and achiness.
       ii. Rotavirus is the most common cause in infants and children, and norovirus (formerly Norwalk virus) is the leading adult cause.
       iii. Although infectious diarrhea in adults is usually viral, it is more likely to be bacterial than in children.
   b. Invasive bacterial infections, such as *Shigella, Salmonella,* and *Campylobacter,* typically present with a prodrome of fever, headache, fatigue, anorexia, and stools that may initially be watery before becoming bloody. Crampy abdominal pain is common. Traveler's diarrhea usually lasts 3–5 days and presents with symptoms similar to viral gastroenteritis. Toxigenic *Escherichia coli* is a common cause of traveler's diarrhea.
6. Severe abdominal pain associated with acute diarrhea in an older patient suggests the possibility of an ischemic bowel. Other noninfectious causes of acute diarrhea include fecal impaction, diverticular disease, acute presentation of inflammatory bowel disease and, rarely, colonic neoplasm.
C. Chronic diarrhea has the following features.
   1. The differential diagnosis for chronic diarrhea is extensive (Figs. 12.1 and 12.2). However, the diagnosis can be broken down into major groups based on stool characteristics: watery, inflammatory (bloody), and fatty. Watery diarrhea is further divided into secretory and osmotic diarrhea.

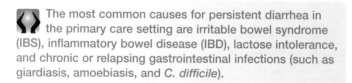 The most common causes for persistent diarrhea in the primary care setting are irritable bowel syndrome (IBS), inflammatory bowel disease (IBD), lactose intolerance, and chronic or relapsing gastrointestinal infections (such as giardiasis, amoebiasis, and *C. difficile*).

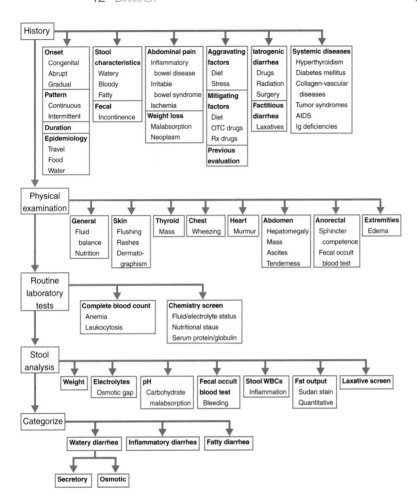

FIGURE 12.1 Workup of chronic diarrhea, part 1. *(Reprinted from Gastroenterology, Vol 116, Issue 6, Kenneth D. Fine and Lawrence R. Schiller, AGA Technical Review on the Evaluation and Management of Chronic Diarrhea, Pages 1464–1486, Copyright 1999, with permission from Elsevier.)*

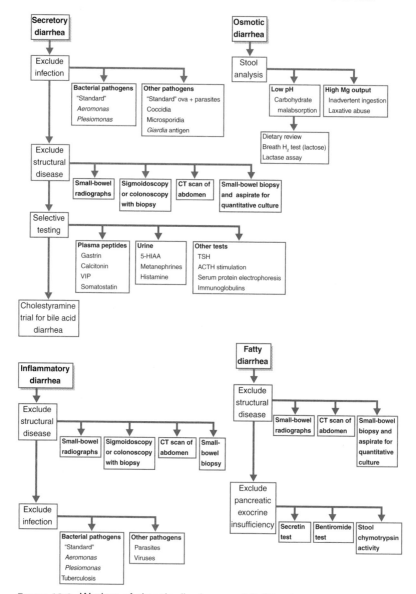

FIGURE 12.2 Workup of chronic diarrhea, part 2. (*Reprinted from Gastroenterology, Vol 116, Issue 6, Kenneth D. Fine and Lawrence R. Schiller, AGA Technical Review on the Evaluation and Management of Chronic Diarrhea, Pages 1464–1486, Copyright 1999, with permission from Elsevier.*)

2. IBS accounts for about half of the gastrointestinal complaints seen by primary care providers. It typically affects young or middle-aged adults, with a 2:1 female-to-male predominance. Box 12.1 lists criteria for IBS.

3. IBD refers either to ulcerative colitis or to Crohn disease.

   a. IBD has a bimodal age distribution for both ulcerative colitis and Crohn disease. The largest peak occurs in the third decade of life, with a smaller peak in the sixth decade of life.

   b. Table 12.1 lists some of the characteristics that differentiate ulcerative colitis from Crohn disease.

BOX 12.1 Criteria for Irritable Bowel Syndrome

1. Continuous or recurrent symptoms associated with abdominal pain relieved by defecation or associated with a change in frequency or stool consistency.
2. A varied pattern of disturbed defecation occurring 25% of the time and consisting of two or more of the following:
   - Change in frequency or consistency of stool
   - Needing to strain to pass stool
   - Feeling an urgent need to defecate
   - Bloating
   - Passing mucus in the stool
   - Feeling incomplete evacuation

TABLE 12.2 Comparison of Ulcerative Colitis and Crohn Disease

Feature	Ulcerative Colitis	Crohn Disease
Clinical diarrhea	Common	Common
Rectal bleeding	Common	Common
Abdominal pain	Less prominent	Prominent
Abdominal mass	Rare	Common
Perianal disease	Uncommon	Common
Fistula	Rare	Common
Weight loss	Occasional	Common
Risk of malignancy	Increased	Slightly increased
Distribution of lesions	Continuous	Skip lesions
Rectal involvement	Almost 100%	Occasionally occurs

4. Lactose intolerance is common and to some extent affects more than half the world's population. There are three categories: congenital, primary with delayed onset, and secondary.
   a. The most common type is delayed onset, in which as individuals age the level of the enzyme lactase decreases.
   b. A secondary deficiency occurs when enzyme activity decreases because of a diffuse intestinal insult, such as in Crohn disease.
5. *Giardia* and other parasitic infections can present with chronic diarrhea. Recent travel to an area where these organisms are endemic increases the likelihood of these infections.
6. Stools that contain fat globules suggest malabsorption, often due to pancreatic insufficiency. Infections, enzyme deficiencies (e.g., lactose intolerance), and mucosal abnormalities such as those seen in celiac disease are among the other most common causes of malabsorption in the primary care setting. Once thought to be rare, celiac disease (due to an abnormal immune response to gluten, a protein found in wheat, barley, and rye) has been estimated to affect 1 in 133 Americans. It is most common in those of European ancestry.

II. Evaluation
A. Acute diarrhea

 Most cases of acute diarrhea are mild, self-limiting illnesses, and diagnostic testing is unnecessary.

1. Box 12.2 lists indications suggesting a need for a more detailed evaluation.
2. Examining the stool for leukocytes and occult blood is a useful first test.
   a. A stool specimen that has fewer than three to four white blood cells per high-powered field reflects a noninflammatory process that is usually self-limited and requires no further investigation.
   b. The presence of more than five fecal leukocytes per high-powered field suggests an inflammatory process; when combined with a history of an abrupt onset of more than four stools per day and no vomiting before the onset of diarrhea, it has a positive predictive value of 60%–70% for bacterial diarrhea (*Shigella, Salmonella, Campylobacter.*)

BOX 12.2

Indications for Evaluation of Acute Diarrhea

- Evidence of dehydration
- More than six stools per 24 hours
- No improvement after 48–72 hours
- Presence of bloody stool
- Temperature higher than 38.5°C (101°F)
- Severe abdominal pain
- Diarrhea in an older or immunocompromised individual

      i. If an inflammatory process is suspected, stool cultures should be sent to detect *Salmonella, Shigella, Campylobacter,* and Shiga-toxin producing *E. coli* (such as O157:H7).

     ii. Stool examinations for ova and parasites have been recommended for patients at risk for *Giardia* or other parasitic infections; however, enzyme immunoassays are now considered to be more sensitive.

B. Chronic diarrhea

  1. The workup for chronic diarrhea should be individualized. Reviewing stool characteristics, past medical illnesses and surgeries, travel history, diet, and medications helps focus the approach.

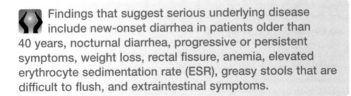

Findings that suggest serious underlying disease include new-onset diarrhea in patients older than 40 years, nocturnal diarrhea, progressive or persistent symptoms, weight loss, rectal fissure, anemia, elevated erythrocyte sedimentation rate (ESR), greasy stools that are difficult to flush, and extraintestinal symptoms.

  2. For patients who have no "red flags" to suggest serious illness and whose physical examination suggests a benign illness, only a limited diagnostic evaluation may be needed.

    a. For example, patients suspected of having lactose intolerance that responds to a lactose-free diet need no further testing.

  3. Look for offending foods or drugs.

As many as 4% of cases of chronic diarrhea may be due to medications and food additives.

a. Box 12.3 lists several medications that may cause diarrhea. Generally, no further evaluation is needed in those patients whose diarrhea responds to decreasing or stopping a medication.

4. For patients with chronic diarrhea whose cause is not readily apparent from the history and physical examination, an initial evaluation consists of a complete blood count (CBC), ESR, and checking the stool for occult blood, leukocytes, ova, and parasites.

a. An assay for *C. difficile* toxin is indicated for patients with recent antibiotic exposure.

b. For patients with associated left lower quadrant pain or bloody diarrhea, early sigmoidoscopy examination to detect mucosal ulcerations, friability, and masses and to biopsy for suspected IBD is indicated.

c. If an amoebic infection is suspected, mucosal smears obtained during sigmoidoscopy can be examined for amoeba.

d. Biopsy can also detect less common diseases such as amyloidosis and collagenous colitis.

BOX 12.3

Medications That May Cause Diarrhea

Alpha-glucosidase inhibitors
Antacids
Antibiotics
Antidepressants
Colchicine
Lactulose
Laxatives
Loop diuretics
Proton pump inhibitors
Quinidine
Theophylline
Thyroxine

5. Blood tests have the following features.

 Blood tests may be useful but are rarely diagnostic.

   a. A CBC can detect anemia or leukocytosis.
   b. Serum electrolytes can detect abnormalities associated with fluid loss.
   c. Tests for celiac disease include IgA antiendomysial antibody and antitissue transglutaminase (tTGA). In cases of immunoglobulin A deficiency, antigliaden IgG improves sensitivity.
6. Often cases with chronic diarrhea of unclear etiology or suspected IBD need referral to a gastroenterologist for evaluation.

III. Management

Fluid therapy, an alteration in diet, and monitoring the patient for resolution of symptoms are sufficient for most patients with acute diarrhea.

A. Oral rehydration is usually adequate.
   1. Commercial rehydration solutions such as Pedialyte and Ricelyte are designed for fluid and electrolyte replacement and are most commonly used for infants and children.
   2. Sports drinks, fruit drinks, and flavored soft drinks augmented with crackers, soup, or broth are usually adequate to replace fluids in adults or older children with diarrhea.
B. More severely dehydrated individuals may require intravenous fluids.
C. Other diet tips comprise the following.
   1. Avoiding milk products and caffeine-containing foods may be helpful.
   2. Boiled starches (potatoes, rice, and noodles) with some salt are good foods for patients with acute diarrhea.
   3. For children, a BRAT diet (bananas, rice, apples, and toast) is commonly recommended, although there is limited evidence documenting the effectiveness of this strategy.
   4. Lactose intolerance options follow.

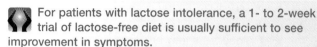

For patients with lactose intolerance, a 1- to 2-week trial of lactose-free diet is usually sufficient to see improvement in symptoms.

    a. Taking lactase capsules orally before consuming dairy products is also an effective treatment.

D. Medications consist of the following.

    1. Several preparations are available for symptomatic treatment. Preparations containing kaolin and pectate (Kaopectate) are available over the counter; however, despite wide usage their efficacy is uncertain. Bismuth subsalicylate (Pepto-Bismol) is also used for diarrhea and may have an antisecretory effect.

    2. The antimotility drugs, such as loperamide, are the drugs of choice for most nonspecific treatment. These medications slow gut motility, facilitating intestinal absorption. They should not be used in febrile patients with inflammatory infectious diarrhea.

    3. Specific management depends on the underlying cause of the diarrhea. For patients with bacterial diarrhea, the use of antibiotics depends on the organism, health of the individual, and systemic symptoms. All cases of *Shigella* should be treated with either a fluoroquinolone or trimethoprim-sulfamethoxazole (TMP-SMZ). *Salmonella* infections causing mild to moderate symptoms should generally not be treated because antibiotics may prolong the carrier state. Patients with salmonella who have severe symptoms or those at risk for bacteremia (e.g., HIV-infected patients or elderly individuals) should be treated with a fluoroquinolone.

    4. Treating patients with a culture-proven *Campylobacter* infection shortens the duration of the illness if symptoms are still present when the culture results become available. Erythromycin is the drug of choice, but quinolones are also effective. *E. coli* causes a wide spectrum of disease. Invasive *E. coli* with bloody diarrhea should be treated with a fluoroquinolone or TMP-SMZ. Traveler's diarrhea due to toxigenic *E. coli* responds to either a short course of a fluoroquinolone or TMP-SMZ. *C. difficile* infection should be treated with metronidazole; an alternative is oral vancomycin. *Giardia* is also treated with metronidazole.

E. Patients with IBS whose predominant symptom is diarrhea should do the following.

1. Using an antimotility agent such as loperamide (Imodium), 2–4 mg up to four times a day, or diphenoxylate hydrochloride with atropine (Lomotil), 10–20 mg up to four times per day, may provide relief.

2. Antispasmodics such as dicyclomine (Bentyl) 10–20 mg before meals may benefit patients with associated abdominal cramping and pain. A high-fiber diet is helpful for IBS patients with diarrhea alternating with constipation. (New FDA restricted use only severe refractory cases.)

F. Patients with celiac disease must follow a lifelong gluten-free diet. Foods and beverages that contain wheat, barely, rye, and possibly oats should be eliminated completely.

G. Management goals for IBD are to control active disease, maintain remission, detect complications, and refer to surgery when appropriate. Most patients should be co-managed by a gastroenterologist experienced in managing IBD.

 MENTOR TIPS DIGEST

- Antibiotic use within 2 weeks suggests that diarrhea may be from either an alteration of bowel flora or *Clostridium difficile* infection.
- Viral gastroenteritis accounts for most cases of acute infectious diarrhea.
- The most common causes for persistent diarrhea in the primary care setting are IBS, IBD, lactose intolerance, and chronic or relapsing gastrointestinal infections (such as giardiasis, amoebiasis, and *C. difficile*).
- Most cases of acute diarrhea are mild, self-limiting illnesses, and diagnostic testing is unnecessary.
- Findings that suggest serious underlying disease include new-onset diarrhea in patients older than 40 years, nocturnal diarrhea, progressive or persistent symptoms, weight loss, rectal fissure, anemia, elevated ESR, greasy stools that are difficult to flush, and extraintestinal symptoms.
- As many as 4% of cases of chronic diarrhea may be due to medications and food additives.
- Blood tests may be useful but are rarely diagnostic.
- Fluid therapy, an alteration in diet, and monitoring the patient for resolution of symptoms are sufficient for most patients with acute diarrhea.

- **For patients with lactose intolerance, a 1- to 2-week trial of lactose-free diet is usually sufficient to see improvement in symptoms.**

Resources

American Gastroenterological Association: American Gastroenterological Association medical position statement: Guidelines for the evaluation and management of chronic diarrhea. Gastroenterology 116:1461–1463, 1999.
Even almost 10 years after they were produced, these guidelines for chronic diarrhea are useful.

Camilleri M. Therapeutic approach to the patient with irritable bowel syndrome. American Journal of Medicine 107:275–325, 1999.
IBS is one of the most common problems seen in primary care. The article reviews the diagnostic criteria for IBS and the evidence to support current therapies.

Schmulson MW, Chang L. Diagnostic approach to the patient with irritable bowel syndrome. American Journal of Medicine 107:205–265, 1999.

Thielman NM, Guerrant RL. Clinical practice: Acute infectious diarrhea. New England Journal of Medicine 350:38–47, 2004.
A concise, clinically oriented review of the diagnosis and management of acute infectious diarrhea.

Wilson JF. Irritable bowel syndrome. Annals of Internal Medicine 147: ITC1–ITC17, 2007.

Chapter Self-Test Questions

Circle the correct answer. After you have responded to the questions, check your answers in Appendix A.

1. Acute diarrhea is:

a. Explosions of flatus accompanying defecation.

b. A watery loose stool.

c. More than three loose bowel movements in 24 hours.

d. More than five formed or unformed stools in 24 hours.

2. Types of acute diarrhea are differentiated by:

    a. Greater or less than 1 L in 24 hours.

    b. Presence of white blood cells in feces.

    c. Phosphorus concentration in feces.

    d. Litmus paper measurement of pH.

3. Diarrhea associated with antibiotic usage commonly features:

    a. *Clostridium difficile* toxin.

    b. *Clostridium difficile* mucosal invasion.

    c. *Candida albicans* mucositis.

    d. Crohn disease.

 See the testbank CD for more self-test questions.

13

MUSCULOSKELETAL PAIN

Marianne M. Green, MD, and Stephen L. Adams, MD

I. Introduction

A. Musculoskeletal pain is a very common presenting symptom.

B. It is among the most frequent chief complaints during office visits to the primary care physician.

C. Etiologies are myriad. Symptoms may be due to trauma (either acute or chronic), overuse, mechanical problems, metabolic disorders, or infection.

> ◆ The physician must ascertain the circumstances behind an acute musculoskeletal injury.

1. Ask all patients about a history of trauma.

2. Fever and chills suggest an infectious cause.

3. Weight loss or prior history of cancer suggests an underlying malignancy.

4. The age of the patient can be very useful in estimating likelihood of certain diagnoses. For example, an elderly person is more at risk for an osteoporotic fracture than is a young person.

> ◆ For a persistent pain (>1 month) especially in patients over age 50, consider malignancy as a possibility, and imaging may be needed.

D. The diagnostic approach after the appropriate tailored history and physical may include radiographic studies, examination of joint aspirate to look for infection or crystals, or nerve conduction studies when neuropathy is a consideration.

E. Treatment for most acute musculoskeletal injuries includes rest, ice, compression, and elevation (the RICE protocol).

Always consider the possibility of referred pain, such as atypical angina presenting as shoulder pain or an abdominal aortic aneurysm presenting as low back pain.

F. This chapter will review several of the most common conditions: shoulder pain, carpal tunnel syndrome, osteoarthritis, low back pain, and patellofemoral syndrome.

II. Shoulder Pain

  A. Pathophysiology

  1. Inflammation or injury to the rotator cuff causes most shoulder pain.

    a. The muscles of the rotator cuff can be remembered using the SITS mnemonic: Supraspinatus, Infraspinatus, Teres Minor, and Subscapularis.

    b. The major function of the first three muscles is externally to rotate the humerus. The supraspinatus also abducts the humerus. The subscapularis serves as an internal rotator of the shoulder.

 A complete rotator cuff tear is unlikely in patients younger than 30 years unless they are major athletes or have sustained significant trauma.

  2. Other causes of shoulder pain include biceps tendonitis, deltoid bursitis, adhesive capsulitis (frozen shoulder), glenohumeral instability, acromioclavicular (AC) injury, fracture, and metabolic and infectious causes.

  B. Epidemiology

  1. Younger patients are most susceptible to traumatic injuries, such as AC joint subluxation and glenohumeral instability.

  2. Rotator cuff injury is the most common shoulder problem seen in athletes. **Impingement** of the rotator cuff tendons beneath an arthritic AC joint may be the presenting problem in the elderly.

    a. The supraspinatus is the muscle involved in the majority of rotator cuff injuries.

  3. The proximal humerus is a bone commonly fractured in elderly women with osteoporosis.

4. Conditions that increase in frequency with age are impingement syndrome, adhesive capsulitis, and rotator cuff tear.

C. Patient history

1. Elicit a history of chronic overuse, acute trauma, or both.

    a. Patients may not recall a specific causal incident.

    b. Patients may report a history of glenohumeral instability ("I dislocated my shoulder").

2. Pain is the predominant complaint, often worse at night.

    a. Most patients have pain in the lateral or anterior shoulder.

 Posterior shoulder pain is rare and is usually due to cervical spine disease.

3. Patients may complain of weakness, especially if there is a tear in the rotator cuff.

D. Physical examination

1. Inspection

    a. May reveal atrophy of the rotator cuff muscles

    b. With the patient in the seated position and arm at the side, traction on humerus may cause posterior gap between humerus and acromion; this "sulcus sign" may be present in patients with glenohumeral dislocation

    c. If present, note superficial signs of inflammation, e.g., erythema, swelling

2. Palpation

    a. Palpate all bones surrounding the shoulder.

    b. Deltoid bursa and biceps tendon should be specifically located and palpated for tenderness.

    c. Tenderness of the AC joint seldom occurs in impingement syndrome.

    d. Assess neurovascular integrity.

3. Range of motion

    a. Test abduction by asking the patient to make the touchdown sign: raising both arms in the plane of the body.

    b. To assess adduction, perform the "drop arm test." If the test result is positive, the patient is unable to control slowly lowering the involved arm back to the sides. This is an insensitive but very specific test for a complete supraspinatus tear.

    c. Test internal rotation by having the patient reach over the head to touch the back. Inability to reach the thoracic spine is abnormal.

d. Test external rotation with elbow flexed and upper arm at the side. First passively, then actively, rotate the hand and arm away from the body at both 0 and 90 degrees.

e. Compare the affected and unaffected arms' internal and external rotation.

> Adhesive capsulitis, also called frozen shoulder, is present when there is loss of both active *and* passive range of motion.

4. Special maneuvers

    a. Tests for impingement (rotator cuff impingement due to decreased subacromial space) include the Neer and Hawkins tests.

        i. **Neer test.** Internally rotate the patient's arm at the side; then bring the arm forward in flexion until it is straight up. Press down on the affected AC joint to prevent scapula motion. The test result is positive if the maneuver causes pain (Fig. 13.1).

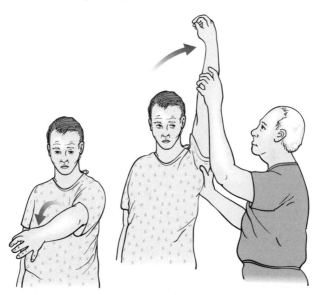

FIGURE 13.1 **Neer test.** *(Redrawn from Woodward TW, Best TM: The painful shoulder: part I. Clinical evaluation. Am Fam Physician 2000;61(10):3079–3088, Figure 5.)*

    ii. **Hawkins test.** Flex the patient's elbow and arm, holding the arm in the horizontal position. The test result is positive if internal rotation causes pain with impingement (Fig. 13.2).

  b. Perform the **apprehension test** with the patient supine or seated, raising the arm to 90 degrees flexion. While pressing on the anterior glenohumeral joint, externally rotate the arm. Patients with glenohumeral instability report pain or apprehension that the shoulder would dislocate (Fig. 13.3).

5. Strength testing

  a. Supraspinatus is tested with the **"empty can" test.** Abduct both patient arms to 90 degrees, positioned 30 degrees anterior to the coronal plane of the body and pronated with the thumb pointing down as if emptying a can. Push down on both arms while the patient resists. Weakness in the affected arm is a positive test result (Fig. 13.4).

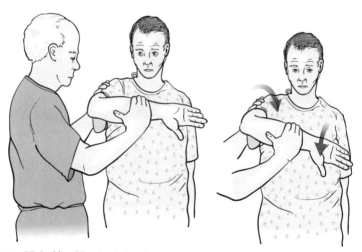

FIGURE 13.2 Hawkins test. *(Redrawn from Woodward TW, Best TM: The painful shoulder: part I. Clinical evaluation. Am Fam Physician 2000;61(10):3079–3088, Figure 6.)*

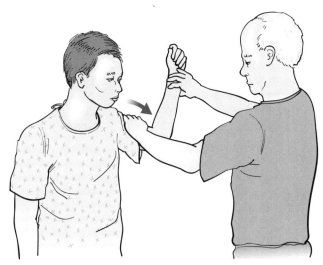

FIGURE 13.3 **Apprehension test.** *(Redrawn from Woodward TW, Best TM: The painful shoulder: part I. Clinical evaluation. Am Fam Physician 2000;61(10): 3079–3088, Figure 8.)*

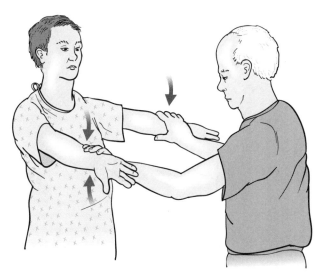

FIGURE 13.4 **Supraspinatus examination ("empty can" test).** *(Redrawn from Woodward TW, Best TM: The painful shoulder: part I. Clinical evaluation. Am Fam Physician 2000;61(10):3079–3088, Figure 3.)*

  b. The infraspinatus and teres minor muscles are external
  rotators. Position the patient's arms at the side with elbows
  flexed. Decreased strength in external rotation against
  resistance (Fig 13.5) reflects weakness of these muscles
  of the rotator cuff.
  E. Differential diagnosis
    1. To evaluate possible infectious or metabolic cause of shoulder
    pain, perform arthrocentesis of joint for cell count, culture,
    crystal analysis
    2. Radiography

 Plain radiographs are required if there is a history of
trauma.

  3. Shoulder MRI necessary to evaluate for surgical repair of a
  rotator cuff or if diagnosis unclear

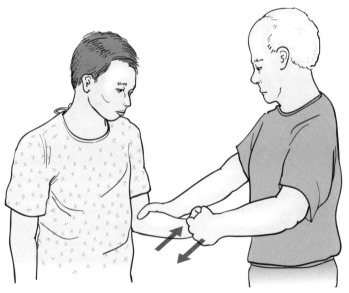

FIGURE 13.5 Infraspinatus/teres minor examination. *(Redrawn from Woodward
TW, Best TM: The painful shoulder: part I. Clinical evaluation. Am Fam Physician
2000;61(10):3079–3088, Figure 4.)*

F. Management
   1. Nonsurgical treatment modalities for acute and chronic inflammation of the rotator cuff include nonsteroidal anti-inflammatory drugs (NSAIDs), ice, and a program of physical therapy.
   2. Impingement and adhesive capsulitis may respond to physical therapy, although orthopedic referral for severe or refractory cases is necessary.
   3. Refer rotator cuff tears to orthopedists for consideration of surgical repair.
   4. Metabolic or infectious etiologies of shoulder pain require specific treatment.

III. Carpal Tunnel Syndrome
   A. Pathophysiology
   1. The carpal tunnel contains the median nerve and nine flexor tendons that course through the wrist. The carpal bones and flexor retinaculum, also known as the transverse carpal ligament, form the carpal tunnel.
   2. Flexor tenosynovitis causes swelling that compresses the median nerve as it traverses the carpal tunnel.
   3. The median nerve is on the palmar side of the wrist and provides sensory innervation to part of the thumb, the second and third fingers, as well as to the radial aspect of the fourth finger. It provides the sole motor innervation to the abductor pollicis brevis.
   B. Epidemiology
   1. Carpal tunnel syndrome is the most common entrapment neuropathy.

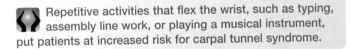
Repetitive activities that flex the wrist, such as typing, assembly line work, or playing a musical instrument, put patients at increased risk for carpal tunnel syndrome.

   2. Associated conditions include rheumatoid arthritis, history of Colles fracture, pregnancy, and hypothyroidism.
   3. There is a genetic predisposition to carpal tunnel syndrome.
   C. History
   1. Ask patient about a history of repetitive wrist flexion.
   2. The patient often complains of paresthesia in the median nerve distribution. These symptoms are often worse at night.

3. More severe compression can cause radiation of pain into the forearm.

4. Ask about a history of thyroid disease or symptoms of hypothyroidism.

D. Physical examination

   1. Examination results may be normal early in the course of disease.

   2. Sensory examination may reveal a diminished response to pinprick over the palmar aspect of the median nerve distribution.

   3. Thumb abduction may be weak, and thenar atrophy may be present.

   4. Phalen sign and Tinel sign

 These are two classic physical examination signs. Their sensitivity is only 20%–50%.

     a. Phalen sign. With the patient's elbows resting on the table, let the wrists fall freely into maximum flexion. This results in passive hyperflexion of the wrist. A positive test result occurs when the patient develops symptoms of pain, numbness, and tingling within 3 minutes.

     b. Tinel sign. Tap over the route of the median nerve on the volar side of the patient's wrist at the distal wrist crease. A positive test result occurs when this provokes paresthesia in the median nerve sensory distribution.

E. Differential diagnosis

   1. Cervical radiculopathy, thoracic outlet syndrome, generalized neuropathy, and syringomyelia.

 Nerve conduction velocity (NCV) and electromyography (EMG) studies may be necessary to differentiate conditions.

F. Management

   1. Early treatment includes rest and modification of the activity related to wrist flexion.

   2. Wearing a wrist splint initially at night places the wrist in a neutral position.

   3. Inject corticosteroid into or near the carpal tunnel.

4. Systemic corticosteroids may be effective.

5. Severe cases may require surgery to divide the transverse carpal ligament.

IV. Osteoarthritis (OA)

A. Pathogenesis

    1. OA results from a complex mixture of biomechanical and biochemical causes.

    2. Although idiopathic OA with no known predisposing factors is the most common form, OA occurs most often in weight-bearing joints as a result of "wear and tear" on the articulations caused by joint injury, obesity, laxity of the joints, and muscle weakness.

    3. Genetics and dietary factors may play a role.

    4. There are various patterns of joint involvement.

 The interphalangeal joints are most commonly affected in idiopathic OA.

    a. Other affected joints besides the hip and the knee include the base of the thumb and the spine. Idiopathic OA rarely affects the elbows, wrists, and ankles.

    b. In generalized OA more than three joints are affected.

    5. OA does not have systemic manifestations.

B. Epidemiology

 The National Health and Nutrition Examination Survey reported the prevalence of OA as 0.1% in 25–34-year-olds and >80% in people over the age of 55.

    1. Age, female sex, obesity, occupation, prior injury, genetics, and history of sports activities all increase risk.

    2. OA of the hip and knee is the most common reason for total knee and hip replacement.

C. History

    1. OA causes pain that is localized to the involved joint and is described as a deep ache.

    2. An early manifestation of OA is pain that is worse during use of the joint and relieved with rest. As the disease progresses, the pain may occur earlier in onset with joint use and may persist even with the joint at rest.

D. Physical examination

1. Heberden nodes are bony enlargements of the distal interphalangeal (DIP) joints.
2. Bouchard nodes are bony enlargements on the proximal interphalangeal joints (PIP).
3. There is usually tenderness over the joint lines of involved joints.
4. There may be crepitus with movement of the joint, especially in the knee.
5. There is restricted range of motion of involved joints.
6. There is pain with passive range of motion.

E. Differential diagnosis

> Obtain erythrocyte sedimentation rate, rheumatoid factor, and synovial fluid analysis in all patients in whom the diagnosis is not certain.

1. Calcium pyrophosphate deposition (CPPD), rheumatoid arthritis, and infection all are alternative considerations.
2. X-rays of the affected joint may show joint space narrowing and osteophyte formation, but their presence does not prove that OA is the cause of the patient's pain.

F. Management

1. Treatment is both nonpharmacologic and pharmacologic in an effort to keep the patient pain-free.
2. Muscle conditioning and aerobic exercise can help slow down progression of disease.
3. More advanced cases may require physical therapy as well as assistance with daily living activities.
4. Acetaminophen or an NSAID is appropriate initial analgesia. Topical NSAIDs and capsaicin are useful adjunctive therapy.
5. Many patients will use alternative therapies such glucosamine/chondroitin and acupuncture.
   a. Two meta-analyses failed to show effectiveness of glucosamine/chondroitin.
   b. Acupuncture may be effective for some types of osteoarthritis.
6. Joint replacement is an option for severe cases.

V. Low Back Pain

A. Pathophysiology

  1. Etiology is myriad, varying from seemingly minor strains or spasms to metastatic spread of malignant tumors.

  2. Specific problems of the lumbar spine include spondylosis (stress injury of the pars interarticularis), spondylolisthesis (the sliding of one vertebra over another), herniated nucleus pulposus, spinal stenosis, vertebral fractures, and ankylosing spondylitis.

  3. Infectious causes such as osteomyelitis and epidural abscess are possible in the right setting.

  4. Referred pain has the following feature.

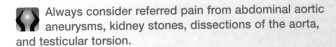

Always consider referred pain from abdominal aortic aneurysms, kidney stones, dissections of the aorta, and testicular torsion.

B. Epidemiology

  1. Some studies estimate that 2.5 % of all outpatient visits to the primary care office are due to low back pain.

  2. Low back pain is second only to the common cold as a major cause of lost work time.

  3. Some data suggest that 60%–80% of all adults will experience low back pain during their adult lives.

C. Patient history

The primary goal of the clinical examination is to identify patients who require an immediate surgical evaluation and those whose symptoms suggest a more serious underlying condition such as malignancy or infection.

  1. The onset and timing of the pain are essential. A history of trauma or onset while trying to lift a heavy load is helpful in developing a likely cause of the pain.

  2. Ask about radiation of the pain into the extremities, which suggests a radicular component and increases the likelihood of disc herniation.

  3. Ask about the presence of paresthesia, numbness, or weakness in the lower extremities. Bowel or bladder incontinence suggests a serious underlying neurologic involvement and should result in immediate imaging and referral.

4. A history of cancer or fever often lowers the threshold for imaging.

5. A detailed psychosocial history may predict outcome in chronic low back pain because concurrent issues can affect pain or perception.

D. Physical examination

1. Examination includes vital signs and thorax, abdomen, lower extremities, and vascular and neurologic evaluation.

2. Inspect the back, looking for abnormality in curvature and in range of motion.

3. Palpate each of the lumbar vertebrae and paraspinous muscles for signs of bony or soft-tissue involvement.

4. Neurologic evaluation includes a good sensory examination including over the medial foot (L4), the web space between the great and the second toe (L5), and the lateral foot (S1).

5. Evaluate deep tendon reflexes for evidence of nerve root involvement.

6. Motor examination includes evaluation of hip flexors and adductors (L2–L3), knee extension (L3–L4), and foot dorsiflexion, inversion, and plantar flexion (L4–L5, S1).

7. Perform straight leg raise test to assess compression or irritation of the nerve roots.

8. Assess heel walking and toe walking. Inability to walk on the heels indicates weakness in L5, the foot dorsiflexors, and inability to walk on the toes indicates an S1 root involvement.

9. Watching a patient pick up a piece of paper from the floor can be very helpful in confirming poor bending technique, even in patients who say they "know" to bend their knees.

E. Imaging

> Most patients presenting with acute low back pain will not require immediate imaging because conditions requiring immediate intervention are rare.

1. The American College of Radiology has developed guidelines for imaging patients presenting with low back pain.
   a. Plain radiography

There is no evidence that routine plain radiography of patients with nonspecific low back pain results in improved outcomes.

    i. Plain radiography is recommended for patients with:
      (1) Possible vertebral compression fractures (history of osteoporosis or corticosteroid use).
      (2) Unexplained weight loss.
      (3) Significant trauma.
      (4) Failure to improve after 1 month.
      (5) Age over 50 years.
      (6) History of cancer.
      (7) Unrelenting night pain or pain at rest.
  b. Magnetic resonance imaging (MRI)

 MRI is the preferred imaging for patients with severe or progressive neurologic defects or when underlying conditions such as infection or malignancy are likely. Perform MRI when back pain has persisted and patients are candidates for intervention such as surgery or epidural corticosteroid injection.

F. Treatment

 Most patients with acute back pain, with or without sciatica, improve within 1 month with noninvasive management.

  1. Self-care management that has been shown to be effective includes:
    a. Remaining active.
    b. Education booklets and handouts.
    c. Application of heat to area.
  2. Medication options include acetaminophen, NSAIDs muscle relaxants, and opioid analgesics.
  3. Studies fail to show systemic corticosteroids benefit treatment of low back pain, with or without radicular symptoms.
  4. Physicians should consider the following treatments with proven benefit for patients who do not improve with self-care.

    a. Physical therapy
    b. Acupuncture
    c. Massage therapy
    d. Yoga
    e. Cognitive behavioral therapy
    f. Spinal manipulation
    g. Tricyclic antidepressants
    h. Gabapentin

5. Reserve surgery for patients who have severely debilitating neurologic deficits or pain that has persisted despite noninvasive therapies.

VI. Patellofemoral Syndrome

A. Pathophysiology

    1. The patella is a sesamoid bone that protects the knee from direct trauma and serves as a fulcrum for the quadriceps in extension. It articulates with the trochlear groove of the femur.

    2. Irritation and inflammation in the patellofemoral groove cause pain in this syndrome. Implicated causes include overuse, biomechanical problems (e.g., widened Q angle of the hips, abnormal pronation of the foot), and muscular dysfunction.

B. Epidemiology

    1. Anterior knee pain is one of the most common musculoskeletal complaints in physically active persons.

    2. Up to 25% of runners may have symptoms of anterior knee pain at one time or another.

    3. One study noted over 10% of musculoskeletal problems presenting to primary care were for anterior knee pain.

C. History

    1. Patients may describe a dull, aching discomfort and stiffness in the anterior knee. Symptoms are often bilateral.

    2. The condition is often exacerbated by prolonged sitting and knee flexion ("theatre sign").

    3. A history of trauma is usually absent.

    4. A family history of anterior knee pain may be present.

    5. Consider "locking" or "giving out."

 Ask all patients with knee pain about these signs. They may indicate a meniscus or ligament problem.

D. Physical examination
1. Physical examination may show swelling, effusion, and crepitus below the patella.
2. A "grind test" result is positive when the examiner puts pressure on the patella, pushing it into the femoral groove, and elicits pain.

E. Differential diagnosis
1. "Locking" often indicates meniscus injury, although this usually presents with medial or lateral knee pain.
2. "Giving out" indicates a ligament injury. Anterior cruciate ligament (ACL) rupture presents with anterior knee pain, but more swelling and a history of trauma will be present.
3. Other causes of anterior knee pain include patellar tendonitis, bursitis, overuse syndrome, plica, Osgood-Schlatter disease, Legg-Calvé-Perthes disease, infections, neoplasm, and inflammatory disease.
4. Plain radiography is not usually helpful unless there is a history of trauma.
5. For prolonged symptoms that do not respond to treatment, MRI can aid in making the diagnosis.

F. Treatment
1. Modification of activities that increase patellofemoral pressure, such as squatting and kneeling, may be helpful.
2. Short periods of ice applied to the knee reduce symptoms.
3. Exercise, including strengthening of the vastus medialis oblique muscle, is useful.

 MENTOR TIPS DIGEST

General
- The physician must ascertain the circumstances behind an acute musculoskeletal injury.
- For a persistent pain (>1 month) especially in patients over age 50, consider malignancy as a possibility, and imaging may be needed.
- Always consider the possibility of referred pain, such as atypical angina presenting as shoulder pain or an abdominal aortic aneurysm presenting as low back pain.

Shoulder Pain
- A complete rotator cuff tear is unlikely in patients younger than 30 years unless they are major athletes or have sustained significant trauma.

- Posterior shoulder pain is rare and is usually due to cervical spine disease.
- Adhesive capsulitis, also called frozen shoulder, is present when there is loss of both active *and* passive range of motion.
- Plain radiographs are required if there is a history of trauma.

Carpal Tunnel Syndrome

- Repetitive activities that flex the wrist, such as typing, assembly line work, or playing a musical instrument, put patients at increased risk for carpal tunnel syndrome.
- Two classic physical examination signs are the Phalen sign and Tinel sign. Their sensitivity is only 20%–50%.
- NCV and EMG studies may be necessary to differentiate conditions.

Osteoarthritis

- The interphalangeal joints are most commonly affected in idiopathic OA.
- The National Health and Nutrition Examination Survey reported the prevalence of OA as 0.1% in 25–34-year-olds and >80% in people over the age of 55.
- Obtain erythrocyte sedimentation rate, rheumatoid factor, and synovial fluid analysis in all patients in whom the diagnosis is not certain.

Low Back Pain

- Always consider referred pain from abdominal aortic aneurysms, kidney stones, dissections of the aorta and testicular torsion.
- The primary goal of the clinical examination is to identify patients who require an immediate surgical evaluation and those whose symptoms suggest a more serious underlying condition such as malignancy or infection.
- Most patients presenting with acute low back pain will not require immediate imaging because conditions requiring immediate intervention are rare.
- There is no evidence that routine plain radiography for patients with nonspecific low back pain results in improved outcomes.
- MRI is the preferred imaging for patients with severe or progressive neurologic defects or when underlying conditions such as infection or malignancy are likely. Perform MRI when

back pain has persisted and patients are candidates for intervention such as surgery or epidural corticosteroid injection.
- Most patients with acute back pain, with or without sciatica, improve within 1 month with noninvasive management.

Patellofemoral Syndrome
- Ask all patients with knee pain for the presence of "locking" or "giving out." These may indicate a meniscus or ligament problem.

Resources

Chou R, et al. Diagnosis and treatment of low back pain: A joint clinical practice guideline from the American College of Physicians and the American Pain Society. Annals of Internal Medicine 147:478–491, 2007.

Chou R, Huffman L. Nonpharmacological therapies for acute and chronic low back pain: A review of the evidence for an American Pain Society/ American College of Physicians clinical practice guideline. Annals of Internal Medicine 147: 492–504, 2007.

D'Arcy CA, McGee S. Does this patient have carpal tunnel syndrome? Journal of the American Medical Association 283:3110–3117, 2000.

Deyo RA, Weinstein JN. Low back pain. New England Journal of Medicine 344:363–370, 2001.

Hunter DJ. In the clinic: Osteoarthritis. Annals of Internal Medicine. 147:ITC8-1-ITC8-16, 2007.

Woodward TW, Best TM. The painful shoulder, part 1: Clinical evaluation. American Family Physician 61, 2000.

Chapter Self-Test Questions

Circle the correct answer. After you have responded to the questions, check your answers in Appendix A.

1. A 45-year-old male carpenter has leg pain and fever. On examination, passive and active movements of the knee cause pain. Based on this information, what is the most likely cause of his leg pain?

   a. Osteoarthritis

   b. Rheumatoid arthritis

c. Gout

    d. Septic arthritis

2. A 45-year-old male carpenter has leg pain and 25 pound unexplained weight loss in the past month. On examination, the hip and knee are normal, but there is tenderness on palpation of the mid-femur. Based on this information, what is the most likely cause of his leg pain?

    a. Malignancy

    b. Osteoarthritis

    c. Tenosynovitis

    d. Gout

3. A 45-year-old male carpenter has low back pain. He admits to having similar pain in the past, usually lasting for weeks. This episode started with bending at work. On examination, there is tenderness on palpation of lumbar paraspinous muscles; knee jerk reflexes are 1+ and bilaterally symmetric; ankle jerks are absent. The straight leg raising test produces posterior thigh pain with both legs. Which is the most appropriate diagnostic test?

    a. MRI of lumbosacral spine

    b. Plain x-ray of lumbosacral spine

    c. EMG of lower legs

    d. No test

 See the testbank CD for more self-test questions.

CHAPTER 14

DERMATOLOGY IN PRIMARY CARE

Cynthia A. Lagone, MD

I. Overview

A. The skin is the largest organ of the body. Diseases of the skin can be a primary disorder or a secondary disorder as a manifestation of a systemic disease. The most common primary skin disorders are discussed in this chapter.

B. General principles consist of the following.

    1. History

        a. Obtain a directed history, including onset, duration, location, and associated symptoms.

        b. Occupation and new exposures are important.

        c. Any previously prescribed treatments should be noted.

        d. Review medications, including any over-the-counter (OTC) medicines.

        e. A brief past medical history and family history should be included when appropriate.

    2. Physical

        a. It is important to have a patient disrobe to perform a thorough examination.

        b. Examine the skin, noting characteristics and distribution of lesions.

> Dermatology is a morphologically oriented specialty. It is very important to identify and be able to describe the lesions accurately.

        c. Tables 14.1 and 14.2 define common terms used in the description of skin lesions.

TABLE 14.1
Primary Lesions

Primary Lesion	Description
Macule	A flat, circumscribed discoloration
Papule	An elevated, solid lesion up to 5 mm
Nodule	A palpable, solid lesion greater than 5 mm
Plaque	A superficial, circumscribed, elevated flat lesion greater than 5 mm
Wheal	A transient, slightly edematous lesion with a characteristic pale red color
Vesicle	A circumscribed collection of free fluid less than 5 mm
Bulla	A circumscribed collection of free fluid greater than 5 mm
Pustule	A circumscribed, superficial cavity of the skin that contains purulent material
Petechia	A visible collection of red blood cells less than 5 mm
Purpura	A visible collection of red blood cells greater than 5 mm
Telangectasia	Dilated superficial blood vessels

TABLE 14.2
Secondary Lesions

Secondary Lesion	Description
Scale	Thickened, loose excess stratum corneum that sheds readily
Crust	Dried exudate; a scab
Excoriation	An often linear erosion caused by scratching
Ulcer	A focal loss of epidermis and dermis
Fissure	A linear loss of epidermis and dermis, with sharp vertical walls
Lichenification	An area of thickened skin with accentuated lines, giving the skin a washboard appearance
Scar	An abnormal collection of connective tissue from dermal damage
Atrophy	Thinning of the epidermis or dermis, resulting in a depression of the skin

3. Develop differential diagnosis based on data gathered
4. Testing
   a. For most skin diseases, testing is minimal. The diagnosis is made by history and appearance.
   b. Lesions can be scraped with a scalpel and examined with potassium hydroxide (KOH) or saline.
   c. A skin biopsy can be performed.
   d. Serum testing for infectious or autoimmune processes may be done.
5. Initiate treatment; monitor lesions for improvement
C. There are literally hundreds of different skin disorders. The rest of this chapter focuses on those most commonly seen in primary care.

II. Acne Vulgaris

A. Pathophysiology
   1. Acne vulgaris is an inflammation of the pilosebaceous units of the skin. The pilosebaceous unit consists of a small hair follicle associated with a large sebaceous gland.
   2. Acne begins in predisposed patients when sebum production is increased. Sebum is partly controlled by androgen stimulation—thus the emergence of acne in adolescence. Increased sebum causes a change in the lining of the follicle, and a plug develops. Behind this blockage, there is an overgrowth of the bacterium *Propionibacterium acnes*.
   3. Irritation and inflammation develop, which provokes an immune response. Inflammatory mediators lead to follicular rupture and leakage of lipids, bacteria, and fatty acids into the dermis.
B. Epidemiology
   1. Acne is the most common skin disease. It affects almost everyone in varying amounts in their lifetime.
   2. It is most common during adolescence, affecting 80%–85% of all teenagers. It can persist into the second and third decades.
   3. Acne tends to be more frequent and severe in males.
   4. Extrinsic factors can aggravate acne.
      a. Emotional stress
      b. Mechanical pressure
         i. Straps from sports helmets or just pressure from leaning face on hand can trigger outbreaks.
         ii. Friction from frequent and overzealous washing worsens acne. Many laypersons think that more or better washing is the cure for acne. Explain to patients that there are

histologic reasons for acne that harder scrubbing does not
negate.
   c. Occlusive products (e.g., cosmetics)
   d. Endocrine factors that increase androgens, e.g., normal fluctuations in menstrual cycle, polycystic ovarian syndrome
   e. Medications
      i. Glucocorticoids
      ii. Anabolic steroids
      iii. Progestin-only birth control pills
   f. Diet
      i. Many patients insist that their acne is exacerbated by
      certain foods.
      ii. There is no conclusive evidence that diet plays a role.
C. History and physical examination
   1. Determine the onset, and ask about possible aggravating factors.
   2. Review current or previous treatments, including OTC treatments.
   3. On physical examination, note the characteristics and distribution.
      a. Acne is most common in areas with a dense population of
      pilosebaceous units such as the face, chest, and back.
      b. Acne characteristically presents as closed comedones (white-
      heads), open comedones (blackheads), papules, pustules and,
      in severe cases, nodules, cysts, and scarring.
      c. Acne is typically graded as mild, moderate, or severe
      (Table 14.3).
D. Differential diagnosis
   1. Acne rosacea, folliculitis, perioral dermatitis, pseudofolliculitis
   barbae, drug eruption

TABLE 14.3	Acne Grades
Acne Grade	**Principal Lesion**
Mild	Comedones
Moderate	Comedones
	Papules
	Pustules
Severe	Papules
	Pustules
	Nodules
	Cysts

E. Laboratory tests

 Laboratory tests are generally not helpful for acne.

F. Treatment
   1. General principles
      a. Treatment is chosen based on acne severity (Table 14.4).
      b. Treatment is tailored depending on side effects.
         i. Many therapies cause dryness and skin irritation.

Topical preparations come in several forms. For dry skin use a cream or lotion. For oily skin choose a gel or solution.

   c. Treatment takes time.

All acne therapies can take weeks for results to be apparent. Patients must be counseled regarding realistic expectations.

   2. Specific treatments
      a. Topical retinoids

 Retinoids are widely used and very effective.

         i. Mechanism is via anti-inflammatory effect and promoting normal keratinocyte desquamation

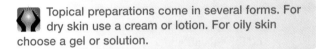

TABLE 14.4	Acne Management
Acne Grade	**Management**
Mild	Topical treatments (antibacterials, benzoyl peroxide, retinoids)
Moderate	Topical therapies, systemic antibiotics, hormones
Severe	Isotretinoin

    ii. Tretinoin, adapalene, tazarotene are examples

    iii. Primary limiting factors are their irritant potential and that they are degraded by light and benzoyl peroxide (BP)

    iv. Best applied at night

b. BP

 BP should be part of most patients' treatment.

    i. Mechanism is via comedolytic activity and antibacterial activity against *P. acnes*

    ii. Primary limiting factor is irritant potential

c. Topical antibiotics

    i. Mechanism is via antibacterial activity against *P. acnes*

    ii. Clindamycin and erythromycin are available agents

 The limiting factor in the use of topical antibiotics is increasing resistance.

    iii. Resistance minimized by combining with BP.

d. Systemic antibiotics

    i. Mechanism is via antibacterial activity against *P. acnes* and possibly anti-inflammatory effect.

    ii. Erythromycin, clindamycin, and tetracycline and its derivatives have been used.

      (1) Erythromycin is rarely used given rising resistance rates.

      (2) Systemic clindamycin is generally avoided given its propensity to cause pseudomembranous colitis.

      (3) Tetracycline and its derivatives are the preferred agents.

        (A) Use of tetracycline is limited given gastrointestinal (GI) side effects, need for frequent dosing, and less overall effectiveness than newer agents.

        (B) Doxycycline is a good option; however, use may be limited by photosensitivity (dose 50–100 mg once to twice daily).

Minocycline is the preferred agent given its lower risk of GI side effects and photosensitivity (dose 50–100 mg once or twice daily).

e. Hormonal therapy: oral contraceptive pills (OCPs)
  i. They work by antagonizing the actions of circulating androgens.
  ii. Up to 83% of patients will have clinical improvement in their acne symptoms.
  iii. Most OCPs should act similarly to reduce acne lesions, although only Ortho Tri-Cyclen and Estrostep have received U.S. Food and Drug Administration approval for the treatment of acne.
f. Systemic retinoid

 Isotretinoin is the most effective treatment for acne.

  i. Mechanism is by reducing sebum production, normalizing keratinization, and anti-inflammatory effects
  ii. Only medication that is curative; up to 60% of patients will have prolonged remission after treatment course
  iii. Limited by its side-effect profile
    (1) It has skin irritant properties. It may cause leucopenia or transaminitis as well as lipid abnormalities.
    (2) The principal concern is teratogenicity.

 Isotretinoin is potently teratogenic.

    (A) Most physicians recommend two forms of birth control in young women taking isotretinoin.
    (3) More recent concerns have been associations of isotretinoin with mood disorders.

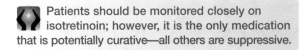 Patients should be monitored closely on isotretinoin; however, it is the only medication that is potentially curative—all others are suppressive.

III. Eczema

A. Overview

1. The terms "eczema" and "dermatitis" are often used interchangeably.

2. Erythema, scale, and vesicles characterize eczematous inflammation.

3. There are three stages of eczema/dermatitis: acute, subacute, and chronic.

    a. Acute dermatitis has an inflamed, oozing epidermis. On biopsy there is an area of edema in the epidermis that pushes apart keratinocytes and causes vesicles and small blisters.

    b. Subacute dermatitis has a visible scale and crust associated with inflamed skin. On biopsy there are scaling and epidermal infiltration of lymphocytes among the keratinocytes.

    c. Chronic dermatitis has a thickened, often violaceous, plaque. On biopsy there is epidermal acanthosis or thickening with a lymphocytic infiltrate in the papillary dermis.

4. The most common disorders in this group are atopic dermatitis, contact dermatitis, and seborrheic dermatitis.

B. Contact dermatitis

1. Pathophysiology

    a. It is inflammation secondary to substances that come in direct contact with the skin.

    b. It can be either allergic or irritant.

      i. Allergic contact dermatitis occurs in patients who have been previously sensitized with a contact allergen. It is a classic, delayed, cell-mediated hypersensitivity reaction.

 The most common triggers in North America are poison ivy and poison oak.

      (1) Other common triggers are nickel perfumes and topical medicine such as neomycin.

      ii. Irritant dermatitis occurs when the substance directly damages the skin.

2. Clinical manifestations

 It is typically an intense pruritic rash.

    a. Erythematous, edematous papules and plaques are characteristic. Blisters and vesicles may be involved.

    b. The location may be a clue to the trigger; e.g., around the neck from nickel jewelry, in a line along the legs with poison ivy.

  3. Differential diagnosis

    a. Atopic dermatitis, seborrheic dermatitis, fungal infections, psoriasis, nummular eczema

  4. Laboratory testing

    a. Skin biopsy may be helpful but is usually not necessary.

    b. Patch testing may be helpful to help identify the offending allergen.

  5. Treatment

    a. Identify and remove the offending agent.

    b. Topical treatment includes cold, wet dressing or topical corticosteroids.

    c. Oral antihistamines may be helpful.

    d. In severe cases oral steroids may be used.

      i. 20–40 mg of prednisone daily, tapered over 1–2 weeks

C. Atopic dermatitis

  1. Pathophysiology

    a. The exact mechanism in atopic dermatitis is incompletely understood. It appears to be IgE-mediated with allergic triggers generating an immune response.

    b. Most patients have a personal or family history of asthma, allergic rhinitis, or atopy.

    c. Patients often have immediate positive skin tests in response to a number of food and environmental allergens.

    d. Patients have decreased cell-mediated immunity, a decreased number of immunoregulatory T cells, and usually increased serum IgE.

  2. Clinical manifestations

    a. It presents as red scaling and crusting lesions. In adults the lesions may be thickened or lichenified.

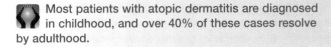

Most patients with atopic dermatitis are diagnosed in childhood, and over 40% of these cases resolve by adulthood.

    b. Patients always have dry skin that is pruritic.

    c. Atopic dermatitis flares in dry winter months and improves in the summer.

    d. Atopic dermatitis has a predilection for elbow, knee, and buttock flexures; the ankles; neck; wrists; and the dorsa of feet and hands.

    e. Secondary bacterial and fungal infections are a common complication.

3. Differential diagnosis: contact dermatitis, seborrhea, psoriasis, fungal infections

4. Laboratory testing

    a. No specific test is usually required to confirm the diagnosis.

    b. Radioallergosorbent test (RAST) and skin testing may be helpful in certain cases.

5. Treatment

    a. Patient education is extremely important.

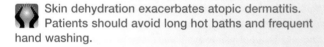 Skin dehydration exacerbates atopic dermatitis. Patients should avoid long hot baths and frequent hand washing.

      i. Emollients are key and should be used daily.

      ii. Excessive rubbing and scratching can lead to lichenification and refractory lesions.

    b. Oral antihistamines are helpful in treating the pruritus.

    c. Mild-to-moderate atopic dermatitis should be treated with topical steroids. Initially, higher potency is used for the acute flare, then a lower-to-intermediate strength is used two to three times a week for maintenance.

    d. Topical calcineurin inhibitors are helpful in moderate flares and for maintenance.

      i. Their advantage is that there is no skin atrophy.

      ii. They are equivalent to low-potency steroids.

      iii. There is some concern that they induce cancers.

      iv. Two examples are tacrolimus and pimecrolimus.

    e. Ultraviolet light therapy is helpful.

    f. Severe cases are treated with oral cyclosporine or other immunosuppressants, such as methotrexate, azathioprine, and mycophenolate.

D. Seborrheic dermatitis
   1. Pathophysiology
      a. It is a common, chronic dermatosis with scaling and erythema. It occurs in areas where sebaceous glands are most active, such as the scalp, face, and body folds.
      b. Biopsy results show mounds of parakeratotic scale around hair follicles with mild superficial inflammation and lymphocytes.

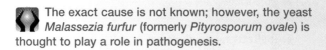 The exact cause is not known; however, the yeast *Malassezia furfur* (formerly *Pityrosporum ovale*) is thought to play a role in pathogenesis.

   2. Clinical manifestations
      a. It has a gradual onset.
      b. It can occur in infants (cradle cap) or adults.
      c. The condition is worse in the winter and improves in the summer.
      d. The scales are frequently yellow or oily in appearance. There is underlying erythema. Pruritus is not characteristic.
      e. Skin lesions can be diffuse, such as on the scalp, or scattered and discrete on the face and trunk.
   3. Differential diagnosis
      a. Psoriasis, contact dermatitis, pityriasis versicolor, tinea, subacute lupus erythematosus
   4. Laboratory testing
      a. Laboratory testing is usually not necessary.
   5. Treatment
      a. Mild scalp involvement is treated with over-the-counter shampoos containing tar preparations, selenium sulfide, or zinc.

 The shampoo should be left on the scalp for 3–5 minutes before rinsing.

      i. Examples are Selsun Blue, Head and Shoulders, and T/Gel.
      b. Antifungal shampoo with ketoconazole or ciclopirox can be used.
      i. These can also be lathered onto the face and body.
      c. Topical ketoconazole cream and intermittent low-potency corticosteroid creams are effective for nonscalp seborrheic dermatitis.

    d. Seborrheic blepharitis, which is seborrhea of the eyelids, is treated by gently removing the scales once a day with a diluted solution of baby shampoo on a cotton ball.

IV. Psoriasis

  A. Overview

 Psoriasis is a common skin disease affecting about 1%–3% of the population.

    1. It affects men and women equally, with a bimodal distribution in adolescence and age 50–60 years.

    2. It is a lifelong condition with recurrent exacerbations and remissions.

Although most patients with psoriasis have a normal life span, the disease can be highly disabling emotionally. Patients often shun outdoor activities and intimacy because they are self-conscious of their appearance.

    3. There are several types: plaque (most common), guttate, pustular, and nail.

    4. Approximately, 5%–10% of patients have accompanying arthritis. This tends to be more common in young women and in those with nail involvement.

  B. Pathophysiology

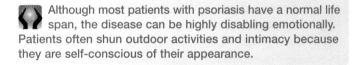 The principle abnormality is abnormal cell proliferation. The epidermal cells have a shortened cycle time with 36 hours as compared with over 300 hours in normal skin. This results in significant increase in the normal production of epidermal cells and keratinization. The result is scaling.

    1. The dermis has large tortuous capillaries that are close to the surface and give plaques their characteristic red hue.

    2. Etiology of abnormal cell proliferation is unknown; however, psoriasis is genetically linked with a higher incidence in families, and there is some association with the human leukocyte antigen (HLA) system.

C. Clinical manifestations

1. Psoriasis is characterized by red scaling papules that coalesce to form plaques. The scale is silvery white and can become very thick.

 When the scale is removed there is pinpoint bleeding characteristic of psoriasis that is called the Auspitz sign.

2. Psoriasis can present anywhere but has a predilection for the elbows, knees, scalp, and gluteal cleft.
3. In the skin folds, the plaques appear smooth and red.
4. Nail findings are pitting, hyperkeratosis, and onycholysis.

D. Triggers of exacerbations

1. Triggers are stress, infection, ethanol, and medications. Lithium, beta blockers, and antimalarials are well documented triggers and should be avoided in a patient with psoriasis.

 Psoriasis can develop in traumatic sites such as scars, sunburns, and scratches. This is known as the Koebner phenomenon.

E. Laboratory testing

1. Diagnosis is usually made by physical examination and history.

F. Differential diagnosis

1. Lichen planus, seborrheic dermatitis, secondary syphilis, pityriasis rosacea, mycosis fungoides, systemic lupus erythematosus

G. Treatment

1. Treatment is lifelong, avoiding triggers and treating exacerbations.
2. Mild disease (which is defined as involving <20% of the body) is treated as summarized in Table 14.5. Topical steroids and creams, such as calcipotriol, tazarotene, anthralin, and tar, can be used with or without ultraviolet light.
3. Localized plaques can be treated with intralesional steroids.
4. Patients with more diffuse disease (>20% body) are treated with a number of different therapies: ultraviolet light B (UVB) phototherapy and tar, psoralen and ultraviolet light A (PUVA), methotrexate, acitretin, cyclosporine, and biologic agents: infliximab, etanercept, alefacept.

TABLE 14.5

Therapeutic Options for Persons With Psoriasis on Less Than 20% of the Body

Treatment	Advantages	Disadvantages	Comments
Topical steroids	Rapid response, controls inflammation and itching, best for intertriginous areas and face, convenient, not messy	Temporary relief (tolerance occurs), less effective with continued use, atrophy and telangiectasia occur with continued use, brief remissions, very expensive	Best results occur with pulse dosing (e.g., 2 weeks of medication and 1 week of lubrication only), plastic occlusion is very effective
Calcipotriol (Dovonex)	Well tolerated, long remissions possible	Burning, skin irritation, expensive	Best for moderate plaque psoriasis
Tazarotene (Tazorac)	Effective, long remissions possible	Irritating, expensive	Topical steroids can control irritation and enhance effectiveness
Anthralin	Convenient short contact programs, long remissions, effective for scalp	Purple-brown staining, irritating, careful application (only to plaque) required	Used on chronic (not inflamed) plaques, best results occur when used with UVB light
Tar	New preparations are pleasant	Only moderately effective in a few patients	Most effective when combined with UVB light (Goeckerman regimen)
UVB and lubricating agents or tar	Insurance may cover part or all of treatment, effective for 70% of patients, no need for topical steroids	Expensive, office-based therapy	Used only on plaque and guttate psoriasis, travel and time required

Therapeutic Options for Persons With Psoriasis on Less Than 20% of the Body (Continued)

Treatment	Advantages	Disadvantages	Comments
Tape or occlusive dressing	Convenient, no mess	Expensive, only for limited disease	May be used to occlude topical steroids
Intralesional steroids	Convenient, rapidly effective, long remissions	Only for limited areas, atrophy and telangiectasia occur at injection site	Ideal for chronic scalp and body plaques when small and few in number

From Habif TP: Clinical Dermatology: A Color Guide to Diagnosis and Therapy, 4th ed. Mosby, 2003.

5. Those with psoriatic arthritis are treated with nonsteroidal anti-inflammatory drugs (NSAIDs): methotrexate, sulfasalazine, cyclosporine, and the biologic agents.
6. Patients treated with UV therapy should be monitored for skin cancer due to increased incidence.

V. Superficial Fungal Infections

A. Overview
1. Dermatophytes are fungi that infect and survive on dead keratin.
2. Dermatophytes cause skin infections called tinea and are further categorized by their location (i.e., tinea pedis, tinea capitus)
3. Dermatophytes are ubiquitous and routinely infect healthy people. However, patients with a compromised immune system are more susceptible.
4. Infections are spread by human-to-human contact or by animal-to-human.
5. Three types of dermatophytes are responsible for the majority of skin infections: Epidermophyton, Trichophyton, and Microsporum.

B. Pathophysiology

 Dermatophytes produce keratinases that digest keratin and sustain their existence on skin structures.

   1. There may be genetic susceptibility, but host factors that facilitate infection are atopy, steroids, and diabetes. Local factors that promote infection are sweating and occlusion.

C. Clinical manifestations

   1. The rash appearance can vary based on the area of the body infected.

   2. The rash may be pruritic.

   3. The infection is usually an erythematous, scaling, well-demarcated patch with a distinct border when it occurs on the trunk, face, or extremities. There may be central clearing of the rash.

   4. Tinea pedis appears as painful, erythematous vesicular lesions between the toes and on the soles.

D. Differential diagnosis

   1. Differential diagnosis is often based on location. Consider contact dermatitis, and atopic dermatitis, pityriasis infection, erythema migrans, and subacute lupus.

E. Laboratory testing

> The best tool for diagnosis is visualization of branching hyphae under the microscope. Scrape the scale from the active border, and place it on a slide with 10% KOH solution.

   1. A fungal culture may also be obtained in cases where the diagnosis is less clear.

   2. Dermatophyte infections of the hair shaft infected by *Microsporum canis* show a diagnostic brilliant green when examined under the Wood lamp.

F. Treatment

   1. Most dermatophyte infections of the skin can be treated successfully with topical antifungals.

   a. Topical polyene and azoles have been mainstays of therapy, but there is emerging resistance.

      i. Examples: nystatin and ketoconazole

   b. Terbinafine is an allylamine that is fungicidal as well as fungistatic.

> Terbinafine 1% applied one to two times daily has higher cure rates than older azole agents and has fewer side effects.

2. Oral agents are usually necessary to treat hair and nail infections. They can also be used on patients with extensive skin involvement. These include griseofulvin, ketoconazole, itraconazole, and terbinafine. They are all associated with potential side effects and should be used with caution.

   a. Terbinafine has fewer side effects and for most infections is more effective.

G. Special considerations

1. Candidiasis is a cutaneous yeast infection that can occur on moist skin sites, including the mucous membranes. *Candida albicans* is the most common cause of candidiasis in humans. It lives on the normal flora of the mouth, vagina, and GI tract. It can become pathogenic in a number of conditions including areas of increased moisture, pregnancy, diabetes, and oral contraceptive pills. It is usually treated with controlling the exacerbating factors and topical imidazoles. Oral agents can be used for severe infections.

2. Pityriasis versicolor is an asymptomatic fungal infection of the trunk due to *M. furfur*. The lesions have a fine scale. On pale skin the lesions are hyperpigmented. On dark skin the lesions are depigmented. Topical antifungals work well, but recurrence is common.

3. Onychomycosis is a nail infection caused by any fungus, including yeasts and nondermatophyte molds.

   a. KOH examination of nail scrapings can be diagnostic, but often a fungal culture of subungual debris or nail clippings is needed to make the diagnosis. In proximal infections, a nail plate biopsy may be needed.

   b. Treatment consists of the following.

      i. Oral treatment includes terbinafine and itraconazole, which are more effective then griseofulvin.

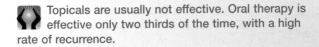
Topicals are usually not effective. Oral therapy is effective only two thirds of the time, with a high rate of recurrence.

Treat onychomycosis of the fingernails for a minimum of 6 weeks and the toenails for 12 weeks. Terbinafine 250 mg daily is a good option.

VI. Skin Cancer

A. Overview

1. Skin cancer is the most common type of cancer.

2. A primary care physician must be able to identify suspicious neoplasms and refer for removal when appropriate.

3. The three main types of skin cancer are basal cell, squamous cell, and melanoma.

B. Pathophysiology

1. Studies clearly show a relationship between early childhood sun exposure and the development of skin cancer.

2. Genetic factors also play a role, especially in melanoma.

C. Basal cell carcinoma

1. This is the most prevalent type of skin cancer.

2. Risk factors include fair skin and sun exposure. It is most commonly found on the face and skin appendages.

3. It is locally invasive, destructive, and aggressive, but it rarely metastasizes.

4. Appearance:

> The typical appearance is a pearly white, pink, or red, dome-shaped papule with characteristic fine telangiectasia. The center frequently ulcerates and bleeds, causing a crust or scale.

5. Treatment is usually surgery, although cryotherapy and radiation are used in certain situations. Mohs surgery is a microscopic, tissue-sparing technique especially useful on the face.

D. Squamous cell carcinoma (SCC)

1. This lesion is a malignant tumor arising from the keratinocytes.

2. It usually develops in sun-damaged skin, often in an actinic keratosis (AK).

   a. AK is a SCC confined to the epidermis.

   b. Almost all AKs are considered to be from sun damage.

   c. AKs can be treated with topical 5-fluorouracil or Imiquimod.

3. SCC usually presents as a hyperkeratotic ulcerated or expanding nodule. It has the potential to metastasize to local lymph nodes.

4. Treatment is generally the same as for basal cell carcinoma: surgery, cryotherapy, or radiation.

E. Malignant melanoma (MM)
1. MM is one of the most dangerous forms of cancer, and its incidence is rapidly increasing.
2. It can occur at any age and on any area of the skin, and it can metastasize to any organ.
3. The goal is early recognition; a thorough skin examination is extremely important.
4. Remember the ABCDs of malignant melanoma recognition.
   a. Asymmetry—two halves of the lesion not identical
   b. Border—irregular, notched, or poorly circumscribed
   c. Color—pure black or haphazard display of red, blue, brown, or black
   d. Diameter—greater than 6 mm (size of a pencil eraser)
5. MM can begin de novo or in a preexisting mole; this is why any changing mole needs to be taken seriously.
6. The diagnosis is made with excisional biopsy. The patient should be referred to a specialist for staging and treatment.

 The most important prognostic factor is tumor thickness in millimeters.

 MENTOR TIPS DIGEST

Overview
- Dermatology is a morphologically-oriented specialty. It is very important to identify and be able to describe the lesions accurately.

Acne Vulgaris
- Laboratory tests are generally not helpful for acne.
- Topical preparations come in several forms. For dry skin use a cream or lotion. For oily skin choose a gel or solution.
- All acne therapies can take weeks for results to be apparent. Patients must be counseled regarding realistic expectations.
- Retinoids are widely used and very effective.
- BP should be part of most patients' treatment.
- The limiting factor in the use of topical antibiotics is increasing resistance.
- Among systemic antibiotics, minocycline is the preferred agent given its lower risk of GI side effects and photosensitivity.

- Isotretinoin is the most effective treatment for acne. However, it is teratogenic. Patients should be monitored closely on isotretinoin; however, it is the only medication that is potentially curative—all others are suppressive.

Eczema
- For contact dermatitis, the most common triggers in North America are poison ivy and poison oak.
- It is typically an intense pruritic rash.
- Most patients with atopic dermatitis are diagnosed in childhood, and over 40% of these cases resolve by adulthood.
- Skin dehydration exacerbates atopic dermatitis. Patients should avoid long hot baths and frequent hand washing.
- The exact cause of seborrheic dermatitis is not known; however, the yeast *Malassezia furfur* (formerly *Pityrosporum ovale*) is thought to play a role in pathogenesis.
- The shampoo should be left on the scalp for 3–5 minutes before rinsing.

Psoriasis
- Psoriasis is a common skin disease affecting about 1%–3% of the population.
- Although most patients with psoriasis have a normal life span, the disease can be highly disabling emotionally. Patients often shun outdoor activities and intimacy because they are self-conscious of their appearance.
- The principle abnormality is abnormal cell proliferation. The epidermal cells have a shortened cycle time with 36 hours as compared with over 300 hours in normal skin. This results in significant increase in the normal production of epidermal cells and keratinization. The result is scaling.
- When the scale is removed there is pinpoint bleeding characteristic of psoriasis that is called the Auspitz sign.
- Psoriasis can develop in traumatic sites such as scars, sunburns, and scratches. This is known as the Koebner phenomenon.

Superficial Fungal Infections
- Dermatophytes produce keratinases that digest keratin and sustain their existence on skin structures.

- The best tool for diagnosis is visualization of branching hyphae under the microscope. Scrape the scale from the active border, and place it on a slide with 10% KOH solution.
- Terbinafine 1% applied one to two times daily has higher cure rates than older azole agents and has fewer side effects.
- In onychomycosis, topicals are usually not effective. Oral therapy is effective only two thirds of the time, with a high rate of recurrence.
- Treat onychomycosis of the fingernails for a minimum of 6 weeks and the toenails for 12 weeks. Terbinafine 250 mg daily is a good option.

Skin Cancer

- With basal cell carcinoma, the typical appearance is a pearly white, pink, or red, dome-shaped papule with characteristic fine telangiectasia. The center frequently ulcerates and bleeds, causing a crust or scale.
- With malignant melanoma, the most important prognostic factor is tumor thickness in millimeters.

Resources

DermIS.net Dermatology Information System: www.dermis.net
This Web site also provides a quick reference and color atlas with additional references cited.
Fitzpatrick TB, et al. Color atlas and synopsis of clinical dermatology, 4th ed. New York: McGraw Hill, 2005.
This is a quick reference guide. It has a number of color pictures and lists key points in epidemiology and etiology, history, physical examination findings, differential diagnoses, and treatment plans.
Fyhrquist VN. Contact dermatitis. Dermatological Clinics 25:613–623, 2007.
Habif TP. Clinical dermatology: A color guide to diagnosis and therapy, 4th ed. Mosby, 2003.
Yan, AC. Current concepts in acne management. Adolescent Medicine Clinics 17:613–637, 2006.
Zhang AY. Advances in topical and systemic antifungals. 25:165–183, 2007.

Chapter Self-Test Questions

Circle the correct answer. After you have responded to the questions, check your answers in Appendix A.

1. What is the most common type of skin cancer?

   a. Adenocarcinoma

   b. Squamous carcinoma

   c. Basal cell carcinoma

   d. Melanoma

2. Which type of skin cancer causes the most deaths?

   a. Adenocarcinoma

   b. Squamous carcinoma

   c. Basal cell carcinoma

   d. Melanoma

3. What skin disease has the highest prevalence?

   a. Plantar wart

   b. Acne vulgaris

   c. Psoriasis

   d. Eczema

See the testbank CD for more self-test questions.

15

FATIGUE

Eduard Porosnicu, MD, and Martin J. Arron, MD, MBA

I. Definition

   A. Refers to a perceived decline in a patient's ability to perform physical or mental activity

   B. Subjective: tiredness, malaise, adversity to activity, sensation of exhaustion, weariness

   C. Objective: impaired physical or mental (cognitive and affective) performance

 Fatigue should be distinguished from weakness, hypersomnolence, dyspnea, or apathy.

II. Classification

   A. Acute fatigue: <30 days

   B. Prolonged fatigue: ≥30 days

     1. Chronic fatigue: persistent or relapsing fatigue for a minimum of 6 consecutive months

     2. Chronic fatigue syndrome (CFS): idiopathic chronic fatigue and four or more of the following:

       a. Sore throat

       b. Tender cervical or axillary lymph nodes

       c. Myalgias

       d. Polyarthralgias

       e. New headaches

       f. Unrefreshing sleep

       g. Malaise after exertion

       h. Impaired memory or concentration

III. Epidemiology

    A. Prevalence

 Given the stressful circumstances in life, fatigue is a common symptom occurring in 20%–25% of the population.

        1. 20%–30% of primary care patients report significant fatigue that interferes with their life quality

        2. 5% of primary care patients seek medical advice for fatigue

        3. 50% of primary care patients admit being fatigued when asked (secondary complaint)

        4. Prevalence of CFS in United States is approximately 0.4%, or more than one million people

 CFS accounts for only 1%–9% of patients with chronic fatigue.

        5. CFS is diagnosed in only 20% of those who have the syndrome

        6. Prevalence of chronic fatigue in African Americans and Hispanics is equal to or greater than in the white population

    B. Risk factors

        1. Gender

 Fatigue is twice as common in women as men.

        2. Early childhood psychological abuse, sexual abuse, or physical trauma

        3. Adverse parenting styles

        4. Limited participation in sports during childhood

        5. Middle age, with peak between 40–59 years

        6. Lower income (contrary to popular belief)

        7. History of psychiatric disease

    C. Precipitating factors

        1. Acute medical illness

        2. Acute or chronic psychological stress

    D. Perpetuating factors

        1. Sleep disorders

        2. Physical inactivity

3. Psychiatric disorders
4. Social stress
E. CFS comorbid conditions
  1. Fibromyalgia
  2. Irritable bowel syndrome
  3. Multiple chemical sensitivities
  4. Gulf War syndrome
  5. Temporomandibular joint disorder
  6. Interstitial cystitis
F. Economics of chronic fatigue

 Fatigue is expensive to the overall economy because of impaired productivity.

  1. Total economic cost in the United States is estimated at $9.1 billion annually.
  2. Average lost annual household earning from CFS is $20,000.
  3. Fully 25% of chronically fatigued patients are unemployed or receive disability.

IV. Etiology
A. General

 Fatigue is a symptom associated with a wide variety of acute and chronic medical and psychological disorders.

  1. It is frequently multifactorial in origin.
B. Psychiatric causes are encountered in 60%–70% of cases of chronic fatigue.
  1. Depression
  2. Anxiety
  3. Somatization
  4. Personality disorder
  5. Substance abuse
C. Infections
  1. Viral: Epstein-Barr virus (mononucleosis), cytomegalovirus, HIV
  2. Bacterial: osteomyelitis, endocarditis, abscesses
  3. Mycobacterial: tuberculosis
  4. Systemic fungal infections

D. Medications:
1. Antidepressants: tricyclics, trazodone, nefazodone
2. Antihypertensives: beta blockers, clonidine
3. Immunomodulators: corticosteroids, interferon, tumor necrosis factor, interleukins
4. Sedatives-hypnotics: benzodiazepines, barbiturates
5. Antipsychotics: chlorpromazine, haloperidol
6. Anticonvulsants: phenytoin, valproic acid
7. Antihistamines: hydroxyzine, diphenhydramine
8. Chemotherapy
9. Muscle relaxants: cyclobenzaprine, carisoprodol
10. Antispasmotics: dicyclomine
11. Analgesics: narcotics

E. Endocrine disorders
1. Diabetes mellitus
2. Hypothyroidism and hyperthyroidism
3. Hypocortisolism and hypercortisolism
4. Hyperparathyroidism
5. Hypogonadism

F. Metabolic and fluid-electrolyte imbalance
1. Dehydration
2. Hypercalcemia
3. Hypophosphatemia
4. Hyponatremia or hypernatremia
5. Liver failure
6. Chronic kidney disease

G. Neurologic disorders
1. Parkinson disease
2. Lou Gehrig disease
3. Multiple sclerosis
4. Restless leg syndrome
5. Autonomic failure (e.g., Shy-Drager)
6. Neurally mediated hypotension
7. Postural tachycardia syndrome

H. Pulmonary disease
1. Chronic obstructive pulmonary disease (COPD)
2. Sleep apnea
3. Asthma
4. Interstitial lung disease

I. Cardiac disease
   1. Coronary artery disease
   2. Congestive heart failure
   3. Valvular disease
   4. Cardiomyopathies
J. Connective tissue diseases
   1. Rheumatoid arthritis
   2. Polymyalgia rheumatica
   3. Giant cell arteritis
   4. Sarcoidosis
   5. Systemic lupus erythematosus

V. Pathophysiology

A. General
   1. The pathophysiology of fatigue remains unclear.
   2. Most of the studies have focused on patients with CFS.
   3. Premorbid physical deconditioning may play a role.
   4. Some of the hypotheses to explain chronic fatigue are listed below.
B. Hypofunctional hypothalamic-pituitary-adrenal (HPA) axis
   1. Patients with CFS were found to have a mildly depressed serum cortisol response to stress and abnormally high release of proinflammatory cytokines.
   2. An association exists between CFS and variations in the glucocorticoid receptor gene.
C. Genetic disorders
   1. Studies have demonstrated that variations in certain genes are associated with CFS. One study predicted whether an individual had CFS with 76% accuracy.
   2. Three of the most relevant genes were associated with stress reactions, emotional responses, memory, and other central nervous system activity.
   3. No definitive genetic markers have been identified; the role of genetic profiling in the diagnosis of CFS remains unclear.
D. Brainstem dysfunction
   1. Postulated for postviral fatigue syndromes
   2. Entails viral damage to the dopaminergic pathways and the ascending reticular activating system from brainstem to the cortex

E. Orthostatic intolerance
  1. Some patients with chronic fatigue have postural or neurally mediated hypotension
  2. Reduction in blood pressure when ambulating may result in fatigue, lightheadedness, impaired concentration, and other nonspecific symptoms

VI. Clinical Assessment
  A. General
    1. Physicians may sometimes perceive fatigue as less important because it is diagnostically nonspecific.
    2. Fatigue is an important symptom for the patient and can be disabling.
    3. Chronic fatigue patients can be as debilitated as patients with multiple sclerosis, renal failure, or heart disease.
  B. History

 The history is the most important part of the evaluation.

    1. History should be developed with open-ended, nonjudgmental questions
    2. Fatigue characteristics
      a. Duration
      b. Timing
      c. Triggering factors
      d. Relieving factors
      e. Associated symptoms
    3. Contextual history
      a. Psychosocial history
      b. Sleep history
      c. Sexual history
      d. Recreational drug use
      e. Acute or chronic environmental toxin exposure (e.g., lead, carbon monoxide (CO)
  C. Physical examination

 The physical examination needs to be thorough.

1. The list of possible diagnostic clues to a potential causal illness is extensive
    a. Orthostatic hypotension
    b. Low-grade fever
    c. Skin pallor, jaundice, cyanosis, malar rash, bruises
    d. Oral thrush, mucosal pallor
    e. Lymph node enlargement
    f. Thyromegaly
    g. Breast masses
    h. Cardiac murmurs; jugular venous distention (JVD), S3, pedal edema, rales
    i. Wheezing
    j. Hepatosplenomegaly and/or ascites
    k. Muscle atrophy and/or decreased strength
    l. Clubbing
    m. Joint deformities (swan neck, boutonnière)
    n. Poor balance, coordination
    o. Cognitive defects
D. Diagnostic testing
    1. General
        a. Fatigue is a nonspecific symptom.

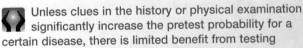

Unless clues in the history or physical examination significantly increase the pretest probability for a certain disease, there is limited benefit from testing beyond age- and gender-appropriate screening.

    2. Suggested battery of routine tests
        a. Complete blood count with differential
        b. Erythrocyte sedimentation rate or reactive protein
        c. Serum urea nitrogen, creatinine, electrolytes
        d. Serum calcium and phosphate
        e. Liver transaminases
        f. Thyroid-stimulating hormone
        g. Fasting blood glucose
        h. Creatine kinase
        i. Urinalysis
        j. Urine pregnancy test (in reproductive-age women)
        k. Globulin and albumin
        l. Antinuclear antibodies and rheumatoid factor

   3. Specialized testing may be indicated if suggested by clinical findings
   a. Polysomnography and other sleep studies
   b. Tilt table testing
   4. Psychiatric referral
   a. Psychiatric or psychological consultation is indicated when such an etiology is suspected or the fatigue remains unexplained despite a thorough medical evaluation by the primary care provider.

VII. Management
   A. General
   1. Idiopathic chronic fatigue can be challenging to treat for both medical and psychological reasons.

 Many patients have preconceived ideas regarding the causes and treatments of their symptoms.

   2. Patients with chronic fatigue may experience more side effects from treatment and may require lower starting doses.
   3. Early intervention may facilitate better outcomes.

 Cognitive behavioral therapy and graded exercise programs are the only proven therapies for chronic fatigue.

   B. Disease-specific therapies
   1. Are directed to the diagnosed condition such as infection, medication side effect, or organ dysfunction
   2. Fatigue due to a psychiatric illness often responds to:
   a. Reassurance.
   b. Stress management.
   c. Sleep hygiene.
   d. Sedative-hypnotic or anxiolytic medications.
   e. Psychotropic medication and/or psychotherapy.
   C. Coping strategies
   1. Develop effective adaptive strategies for improving functioning, limiting symptoms, and increasing quality of life
   2. Helpful strategies include
   a. Acknowledging the disability and establishing reasonable treatment goals

b. Recognizing and addressing counterproductive beliefs
c. Lifestyle management
d. Balanced diet and, if necessary, calorie reduction
e. Graded exercise program
f. Cognitive behavioral therapy
  i. Focuses on the illness experience of patients and the impact the fatigue has on their lives
  ii. Therapy incorporates:
    (1) Cognitive element: focuses on modification of thoughts and beliefs relevant to disease process
    (2) Behavioral element: graded increase in activity.
    (3) A skilled psychotherapist
D. Symptom-specific strategies
  1. For pain
    a. Acetaminophen, nonsteroidal anti-inflammatory drugs (NSAIDs), corticosteroids (avoid opiates, if possible)
  2. For sleep disturbance
    a. Sleep hygiene
    b. Over-the-counter sedatives
    c. Cautious use of hypnotics
  3. For depression
    a. Antidepressants
    b. Psychostimulants
      i. Psychostimulants such as methylphenidate, pemoline, and modafinil have been used in chronic fatigue with varied results.
      ii. In a randomized trial, methylphenidate diminished fatigue and increased concentration significantly in only 17% of CFS patients.
      iii. These medications should be prescribed by experienced clinicians who are familiar with their side effects.
E. Alternative therapies
  1. Many unproven interventions are often tried in chronic fatigue.
  2. Pharmacologic therapy with fludrocortisone, corticosteroids, vitamin B_{12}, and acyclovir has not been proven to be effective.
  3. L-carnitine, coenzyme Q10, monoclonal antibodies, serum immunoglobulins, galantamine, and a variety of herbal remedies have been used without clear evidence of efficacy.
  4. Acupuncture, massage, meditation, and yoga are often prescribed but are of unproven benefit.

VIII. Prognosis

A. Acute fatigue has a good prognosis. It is usually *not* the primary symptom at presentation.

B. Chronic fatigue has a variable course with unpredictable remissions and exacerbations.

C. Patients with idiopathic chronic fatigue may have undiagnosed cancers or other major disorders as a cause of their symptoms.

D. The mortality rate of idiopathic chronic fatigue is low (0.01%).

E. Although the majority of patients improve over time, a significant proportion of patients do not fully recover.

 Children with chronic fatigue have a good chance of recovery (50%–95%). (This is a better rate than seen in adults.) Reassure children and their parents.

MENTOR TIPS DIGEST

- Fatigue should be distinguished from weakness, hypersomnolence, dyspnea, or apathy.
- Given the stressful circumstances in life, fatigue is a common symptom occurring in 20%–25% of the population.
- CFS accounts for only 1%–9% of patients with chronic fatigue.
- Fatigue is twice as common in women as men.
- Fatigue is expensive to the overall economy because of impaired productivity.
- Fatigue is a symptom associated with a wide variety of acute and chronic medical and psychological disorders.
- The history is the most important part of the evaluation.
- The physical examination needs to be thorough.
- Unless clues in the history or physical examination significantly increase the pretest probability for a certain disease, there is limited benefit from testing beyond age- and gender-appropriate screening.
- Many patients have preconceived ideas regarding the causes and treatments of their symptoms.
- Cognitive behavioral therapy and graded exercise programs are the only proven therapies for CFS.
- Children with chronic fatigue have a good chance of recovery (50%–95%). (This is a better rate than seen in adults.) Reassure children and their parents.

Resources

Blockmans D, Persoons P, Van Houdenhove B, et al. Does methylphenidate reduce the symptoms of chronic fatigue syndrome? American Journal of Medicine 119:167.e23–30, 2006.

Chaudhuri A, Behan PO. Fatigue in neurological disorders. Lancet 363:978–988, 2004.

Cornuz J, Guessous I, Favrat B. Fatigue: A practical approach to diagnosis in primary care. Canadian Medical Association Journal 174: 2006.

Goertzel B, Pennachin C, deSouza L, et al: Combinations of single nucleotide polymorphisms in neuroendocrine effector and receptor genes predict chronic fatigue syndrome. Pharmacogenomics. 7:475–483, 2006.

Price JR, Couper J. Cognitive behaviour therapy for chronic fatigue syndrome in adults. Cochrane Database of Systematic Reviews Issue 4, 1998.

Prins JB, van der Meer JW, Bleijenberg G. Chronic fatigue syndrome. Lancet. 367:346–355, 2006.

Reyes M, et al. Prevalence and incidence of chronic fatigue syndrome in Wichita, Kansas. Archives of Internal Medicine 163:1530–1536, 2003.

U.S. Department of Health and Human Services, Centers for Disease Control and Prevention. CFS toolkit for healthcare professionals

Chapter Self-Test Questions

Circle the correct answer. After you have responded to the questions, check your answers in Appendix A.

1. Which of the following suggests objective evidence of fatigue?

   a. Slow, deep tendon reflexes

   b. Diminished deep tendon reflexes

   c. Impaired cognitive performance

   d. Impaired muscle tone

2. What is the approximate frequency of fatigue as the primary complaint in primary care?

   a. 0.5%

   b. 5%

c. 50%

d. 95%

3. Which of these symptomatic complaints are most consistent with fatigue?

a. Excess daytime sleepiness

b. Unremitting weariness

c. Lack of caring about matters that should be important

d. Difficulty breathing at rest

See the testbank CD for more self-test questions.

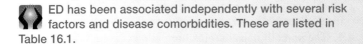

16

ERECTILE DYSFUNCTION

Kevin T. McVary, MD

I. Epidemiology

A. Erectile dysfunction (ED) is defined as the condition when a man cannot acquire or sustain an erection of sufficient rigidity to have sexual intercourse.

B. The estimated prevalence of ED in the United States is approximately 30 million and is associated with approximately $330 million in annual expenditures.

 Both the prevalence and incidence of ED increase with age.

C. ED is not considered a normal part of the aging process.

II. ED Risks

 ED has been associated independently with several risk factors and disease comorbidities. These are listed in Table 16.1.

A. ED may be the presenting symptom of one of the risk factors in Table 16.1, and health-care providers should view ED as a potential symptom of a systemic disease.

III. Erectile Physiology

A. At rest the penis is kept flaccid both through sympathetic outflow onto α_1 receptors as well as through the action of local endothelial factors, which work together to cause tonic contraction of cavernosal smooth muscle.

TABLE 16.1

Risk Factors for Organic ED

Disease	Age-Adjusted Odds Ratio
Diabetes mellitus	4.08
Coronary artery disease	1.79
Hypertension	1.58
Hyperlipidemia	1.63
Peripheral vascular disease	2.63
Alcohol abuse	1.53
BPH/LUTS	2.93
Obesity	1.96
Smoking	1.97–2.45
Metabolic syndrome	33%–40%*
Prior pelvic surgery	25%*
Chronic renal failure	20%–50%*
Endocrine disorders:	
• Hyperthyroid	14.7%*
• Hypothyroid	64.3%*
• Hyperprolactinemia	50%–75%*
Depression	1.82–2.03

*Indicates population prevalence—or not available

B. Erection is initiated by parasympathetic stimulation of penile blood vessels, vascular endothelium, and corpus cavernosal smooth muscle, causing relaxation via a nitric oxide (NO)/cGMP–mediated mechanism.

　1. The smooth muscle relaxation allows increased blood flow and compression of venous outflow by the tunica albugenea.

IV. Pathophysiology of Erectile Dysfunction

Factors contributing to the pathogenesis of ED can be divided into the following six categories: arteriogenic, venogenic, neurogenic, endocrine, psychogenic, and medication-related. More than one category may be involved in an individual patient.

A. Several diseases—diabetes mellitus (DM), metabolic syndrome, chronic renal failure (CRF), benign prostatic hyperplasia

(BPH)—associated with increased risk of developing ED, with underlying pathology as one or several of the six categories
B. Arteriogenic: disturbance in flow of blood into penis
   1. The commonly accepted mechanism involves endothelial cell dysfunction.
   2. Damage to the vascular endothelium can prevent sufficient NO-dependent vasodilation to allow adequate blood inflow. This is often due to atherogenesis for which DM, hypertension (HTN), cardiovascular disease, and smoking are risk factors.

> Prostate Cancer Prevention Trial data demonstrated that men with ED who have no symptoms of vascular disease should be screened for cardiovascular disease and its associated risk factors.

    a. Many consider men with ED and no cardiovascular symptoms to be vascular patients until proved otherwise.
   3. Other causes of arteriogenic ED include pelvic trauma and radiation therapy.
C. Cavernous (venogenic): disturbance in flow of blood out of penis
   1. Insufficient compression of the subtunical venous plexuses allows venous blood to escape and prevents sufficient penile engorgement to attain an erection. No increase in arterial inflow can compensate for the unrestricted venous outflow.
   2. Suggested causes include decreased cavernous smooth muscle content due to smooth muscle cell apoptosis, loss of compliance of venous sinusoids, abnormal vascular structures, degenerative tunical changes, and damage to the tunica albugenea.
D. Neurogenic:
   1. Includes central, peripheral, and iatrogenic causes and may account for up to 20% of all cases of ED
    a. Disorders that affect the sacral spinal cord or the peripheral autonomic fibers to the penis prevent autonomic relaxation of penile smooth muscle.
   2. In patients with spinal cord injury, extent of ED depends on completeness and level of spinal lesion
   3. Other disorders commonly associated with ED include multiple sclerosis and peripheral neuropathy due to DM or alcoholism

   4. Pelvic surgery may result in ED through disruption of autonomic nerve supply leading to smooth muscle cell apoptosis

E. Endocrinologic:

 Androgens contribute to, but are not essential for, normal libido, and their complete role in erectile function remains unclear.

   1. Hyperprolactinemia can result in sexual dysfunction with loss of libido, ED, galactorrhea, gynecomastia, and infertility, as it is associated with low levels of testosterone.
   2. Hypothyroidism and hyperthyroidism are both associated with ED.

F. Diabetes:
   1. In studies using exclusively diabetic populations, the prevalence of ED is estimated anywhere from 35% to 75%.

 Symptoms of ED may be the presenting symptom of diabetes in up to 12% of men.

   2. ED in diabetic men has been most strongly associated with poor glycemic control, insulin dependence, long duration of disease, concurrent smoking ,and diabetic complications such as neuropathy, nephropathy, or retinopathy.
   3. Diabetic ED is a result of a combination of arteriogenic and neurogenic mechanisms.

G. Metabolic syndrome:
   1. The metabolic syndrome is defined by three of the five factors present: 1. abdominal obesity; 2. HTN; 3. glucose intolerance; 4. hypertriglyceridemia; and 5. low HDL cholesterol.
   2. The metabolic syndrome is an independent risk factor for cardiovascular disease and has also been associated with endothelial dysfunction and decreased NO release.

H. Lower urinary tract symptoms (LUTS)/benign prostatic hyperplasia (BPH):
   1. LUTS secondary to BPH have a reported prevalence ranging from 30% in men in their 50s up to 60% in men over the age of 70 years.
      a. Up to 90% of men over the age of 80 years have histologic evidence of BPH on autopsy.

2. Although sexual dysfunction has not been linked definitively to any one specific type of LUTS (obstructive versus irritative versus overall bother), it appears that the overall severity of LUTS is associated with more severe sexual dysfunction.

3. The underlying mechanism is still not clear, but suggested etiologies include increased sympathetic tone, alterations in smooth muscle contraction, endothelial dysfunction, atherosclerosis-induced pelvic ischemia, and age-related hormone imbalances.

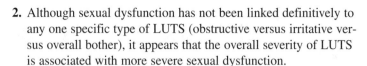 Thus, all men presenting with LUTS/BPH should be evaluated for ED, and all men experiencing sexual dysfunction should be evaluated for LUTS.

I. Chronic kidney disease (CKD):

1. There is a reported prevalence of ED ranging from 20% to 50% in patients with CKD, especially among transplant and dialysis patients.

2. The underlying cause is likely secondary to endothelial damage from underlying vascular disease, diabetes, or prolonged uremia.

J. Psychogenic:

1. It is defined as the persistent inability to achieve or maintain erections satisfactory for sexual performance due predominantly or exclusively to psychological or interpersonal factors.

   a. The most common causes of psychogenic ED are performance anxiety, depression, relationship conflict, loss of attraction, history of sexual abuse, conflicts over sexual preference, or fear of pregnancy or STD.

2. Men who present with ED who have nocturnal erections have at least an element of psychogenic ED, but an underlying organic cause still cannot be ignored (Table 16.2).

 Many cases of ED have some aspect of psychogenic ED involved and are called mixed ED.

3. There are two mechanisms that may be involved in psychogenic ED.

   a. Increased psychogenic stimuli to the sacral cord, which may inhibit reflexogenic erections and prevent the activation of the vasodilator outflow to the penis

TABLE 16.2	
Classification of ED Characteristics	
Organic ED	**Psychogenic ED**
Slow onset	Rapid onset
No situational correlate	Situational dysfunction
Dysfunction constant	Dysfunction comes and goes
Absence of nocturnal and early morning erections	Presence of nocturnal or early morning erections
History of systemic disease, such as diabetes or coronary artery disease, or lifestyle factors	Presence of psychological factors, relationship difficulties, or emotional stressors

     b. Excess of sympathetic outflow or plasma catecholamine levels, which can increase penile smooth muscle tone

  K. Medication and substance-related:

    1. Many patients presenting with ED have a history of prescription drug use.

 There is a consensus that drugs are implicated in a large percentage of ED cases, but the exact mechanisms are complex (Box 16.1).

 Thiazide diuretics and nonselective beta blockers have been implicated most often.

BOX 16.1	
Medications Associated With ED	
Cardiovascular	**Hormones**
Clonidine	GnRH agonists (Leuprolide)
Calcium channel blockers (Verapamil)	Estrogens
Hydralazine	Progesterone
Methyldopa	Corticosteroids
Nonselective beta blockers (Propranolol)	Cyproterone acetate
	5 α-reductase inhibitors

BOX 16.1

Medications Associated With ED (continued)

Reserpine
Guanethidine
Disopyramide
Fibrates (Gemfibrozil)
Amiodarone
Digoxin

Psychiatric

SSRIs (Paroxetine)
Haloperidol
Tricyclic antidepressants
 (Imipramine)
Doxepin
Lithium
MAO inhibitors (Phenelzine)
Trazodone
Phenothiazines (Thioridazine)

Gastrointestinal

H2 blockers (Cimetidine)
Metoclopramide

Anti-inflammatory

Indomethacin
Naproxen

Cytotoxic

Chemotherapy
Sulfasalazine
Methotrexate
Cyclophosphamide
Roferon-A

Genitourinary

Prazosin

Diuretics

Acetazolamide
Thiazides
Spironolactone

Central Nervous System

Opiates
Anticholinergics
Benzodiazepines (Diazepam)
Barbiturates
Carbamazepine
Bromocriptine
Phenytoin

Antiviral

Protease inhibitors

Recreational

Ethanol
Nicotine
Cocaine
Marijuana

2. Antidepressant and antipsychotic agents, particularly neuroleptics, tricyclic antidepressants, monoamine oxidase (MAO) inhibitors, and selective serotonin uptake inhibitors (SSRIs), are associated with erectile, ejaculatory, and sexual desire difficulties.

3. Anti-androgen medications may be associated with decreased sexual desire.

4. Cigarette smoking induces systemic vasoconstriction, is atherogenic, and may directly cause endothelial dysfunction.

 Smoking cessation may decrease the risk of ED.

5. Alcohol causes central sedation, and large amounts can cause liver failure, with longstanding use leading to hyperestrogenemia and ED.

V. Approach to the ED Patient

A. A complete medical and sexual history should be taken during the initial evaluation of any man with ED.

1. Initial questions should focus on the onset of symptoms, progression, and the presence, quality, and duration of erections.

 The absence of nocturnal erections is often a crucial piece of information differentiating organic from psychogenic ED.

a. Organic causes are generally characterized by a gradual and persistent change in rigidity or ability to sustain nocturnal, coital, or self-stimulated erections.

b. Psychogenic ED is often associated with the presence of nocturnal erections, may be situational, and may have an abrupt onset without obvious cause (see Table 16.2).

c. Although a patient may demonstrate symptoms of psychogenic ED, it is important to understand he may also be suffering from an organic cause of ED.

2. Relevant risk factors should be identified (such as DM, lipid disorders, HTN, peripheral vascular disease, smoking, alcoholism, and obesity).

3. It is recommended that the physician administer the International Index of Erectile Function (IIEF) score, or another accepted quantitative form, which measures the severity of the dysfunction and details which domains are affected.

 Decreased libido may be one of the earliest signs of altered testosterone or prolactin.

4. Questions should be asked about whether ejaculation is normal, premature, delayed, or absent.
   a. Retrograde ejaculation is often present in diabetic men with autonomic neuropathy.
5. The patient should also be questioned about the presence of penile curvature or pain with coitus to assess for any structural abnormalities.
6. The patient's surgical history should be probed, with emphasis on bowel, bladder, prostate, or vascular diseases.
7. A complete drug history should be taken, including alcohol consumption and cigarette smoking.
B. The physical examination is a crucial part of the assessment of ED.

 Signs of thyroid, hepatic, hypertensive, cardiovascular, or renal disease should be evaluated.

 Peripheral pulses, reflexes, and visual fields should be examined.

Assess the external genitalia by palpating the penis to check for fibrotic plaques, suggestive of Peyronie disease; also, perform a testicular examination in search of small testes or reduced secondary sexual characteristics, suggestive of hypogonadism.

C. Select laboratory testing is recommended in many cases.
   1. Serum chemistries, complete blood count (CBC), fasting blood glucose, lipid profiles
   2. Measuring free and total testosterone can be important, especially in cases of advanced age, obesity

3. Serum prolactin should be measured, although admittedly low-yield
4. Thyroid function studies should be considered

VI. Indications for Specialty Referral

A. Most patients with ED do not need further workup; some require specialized testing.
B. Situations that support specialized vascular, neurologic, or psychiatric evaluation include the following.
   1. Complicated endocrinopathies
   2. Complicated psychiatric disturbances
   3. Penile abnormalities (e.g., Peyronie disease)
   4. Pelvic/perineal trauma
   5. Necessity of vascular or neurosurgical intervention
   6. Patient wishes a more comprehensive diagnostic evaluation or understanding prior to selection of a treatment
   7. Failure of initial treatment
   8. Presence of medical/legal issues
C. The major classes of diagnostic testing (invasiveness and cost should be weighed) for ED include the following.
   1. Vascular—Duplex Doppler ultrasound, injection of vasoactive substances followed by penile stimulation, dynamic infusion cavernosography/cavernosometry
   2. Neurologic—nocturnal penile tumescence and rigidity, biothesiometry, somatosensory-evoked potentials
   3. Endocrinologic—hypothalamic and/or pituitary function studies, brain magnetic resonance imaging (MRI), thyroid function studies
   4. Psychodiagnostic

VII. Management

A. Patient education
   1. Patient and partner education is essential in the treatment of ED.
   2. Discussion of the treatment options helps clarify how to best offer treatment.
B. Nonpharmacologic therapies
   1. The initial therapy for a patient with obesity, excess alcohol consumption, and cigarette smoking involves lifestyle changes including weight loss and smoking and drinking cessation.
      a. Studies have proved weight loss to be an effective treatment for ED in obese men with no other comorbidities.

2. Review the patient's medications to determine if any are associated with ED.

   a. Consider changing a patient's antidepressant medication to one with fewer sexual side effects, such as bupropion, mirtazapine, sertraline, or fluoxetine.

   b. If the therapeutic benefits of the patient's medication outweigh the sexual side effects, it is appropriate to give a trial of oral phosphodiesterase-5 (PDE-5) inhibitor therapy.

C. Psychosexual therapy

   1. Group therapy, cognitive-behavioral interventions, behavioral desensitization, individual and couples therapy

   2. Psychosexual therapy may help treat organic ED along with first-line pharmacologic or surgical therapy, as there may be mixed disorder

D. Oral PDE-5 inhibitors

   1. PDE-5 inhibitors are oral agents that potentiate the release of NO to enhance erection in men who already have functional NO release.

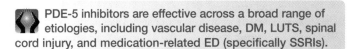

PDE-5 inhibitors are effective across a broad range of etiologies, including vascular disease, DM, LUTS, spinal cord injury, and medication-related ED (specifically SSRIs).

   2. They do not effect ejaculation, orgasm, or sexual drive.

   3. Both vardenafil (Levitra) and sildenafil (Viagra) are semiselective inhibitors of PDE-5 (predominant isoform found in the penis) and have some PDE-6 inhibition (isoform found in the eye), whereas tadalafil (Cialis) inhibits PDE-5 and PDE-11 (isoform found in the prostate, skeletal muscle, and testis).

   4. These three medications show similar efficacy, tolerability, time to onset of action, and side effects.

      a. Tadalafil has a significantly longer half-life, allowing it to be active for up to 36 hours, whereas the other two have a significantly shorter duration of action.

   5. The side effects of these drugs are secondary to inhibition of vascular and smooth muscle PDE-5 and include the following.

      a. Minor side effects such as headaches, facial flushing, dyspepsia, myalgia, nasal congestion

    b. Approximately 7% of men may experience transient altered color vision with sildenafil and vardenafil

    c. Rare but serious side effect of nonarteritic anterior ischemic optic neuropathy (NAION) reported for all three drugs

    d. Vardenafil may cause QT prolongation; contraindicated for patients who take class 1A and III antiarrythmic drugs or who have prolonged QT syndrome

    e. These drugs can potentiate hypotensive effects of nitrates and may result in profound shock and even death; no antidote to nitrate-PDE-5 inhibitor interaction

 These drugs are strictly contraindicated for all men receiving any form of nitrate therapy.

  6. Exercise caution in prescribing these drugs for those with active coronary disease, heart failure, left ventricle low outflow states, and patients on complex antihypertensive regimens because PDE-5 inhibitors have a vasodilatory effect and may cause hypotension.

    a. There is an increase in cardiovascular activity with sexual activity.

    b. PDE-5 inhibitors do not increase the risk of MI or cardiac mortality in patients with known coronary disease or heart failure.

E. Androgen therapy

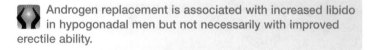 Androgen replacement is associated with increased libido in hypogonadal men but not necessarily with improved erectile ability.

  1. The goals of replacement therapy are to increase sexual interest and desire, attain serum levels close to physiologic levels, and replicate physiologic diurnal rhythm.

  2. Replacement methods include depot intramuscular (IM) injections, oral preparations, and transdermal preparations of testosterone.

    a. The long-acting IM depots of testosterone are the most cost-effective, safe, and practical preparations available.

3. It has not been demonstrated that replicating the diurnal rhythm provides any physiologic advantage.
   a. Oral androgen preparations are associated with increased risk for hepatotoxicity.
   b. The transdermal delivery of testosterone is convenient and reliable and more closely mimics the physiologic testosterone levels.
4. Androgen supplementation in the face of normal testosterone is discouraged because adverse side effects may result without any effect on erectile function.
5. Side effects of unnecessary testosterone administration include infertility, erythrocytosis, hepatotoxicity, worsening of sleep apnea, and dyslipidemia.
6. Hepatic function and a CBC should be measured before and during testosterone therapy.

 Androgen therapy is contraindicated in men with androgen-sensitive cancers.

 It is considered wise to perform a digital rectal examination and measure PSA prior to giving androgens.

F. Intracavernosal self-injection
   1. If oral therapy fails or is contraindicated, the self-injection of intracavernosal vasoactive substances is a reasonable next choice.
   2. There are three different vasoactive medications that are used for intracavernosal injection: alprostadil (prostaglandin E1), papaverine, and phentolamine.
   3. In the long term, anywhere from 13% to 60% of patients discontinue.
   4. The side effects include local adverse events such as prolonged erections, priapism (especially with alprostadil preparations), pain, and fibrosis with chronic use.
      a. It is contraindicated in men with a history of hypersensitivity to the drug or who are at risk for priapism (hypercoagulable states, sickle cell disease).

G. Intraurethral treatments

1. Intraurethral alprostadil (Medicated Urethral System for Erection—MUSE) in a semisolid pellet placed into the urethra is a type of local therapy.

2. Approximately 65% of men receiving intraurethral alprostadil respond with an erection adequate for intercourse when tested in the office, but only 50% of those achieve successful coitus at home.

3. The associated side effects are similar to those of the intracavernous injection (see below), except for a markedly reduced incidence of priapism.

H. Vacuum constriction devices

1. In select situations they are a reasonable treatment alternative for patients who do not desire any of the preceding interventions.

2. The majority of men (68%–83%) who use this device report self- and partner satisfaction even though the primary dropout rate is around 60%.

3. The adverse events include pain, numbness, bruising, and altered ejaculation.

I. Surgery

1. Surgical implantation of a penile prosthesis.

2. Surgical treatments invasive; associated with potential complications and generally reserved for treatment-refractory ED

3. Despite cost and invasiveness, penile prosthesis associated with high rates of patient satisfaction (83% men, 70% partner)

4. American Urological Association Panel on Erectile Dysfunction recommends prosthetic implantation as only surgical standard of care for ED

J. Penile revascularization

1. Has largely fallen out of favor, except for patients who have suffered traumatic injury, and still largely considered experimental surgery

   a. Finding a discrete lesion on penile angiography, especially in a young patient with a history of trauma and no other comorbid vascular risks, is the only indication for revascularization therapy.

2. Venous surgery for dysfunctional cavernosal veno-oclusion possible; has long-term success rate of only 40%–50%.

MENTOR TIPS DIGEST

- Both the prevalence and incidence of ED increase with age.
- ED has been independently associated with several risk factors and disease comorbidities.
- Factors contributing to the pathogenesis of ED can be divided into the following six categories: arteriogenic, venogenic, neurogenic, endocrine, psychogenic, and medication-related. More than one category may be involved in an individual patient.
- Men with ED who have no symptoms of vascular disease should be screened for cardiovascular disease and its associated risk factors.
- Androgens contribute to, but are not essential for, normal libido, and their complete role in erectile function remains unclear.
- Symptoms of ED may be the presenting symptom of diabetes in up to 12% of men.
- All men presenting with LUTS/BPH should be evaluated for ED, and all men experiencing sexual dysfunction should be evaluated for LUTS.
- Many cases of ED have some aspect of psychogenic ED involved and are called mixed ED.
- There is a consensus that drugs are implicated in a large percentage of ED cases, but the exact mechanisms are complex.
- Thiazide diuretics and nonselective beta blockers have been implicated most often.
- Smoking cessation may decrease the risk of ED.
- The absence of nocturnal erections is often a crucial piece of information differentiating organic from psychogenic ED.
- Decreased libido may be one of the earliest signs of altered testosterone or prolactin.
- Signs of thyroid, hepatic, hypertensive, cardiovascular, or renal disease should be evaluated.
- Peripheral pulses, reflexes, and visual fields should be examined.
- Assess the external genitalia by palpating the penis to check for fibrotic plaques, suggestive of Peyronie disease; also, perform a testicular examination in search of small testes or reduced secondary sexual characteristics, suggestive of hypogonadism.
- PDE-5 inhibitors are effective across a broad range of etiologies, including vascular disease, DM, LUTS, spinal cord injury, and medication-related ED (specifically SSRIs).

- These drugs are strictly contraindicated for all men receiving any form of nitrate therapy.
- Androgen replacement is associated with increased libido in hypogonadal men but not necessarily with improved erectile ability.
- Androgen therapy is contraindicated in men with androgensensitive cancers
- It is considered wise to perform a digital rectal examination and measure PSA prior to giving androgens.

Resources

Brown JS, Wessells H, Chancellor MB, et al.: Urologic complications of diabetes. Diabetes Care 28:177, 2005.

Burnett AL: The role of nitric oxide in erectile dysfunction: Implications for medical therapy. Journal of Clinical Hypertension (Greenwich) 8:53, 2006.

Chiurlia E, D'Amico R, Ratti C, et al.: Subclinical coronary artery atherosclerosis in patients with erectile dysfunction. Journal of the American College of Cardiology 46:1503, 2005.

Derby CA, Mohr BA, Goldstein I, et al.: Modifiable risk factors and erectile dysfunction: Can lifestyle changes modify risk? Urology 56:302, 2000.

Jackson G, Rosen RC, Kloner RA, et al.: The second Princeton consensus on sexual dysfunction and cardiac risk: New guidelines for sexual medicine. Journal of Sexual Medicine 3:28, 2006.

Kirby M, Jackson G, Simonsen U: Endothelial dysfunction links erectile dysfunction to heart disease. International Journal of Clinical Practice 59: 225,2005.

Lewis RW, Fugl-Meyer KS, Bosch R, et al.: Epidemiology/risk factors of sexual dysfunction. Journal of Sexual Medicine 1:35, 2004.

Lue TF: Physiology of penile erection and pathophysiology of erectile dysfunction. In Wein AJ, Novick AC, Partin AW (eds), et al.: Campbell-Walsh Urology, 9th ed. Philadelphia: WB Saunders, pp. 718–749, 2007.

Lue TF, Broderick GA: Evaluation and nonsurgical management of erectile dysfunction and premature ejaculation. In Wein AJ, Novick AC, Partin AW, et al. (eds): Campbell-Walsh Urology, 9th ed. Philadelphia: WB Saunders, pp. 750–787, 2007.

McVary KT, Carrier S, Wessells H: Smoking and erectile dysfunction: Evidence-based analysis. Journal of Urology 166:1624, 2001.

Wein AJ, Van Arsdalen KN: Drug-induced male sexual dysfunction. Urology Clinics of North America 15:23, 1988.

Chapter Self-Test Questions

Circle the correct answer. After you have responded to the questions, check your answers in Appendix A.

1. How is ED related to age?

a. Often a congenital disorder manifesting at puberty

b. Prevalence increases with age

c. Normal part of aging process

d. Universal in men older than 80 years

2. What occult cause of ED is common and warrants screening in otherwise healthy men?

a. Colorectal cancer

b. Depression

c. Pituitary hypogonadism

d. Occult *Chlamydia* infection

3. What occult cause of ED is common and warrants screening in otherwise healthy men?

a. Colorectal cancer

b. Pituitary hypogonadism

c. Peripheral vascular disease

d. Osteoarthritis

 See the testbank CD for more self-test questions.

ANXIETY AND DEPRESSION

Douglas R. Reifler, MD

I. Background and Epidemiology

A. Anxiety and depression are very common, affecting 11%–35% of primary care patients, and these disorders can be as debilitating as advanced cardiovascular disease. More patients who have mental disorders visit primary care physicians than visit psychiatrists.

> In spite of their ubiquity, mental disorders are either missed or not addressed in 50% of primary care patients who have them.

B. Mental disorders often coexist with somatic disorders, compounding symptoms and even increasing mortality rates.

C. Point prevalences of common mood and anxiety disorders in primary care patients are as follows.

1. Major depressive disorder: 5%–10%
2. Dysthymia: 2%–4%
3. Bipolar disorder: 1%–2%
4. Panic disorder: 3%–7%
5. Generalized anxiety disorder: 5%–8%
6. Obsessive-compulsive disorder: 1%–2%

D. Twice as many women as men have major depression, but this condition is common in both sexes.

II. Diagnostic Approach

A. Any patient who gives clues of mental distress should be asked about symptoms in a routine and nonjudgmental way.

1. Clues can include overt mention of feeling sad, depressed, or anxious; nonverbal signals such as being tearful or agitated; and subtler hints such as an excessive focus on somatic symptoms.

2. Fatigue, insomnia, or headaches can be somatic manifestations of depression or anxiety. In one study, nearly half of patients referred for Holter monitoring to evaluate palpitations had an underlying mental disorder, including almost 20% with panic disorder.

> The greater the number of somatic symptoms, the more likely the presence of a mental disorder—35% of patients with four or five unrelated symptoms have a mental disorder.

B. The Diagnostic Statistical Manual of Mental Disorders, 4th Edition (DSM-IV) criteria for major depressive disorder and panic disorder are listed in Table 17.1.

TABLE 17.1

DSM-IV Diagnostic Criteria for Major Depressive Episode and Panic Disorder*

Diagnosis	Criteria
Major Depressive Episode	At least five of the following nine symptoms for ≥2 weeks: Depressed mood Anhedonia Weight loss or gain Sleep disturbance Psychomotor retardation or agitation Fatigue Guilt or sense of worthlessness Difficulty concentrating or making decisions Suicidal ideation
Panic Disorder	Recurrent unexpected panic attacks, characterized by sudden intense fear peaking within 10 minutes and at least 4 of the following 13 symptoms: Palpitations Sweats Trembling Dyspnea Choking

continued on page 252

TABLE 17.1	DSM-IV Diagnostic Criteria for Major Depressive Episode and Panic Disorder* (continued)
Diagnosis	**Criteria**
	Chest pain
	Nausea
	Dizziness
	Derealization
	Fear of losing control
	Fear of dying
	Paresthesias
	Chills/hot flushes

*For either diagnosis, symptoms must cause functional impairment and must not be due to a medical illness or substance abuse.

Two brief case-finding questions can exclude or identify depression: "During the past month have you often been bothered by: 1) feeling down, depressed, or hopeless? or 2) little interest or pleasure in doing things? A *no* to both questions makes depression unlikely. A *yes* to one or both should prompt questioning about the full list of DSM-IV criteria for depression.

C. Dysthymia describes less intense but more chronic symptoms of depression, including two or more symptoms of major depression lasting at least 2 years.

D. Generalized anxiety disorder reflects chronic excessive worry that impairs function (accompanied by restlessness, fatigue, difficulty concentrating, irritability, muscle tension, or sleep disturbance) without discrete panic episodes.

E. To identify or exclude bipolar disorder, patients who have depression should be asked about manic episodes—periods of excessive elation with grandiosity, decreased need for sleep, excessive talking, flight of ideas, agitation, or uncontrolled pleasure-seeking (sexual, financial, thrill-seeking, etc.).

F. Anxiety disorders can occur alone or can accompany a mood disorder.

G. Panic disorder symptoms are typically intense, do not have a clear precipitant, peak in under 10 minutes, and then subside.

An alternative explanation should be sought for panic-like symptoms that last longer than 10–15 minutes. Half of all patients who have panic disorder have agoraphobia, or fear of being in public. All patients with panic disorder should be asked about agoraphobia because it can be very debilitating.

H. Patients who have mood or anxiety disorders should always be asked about alcohol and drug use, which can cause, mimic, or worsen symptoms.

I. It is also critical to assess suicidal ideation and risk.

J. Thyroid disorder and occasionally pheochromocytoma can cause some similar symptoms and should be considered in select patients.

III. Treatment

A. Choice of therapy

1. Patients diagnosed with major depressive disorder or panic disorder should be offered psychotherapy, medication, or both. Often the choice depends on patient preference and financial or insurance limitations.

 Randomized trials have proved that certain forms of psychotherapy, particularly cognitive-behavioral therapy and interpersonal therapy, are as effective as antidepressant medication for mild-to-moderate major depressive disorder.

2. Psychotherapy may produce more lasting responses than medication produces for panic disorder.

3. Medication has also proved effective, and the benefit can be additive.

4. Patients who have more severe symptoms should receive both medication and psychotherapy.

5. If impairment is extreme or there is an active risk of suicide or homicide, urgent hospitalization is required.

6. Dysthymia and generalized anxiety disorder are, by definition, more chronic conditions.

7. For some patients, symptoms respond to the medications used for major depression and panic disorder.

8. Certain medications—particularly selective serotonin reuptake inhibitors (SSRIs)—can work for all of these conditions.

9. Patients who have bipolar disorder or obsessive-compulsive disorder should be referred to a psychiatrist for treatment.

B. Medication

1. A variety of effective medications for mood and anxiety disorders can be used in primary care settings (Tables 17.2 and 17.3).

2. The tricyclic antidepressants (TCAs), such as imipramine, desipramine, and nortriptyline, were the most frequently used category several years ago.

TABLE 17.2

Antidepressant Medication Side-Effect Profiles

Medication	Sedation	Postural Hypotension	Sexual Function	Other
SSRIs (citalopram, fluoxetine, paroxetine, sertraline)	Variable (paroxetine > fluoxetine)	→ (except paroxetine ↑)	↓	↑ Anxiety early, headaches, GI upset, ↑↓weight
TCAs (imipramine, nortriptyline, desipramine, others)	↑	↑↑	→	Toxic in overdose, mild ↑ weight, inexpensive
Bupropion	→	→ or ↓	→	↓ Seizure threshold, ↓ smoking urge
Mirtazapine	↑↑	→	→	↑ Weight
Nefazodone	↑↑	↑	→	Many drug interactions
Trazodone	↑↑	↑	Priapism	Mild ↑weight
Venlafaxine	→	↑	↓	Hypertension

Key:
→ little to no change
↑ increase
↓ decrease

TABLE 17.3 Common Medications for Anxiety		
Medication	Advantages	Disadvantages
Benzodiazepines (alprazolam, lorazepam, clonazepam, others)	Immediate-acting, can be used as needed if addiction and suicide risks are low	Sedation, potential addiction, suicide risk
SSRIs	Effective long-term, low suicide risk	↑ (Anxiety early, delayed onset of action
Buspirone	Effective long-term, low suicide risk	Delayed onset of action

The SSRIs are now first-line medications for many conditions because of their simplicity of dosing, relatively fewer side effects, and lower toxicity, particularly in overdose.

3. TCAs are effective for depression, and imipramine has proved effective for panic disorder. TCAs have the advantage of being less expensive.

4. The choice of medication for depression is often based on side-effect profiles, because all antidepressant medications work in about 70% of patients who use them (see Table 17.2).

5. SSRIs as a group have fewer anticholinergic side effects (dry mouth, orthostatic hypotension, sedation) than TCAs.

6. Although SSRIs are generally well tolerated, they can cause gastrointestinal (GI) disturbances, headache, and sexual dysfunction. Their sedating or activating effects are not fully predictable, but paroxetine tends to be the most sedating and fluoxetine the most activating of the SSRIs.

7. Various other antidepressants are also available (see Table 17.2).

8. Before prescribing any antidepressant, a primary physician should become familiar with the side-effect profiles and contraindications.

Bupropion, nefazodone, and mirtazapine cause less sexual dysfunction than SSRIs and can be good alternatives when patients do not tolerate SSRIs for this reason.

9. The antidepressant medications typically require 4–6 weeks to achieve their full beneficial effect.
10. SSRIs are also effective for anxiety disorders, particularly panic disorder, although they can worsen anxiety symptoms in the first 2 weeks.
11. When using SSRIs for panic disorder or depression accompanied by anxiety, the lowest possible dose (10 mg of citalopram, 5 mg of fluoxetine or paroxetine, 12.5 mg of sertraline) should be used at the start.

> Anxiety induced by starting an SSRI can be avoided by concurrent regular doses of a benzodiazepine for a limited time (e.g., alprazolam 0.25 mg three times a day for the first 14 days).

12. Benzodiazepines alone are also effective for anxiety disorders, particularly when medication is needed only intermittently. Because these medications are addictive and are potentially fatal in overdose, the individual patient's risk of addiction and suicide must be weighed against the medication's potential benefit (see Table 17.3).
13. Slow-to-intermediate-onset, long-acting benzodiazepines such as clonazepam tend to have lower addiction risk than shorter-acting ones such as alprazolam or lorazepam. Buspirone is an alternative long-term antianxiety treatment that takes 4–6 weeks to achieve its full effect.

IV. Follow-Up and Referral

A. Patients treated in primary care settings for depression and panic disorder should be seen in follow-up soon after initiation of therapy. They should return at least once in the first 4–6 weeks of therapy—sooner if their symptoms are more severe—to gauge the initial effect of medication and make any necessary adjustments.

> Patients starting an SSRI, TCA, or other antidepressant should be cautioned not to give up on a medication too soon before it has had 4–6 weeks to reach its full beneficial effect.

B. If depression or panic attacks abate with medication, treatment should continue for at least 6 months before an attempt is made to stop the medication.

 Patients whose medication is effective should be cautioned not to stop too soon because their symptoms will return. If symptoms remain in remission for 6–9 months, medication can be gradually tapered off.

C. If an initial antidepressant medication is not working, it is reasonable to try switching medicines, again basing the choice on side-effect profiles. If symptoms do not respond to two treatment attempts, psychiatric referral is warranted. Some patients require two or more agents simultaneously, and psychiatrists are better equipped to manage more complex regimens. Other indications for referral include severe or worsening symptoms.

D. Patients who have multiple recurrences of major depression, panic disorder, or the more chronic conditions of dysthymia and generalized anxiety disorder often require long-term medication to maintain adequate symptom control.

MENTOR TIPS DIGEST

- In spite of their ubiquity, mental disorders are either missed or not addressed in 50% of primary care patients who have them.
- The greater the number of somatic symptoms, the more likely the presence of a mental disorder—35% of patients with four or five unrelated symptoms have a mental disorder.
- Two brief case-finding questions can exclude or identify depres-sion: "During the past month have you often been bothered by: 1) feeling down, depressed, or hopeless? or 2) little interest or pleasure in doing things? A *no* to both questions makes depression unlikely. A *yes* to one or both should prompt questioning about the full list of DSM-IV criteria for depression.
- An alternative explanation should be sought for panic-like symptoms that last longer than 10–15 minutes. Half of patients who have panic disorder have agoraphobia, or fear of being in public. All patients with panic disorder should be asked about agoraphobia because it can be very debilitating.

- Randomized trials have proved that certain forms of psychotherapy, particularly cognitive-behavioral therapy and interpersonal therapy, are as effective as antidepressant medication for mild-to-moderate major depressive disorder.
- The SSRIs are now first-line medications for many conditions because of their simplicity of dosing, relatively fewer side effects, and lower toxicity, particularly in overdose.
- Bupropion, nefazodone, and mirtazapine cause less sexual dysfunction than SSRIs and can be good alternatives when patients do not tolerate SSRIs for this reason.
- Anxiety induced by starting an SSRI can be avoided by concurrent regular doses of a benzodiazepine for a limited time (e.g., alprazolam 0.25 mg three times a day for the first 14 days).
- Patients starting an SSRI, TCA, or other antidepressant should be cautioned not to give up on a medication too soon before it has had 4–6 weeks to reach its full beneficial effect.
- Patients whose medication is effective should be cautioned not to stop too soon because their symptoms will return. If symptoms remain in remission for 6–9 months, medication can be gradually tapered off.

Resources

American Psychiatric Association. Diagnostic and statistical manual of mental disorders, fourth edition. American Psychiatric Association, Washington DC, 1994.
  This reference defines current psychiatric diagnoses. An alternative primary care version of the manual published in 1995 recognizes the more somatic presentations of mental disorders in primary care settings.
Depression Guideline Panel. Depression in primary care: volume 1: Detection and diagnosis. Clinical Practice Guideline, Number 5. Rockville, Md. US Department of Health and Human Services, Public Health Service, Agency for Health Care Policy and Research. AHCPR Publication No. 93-0550. April 1993.
Depression Guideline Panel. Depression in primary care: volume 2: Treatment of major depression. Clinical Practice Guideline, Number 5. Rockville, Md. US Department of Health and Human Services, Public Health Service, Agency for Health Care Policy and Research. AHCPR Publication No. 93-0551. April 1993.

These companion books established federal (Agency for Health Care Policy and Research) clinical guidelines for the diagnosis and treatment of depression in primary care settings.

Spitzer RL, Williams JBV, Kroenke K, et al.: PRIME MD: Primary care evaluation of mental disorders. Pfizer, 1995.

Chapter Self-Test Questions

Circle the correct answer. After you have responded to the questions, check your answers in Appendix A.

1. How common are depression and anxiety disorders in patients seen in primary care practice?

   a. 1 in 100

   b. 1 in 20

   c. 1 in 5

   d. More than half

2. Concerning mental illness, which is most true?

   a. Most patients see psychiatrists.

   b. Relatively few patients with mental disorders ever see a primary care physician.

   c. Most patients with mental illnesses are not recognized by primary care physicians.

   d. All patients with mental illness should have psychiatric referral.

3. Which mental illness diagnosis is most common in primary care practice?

   a. Obsessive-compulsive disorder

   b. Bipolar disorder

   c. Dysthymia

   d. Major depression

See the testbank CD for more self-test questions.

18

SOMATIZATION

Gary J. Martin, MD

I. Pathophysiology

A. *Somatization* is a term that in its broadest sense applies commonly to many people. It is a phenomenon in which unexplained or amplified physical symptoms may be related to psychological factors.

 The process of somatization is commonly involved in many "difficult" patients.

B. Somatoform symptoms have the following features.

1. At one end of the spectrum are ordinary patients who present with a symptom but who appear to worry about it more or focus on it excessively in the setting of additional stressors. These patients are not malingering, and this is different from the rare patient with factitious illness. However, positive reinforcement including a "sick role" can be a contributing factor.

 The process of somatization is very common in patients and in milder forms may just be related to situational stress and not major psychological problems.

2. The amplification of normal bodily processes appears to be part of the pathophysiology. Examples of this amplification might include heightened sensitivity to colon dilatation in patients with irritable bowel syndrome or increased sensitivity to pain in patients with fibromyalgia.

3. Somatic complaints may be an alternative that is more acceptable for a patient to seek help for rather than present for the psychological stressors.

> ◆ A *somatoform symptom* can be defined as a symptom
> that does not have an adequate (based on the physician's clinical judgment) physical explanation to explain its severity and associated disability.

4. Primary care physician's gestalt about a symptom being medically unexplained is quite good. Few patients with symptoms judged to be somatoform are later found to have occult serious physical disorders at follow-up.

5. Childhood illness or illnesses in the family and abuse can also be contributing factors. Family, cultural, and religious norms for expressing pain or emotion may be issues. Major loss and inner conflicts can contribute.

C. Somatoform disorders

1. *Somatoform disorder* is a much more restrictive term (versus *somatoform symptom*) that applies to a much smaller number of patients at one end of the spectrum. Only focusing on the uncommon somatoform disorder misses the much larger important group of patients with an element of somatization who have functional impairment, psychiatric comorbidity, difficult doctor-patient relationships, and increased health-care utilization.

II. Signs and Symptoms

A. Box 18.1 lists verbal and nonverbal clues that should attract the clinician's attention and raise the possibility of somatization as a contributing factor. Many times, patients with somatization are difficult historians. They may be vague and tangential in their answers.

B. These patients may have a "positive review of systems," have dramatic descriptions of their symptoms, may have seen multiple doctors already for their symptoms, and may have failed many therapeutic trials.

C. None of the features in Box 18.1 makes a diagnosis of somatization, but they should raise the clinician's suspicions and lead to additional explorations of the possibility of a psychological component to the patient's problems.

D. Many times these patients will appear more preoccupied with their symptoms than the clinician would expect.

E. At the far end of the spectrum, patients may have seen multiple specialists or had multiple surgeries or be on disability for their problems.

BOX 18.1

Verbal and Nonverbal Clues of Somatoform Symptoms

Verbal

- Vague history
- Multiple prior physicians
- Multiple prior surgeries
- Multiple allergies
- "Positive" review of systems
- Dramatic, emotionally charged description of symptoms
- Excessive research or paper recordings by patient (some of this is commonly done in the current Internet-connected society)
- Patient's concern out of proportion to what you would expect
- Patient's concern much less than what you would expect

Nonverbal

- Poor eye contact
- Sighing
- Depressed or anxious affect
- Who comes with patient to visit
- Inconsistent examination

III. History and Physical Examination

A. Box 18.2 lists questions that are particularly helpful in eliciting additional useful information in the setting of possible somatization.

1. Past medical history including previous physicians' evaluations and family history can be useful.

2. Social history is particularly helpful, including how patients spend their day, who they live with, and how things are going at work and home.

3. Patients who have a relative short history of symptoms may be more open to the possibility of psychological contributions. For these patients, more direct questions about psychosocial stressors can be effective.

4. For patients who have a more chronic presentation and may have already seen other providers for their problems, many of these questions are worked into the social history. This gives patients the perception that they are not being targeted, that the information is a routine part of the social history. For example,

BOX 18.2

Useful Questions for Patients With Suspected Somatoform Symptoms

1. What is going on at home?
2. What new things are coming up in your life?
3. What are you concerned may be the problem?
4. How is this affecting your life?
5. Would you walk me through a typical day?
6. How were things in your family when you were growing up?
7. If there is a window of opportunity: "Things were pretty bad then (pause)"
8. Are there any experiences that you haven't discussed yet that were difficult?
9. It is not uncommon for people to be emotionally, sexually, or physically victimized at some time in their life. Has this ever happened to you?
10. How do you spend your spare time?
11. How do you keep busy?
12. Anniversary dates (for major loss)?

"What do you do for a living?" "Do you smoke? Drink?" "How are things at work?" "Who do you live with?" can all be a routine part of the social history.

5. Time correlations can be helpful. For example, do the patient's symptoms disappear when the patient is on vacation or on weekends? Is there some correlation with a major event like the death of a family member; anniversary of an event?

IV. Differential Diagnosis

A. The process of somatization can occur in many different psychiatric diseases, including major affective disorders such as depression, panic disorder, and even schizophrenia and dementia.

B. At times, patients may be diagnosed with a specific psychiatric condition. For example, a patient might meet the criteria for depression or panic attacks. Disturbed sleep and loss of enjoyment are the two most sensitive questions for detecting depression.

C. Box 18.3 lists the diagnostic criteria for somatoform disorders. Many patients, however, will not be this severe or as well differentiated.

D. The broad collection of patients with unexplained somatic symptoms is quite common and may represent up to 30% to 50% of

BOX 18.3
Diagnostic Criteria for Somatization Disorder

A history of many physical complaints beginning before age 30 that occur over a period of several years and that result in treatment being sought or significant impairment in social, occupational, or other important areas of functioning.

Each of the following criteria must be met, with individual symptoms occurring at any time during the course of the disturbance:
- *Four pain symptoms:* a history of pain related to at least four different sites or functions (e.g., head, abdomen, back, joints, extremities, chest, rectum, during menstruation, during sexual intercourse, or during urination)
- *Two gastrointestinal symptoms:* a history of at least two gastrointestinal symptoms other than pain (e.g., nausea, bloating, vomiting other than during pregnancy, diarrhea, or intolerance of several different foods)
- *One sexual symptom:* a history of at least one sexual or reproductive symptom other than pain (e.g., sexual indifference, erectile or ejaculatory dysfunction, irregular menses, excessive menstrual bleeding, vomiting throughout pregnancy)
- *One pseudo-neurologic symptom:* a history of at least one symptom or deficit suggesting a neurologic condition not limited to pain (conversion symptoms such as impaired coordination or balance, paralysis or localized weakness, difficulty swallowing or lump in throat, aphonia, urinary retention, hallucinations, loss of touch or pain sensation, double vision, blindness, deafness, seizures, dissociative symptoms such as amnesia, or loss of consciousness other than fainting)

Either of the following:
- After appropriate investigation, none of the symptoms can be fully explained by a known general medical condition or the direct effects of a substance (e.g., a drug of abuse, a medication).
- When there is a related general medical condition, the physical complaints or resulting social or occupational impairment are in excess of what would be expected from the history, physical examination, or laboratory findings.
- The symptoms are not intentionally produced or feigned (as in Factitious Disorder or Malingering).

Adapted from American Psychiatric Association. Task Force on DSM-IV. Diagnostic and Statistical Manual of Mental Disorders, 4th ed. Text Revision (DSM-IV-TR). Washington, DC: American Psychiatric Association, 2000.

physician encounters in the primary care setting. It is by no means limited to primary care, and every specialty has examples of this problem. Milder cases occur that do not meet the DSM criteria but that do have significant impairment, difficult relationships, and increased utilization. These can be suspected when patients have ≥3 somatoform symptoms (as defined before) from a list of 15 symptoms: stomach pain, back pain, headache, chest pain, dizziness, faintness, palpitations, shortness of breath, bowel complaints (constipation or diarrhea), dyspeptic symptoms (nausea, gas, or indigestion), fatigue, trouble sleeping, pain in the joints or limbs, menstrual pain or problems, and pain or problems during sexual intercourse.

E. Occasionally patients with certain personality traits and personality disorders may present with somatic complaints.

V. Laboratory Evaluations

A. As a general rule, laboratory evaluations are best used sparingly in this patient population.

B. Classic biomedical diseases can appear in these patients; be careful not to reinforce the "sick role," and avoid testing that leads to false positives and increased anxiety.

C. Questionnaires that screen for anxiety disorders and depression can be used in the office for a subset of these patients, and more formal psychometric testing may be indicated in a small subset.

VI. Management

A. Physicians have learned over the years that relatively frequent visits with follow-up are most helpful for patients with chronic somatization.

1. Visits may need to be as frequent as a week apart initially. This is preferable to having a 3-month return visit scheduled, only to have the patient present to the emergency room or call in the middle of the night with additional symptoms.

Although these patients are not malingering, some of them have noted that a symptom is a "ticket" for an office visit and by scheduling frequent visits a patient does not need to focus on other problems in order to be able to see the physician.

2. Patients' responses to reassurance vary.

  a. Positive response:

 A subset of patients can benefit from reassurance and explanation.

    i. An explanation about the autonomic nervous system and how functional disorders can cause symptoms can be helpful to some patients. The clinician does not dismiss the problem but can explain it as a heightened sensitivity to bodily sensations.

  b. Negative response:

 There is, however, a subset of patients, particularly those with a more chronic presentation, who will respond negatively to reassurance, particularly if given prematurely. These patients need a different approach.

    i. These patients need to understand that you are going to evaluate their problems thoroughly and thoughtfully and without prejudice.

    ii. Typically, after several visits, some rapport will be developed with such patients.

    iii. Two related approaches can then be tried.

      (1) Some psychiatrists recommend offering the patient help with coping with their illness. For example, the patient presents with, e.g., chronic abdominal pain, and in the course of several visits the physician determines that the problem is associated with a great deal of distress in the patient's life, which is interfering with social activities and work. The physician at that point can recommend that the patient return soon again to continue to evaluate the disorder. The physician would also like the patient to get help *coping with* the distress that the problem is causing. The key here is that you are *not* trying to make the point that stress is causing the problem but that the problem is associated with a great deal of disruption in the patient's life. Many patients are willing

to accept seeing a psychiatrist or other mental health worker under those circumstances, particularly if they do not believe that the primary care clinician is dismissing them.

(2) The other approach is that, in the course of several visits and collecting psychosocial information, the clinician may identify the presenting problem but notes that the patient may also have some stress, not drawing any particular relationship between the two. Occasionally, some patients are willing to see a mental health worker for help with the stress in their life without any attempt on the physician's part to link their somatic complaints to their stress. This is particularly likely to happen if the physician keeps close follow-up on the presenting problem so the patient does not feel dismissed.

iv. Many patients over time resolve their somatic problems or greatly minimize them if they are able to connect with a mental health worker using either of the two preceding approaches.

v. Going forward, one of several paths may be best, depending on the individual patient:

(1) Some patients have a specific diagnosis (for example, depression, panic attacks, or generalized anxiety disorder), and a therapeutic trial can be instituted.

(2) Cognitive behavioral therapy may be an option for some patients.

(3) Thorough primary care may continue to be the best option.

> For the rare true somatoform disorder patient, a long-term relationship with a caring physician, including frequent office visits and physical examinations, can be the most cost-effective solution.

(4) The preceding options are preferable to referring the patient to multiple different specialists, all of whom may generate tests and false positives and reinforce a sick role or precipitate complications from downstream testing.

MENTOR TIPS DIGEST

- The process of somatization is commonly involved in many "difficult" patients.
- The process of somatization is very common in patients and in milder forms may just be related to situational stress and not major psychological problems.
- A *somatoform symptom* can be defined as a symptom that does not have an adequate (based on the physician's clinical judgment) physical explanation to explain its severity and associated disability.
- Although these patients are not malingering, some of them have noted that a symptom is a "ticket" for an office visit and by scheduling frequent visits a patient does not need to focus on other problems in order to be able to see the physician.
- A subset of patients can benefit from reassurance and explanation.
- There are, however, a subset of patients, particularly those with a more chronic presentation, that will respond negatively to reassurance, particularly if done prematurely. These patients need a different approach. (Discussed in text.)
- For the rare true somatoform disorder patient, a long-term relationship with a caring physician, including frequent office visits and physical examinations, can be the most cost-effective solution.

Resources

American Psychiatric Association. Task Force on DSM-IV. Diagnostic and Statistical Manual of Mental Disorders, 4th ed, Text Revision (DSM-IV-TR). Washington, DC: American Psychiatric Association, 2000.

Goldberg RJ, Novack DH, Gask L. The recognition and management of somatization: What is needed in primary care training. Psychosomatics 1992;3: 55–61.
Very useful management strategies.

Kroenke K, Spitzer RL, DeGruy FV, et al. A symptom checklist to screen for somatoform disorders in primary care. Psychosomatics 1998;39:263–272.
Useful checklist of symptoms for the more common, less advanced patient.

See the testbank CD for self-test questions.

DIAGNOSIS AND MANAGEMENT OF COMMON CHRONIC ILLNESSES

CONGESTIVE HEART FAILURE

19

Gary J. Martin, MD

I. Overview

A. In the past decade, congestive heart failure (CHF) has become much more prominent. There is greater appreciation of its significance in terms of frequency (particularly with aging of population) and potential severity (given that its 5-year survival can be worse than that of many malignancies).

B. CHF has become one of the most frequent reasons for admission to the hospital, and major disease management programs have been developed to optimize outpatient care to minimize admissions.

   C. Another underappreciated point is that more than half of deaths
      related to heart failure come from asymptomatic patients suffering
      sudden cardiac death.
   D. This highlights the need for earlier diagnosis and treatment.
      Fortunately, in the past few years, there has been a growing num-
      ber of carefully done randomized trials to provide better data for
      treatment of this disease.

II. Approach to CHF Patient

   A. Diagnosis of CHF is made based on a constellation of signs and
      symptoms, including dyspnea on exertion, fatigue, jugular venous
      distention, inspiratory rales, a third heart sound, hepatojugular
      reflux, and edema.
      1. Initial imaging and laboratory tests
         a. Chest x-ray evidence of pulmonary congestion or increased
            heart size is often helpful.
         b. Electrocardiogram may give clues to etiology, showing
            Q waves, left ventricular hypertrophy (LVH), or left bundle
            branch block.
   B. Two key questions must be asked for every CHF patient.

> Always ask yourself: (1) What is the underlying cause of
> the patient's CHF? and (2) What precipitated the current
> exacerbation?

      1. Understanding underlying cause (Box 19.1) can be very important
         in terms of treatment. Coronary artery disease and hypertension
         are the most common causes of underlying CHF. Also important
         are identifying and treating less common etiologies such as
         valvular heart disease or pericardial disease. Symptomatic
         treatment of CHF alone is not appropriate.

BOX 19.1

What Is Underlying Cause of Patient's CHF?

- Hypertension
- Coronary artery disease
- Valvular heart disease
- Cardiomyopathy
- Pericardial disease

2. Box 19.2 lists common causes for exacerbation of CHF. Attention to these can help minimize future exacerbations.
3. Box 19.3 lists clues in the history and physical examination that can be particularly helpful with regard to these two key questions.
4. The single most useful diagnostic test for patients with CHF is the echocardiogram. In general, almost all patients warrant at least one echocardiogram in the evaluation of their condition. An echocardiogram can help sort out systolic from diastolic dysfunction, which has major ramifications for treatment. It can help identify underlying etiology, particularly wall-motion abnormalities suggestive of coronary disease and valvular abnormalities that may not always be detected by auscultation.

III. Management
A. Management can be divided into two broad categories.
 1. *General treatment* to be considered for all patients with CHF
 2. *Etiology-specific treatment*
B. Box 19.4 lists the most validated treatments for CHF.

BOX 19.2

Common Causes of CHF Exacerbation

Factors That Increase Demand on Heart

Increased salt intake or physical activity
Infection, surgery, fluid therapy, transfusions
Pulmonary embolism
Anemia
Hyperthyroidism
Salt- and water-retaining medications (e.g., nonsteroidal anti-inflammatory drugs, steroids)
Pregnancy

Factors That Decrease Cardiac Output

Discontinuation of medications (digoxin, angiotensin-converting enzyme inhibitor [ACEI])
Arrhythmia (e.g., atrial fibrillation, heart block)
Myocarditis or infarction
Toxic substances (e.g., ethyl alcohol [ETOH])
Thiamine deficiency

BOX 19.3

Important Clues About CHF in History and Physical Examination

These clues can help you answer the two key questions:
(1) What is the underlying cause of this patient's CHF (2) What precipitated the current exacerbation?

History of angina or myocardial infarction

History of rheumatic fever, or a recent flu-like illness

History of TB, malignancy (pericardial disease)

Recent pregnancy

Family history of CHF

Dietary indiscretion, lapses in medication, or use of new salt-retaining medications

Evidence of valvular heart on examination (especially aortic or mitral stenosis or regurgitation)

Displaced point of maximum impulse (PMI) suggesting a dilated heart

C. General treatment guidelines follow.

1. *Diuretics* can be the mainstay of symptomatic treatment by relieving pulmonary congestion and edema, particularly when the patient first presents.

2. *Digoxin* has proved to be helpful in symptomatic patients in reducing both symptoms and hospitalizations, which have no overall effect on mortality. For asymptomatic patients with systolic dysfunction it is probably not beneficial.

3. *ACEIs* have become a mainstay in treatment of CHF because of their proven value in reducing symptoms and improving survival. Mortality benefits of over 20% have been well

BOX 19.4

Most Validated CHF Treatments

ACEIs

Beta blockers

Aldosterone antagonists

Revascularization for selected patients with coronary artery disease (CAD)

Implantable defibrillator and cardiac resynchronization in selected patients documented. Aspirin may blunt some of the benefit of ACEI via effect on kinins and probably should be reserved only for patients with known CAD. In long-term trials, ACEI benefits extend to even asymptomatic patients with ejection fractions lower than 40%. Whether *angiotension receptor blockers (ARBs)* are equally efficacious is somewhat controversial, but they are a reasonable substitute for the patient who cannot tolerate ACEI. Data suggest ARBs may have additive benefit on top of ACEIs. *Hydralazine* and *nitrates* may also have additive benefit in the African-American population.

4. In recent years use of *beta blockers* has emerged. In the past these drugs were avoided in patients with CHF because of their negative inotropic effect, but they have been shown to help stop the downhill spiral of CHF pathophysiology involving elevated levels of catecholamines and increased afterload. In this setting, these drugs must be introduced cautiously at doses 5%–10% of ultimate target dose to which they will be titrated. They are initiated when the patient is otherwise optimized and compensated. The majority of data exist for use of metoprolol and carvedilol in this setting. Surprisingly for both ACEIs and beta blockers, ejection fraction may significantly improve over time after these drugs have been instituted. Mortality benefits of beta blockers may also be related to their potential effect at raising the threshold for ventricular fibrillation and preventing sudden cardiac death.

5. *Spironolactone* has recently been added to the multidrug approach to CHF patients. A large randomized trial showed that, in addition to standard therapy, the drug was able to further reduce mortality by approximately 27%. A dose of 25 mg per day was used in this study (RALES study). The mechanism of this benefit is probably less related to its effect on potassium and sodium excretion and more related to decreasing progressive fibrosis.

 ACEIs, beta blockers, and spironolactone have been documented to improve mortality in patients with CHF.

6. *Salt restriction,* using a no-salt-added diet, is a useful adjunct to treatment.

7. *Cardiac rehabilitation* including a carefully tailored exercise program may also benefit CHF patients.

8. If the patient has *atrial fibrillation,* cardioversion should ideally be considered, but if this is not possible, rate control and efforts to prevent embolic disease are important. Rate response in atrial fibrillation may appear to be controlled at rest but frequently is poorly controlled with exercise when digoxin alone is used. Beta blockers or alternatively low doses of verapamil and diltiazem may be necessary to control heart rate to a reasonable level with activity. Warfarin is of proven value in decreasing cardioembolic events in patients with atrial fibrillation, particularly in the setting of CHF. Aspirin at 325 mg per day may be an acceptable alternative of lesser value in patients who cannot take warfarin safely. Tachycardia can contribute to systolic dysfunction, and ejection fraction can improve dramatically over time with cardioversion.

D. Disease-specific treatment guidelines follow.

1. If a patient is found to have CAD contributing to CHF, some type of stratification of risk is appropriate, utilizing treadmill testing with or without additional imaging such as stress echo or perfusion studies including magnetic resonance imaging (MRI) techniques. Pharmacologic stress testing with adenosine or dobutamine may also be necessary. These studies can help select which patients would benefit most from angiography, although some clinicians would recommend angiography in all patients with CHF when CAD is suspected as a significant contributor.

2. *Nitrates and beta blockers* are useful in most patients with symptomatic coronary disease.

3. *Aspirin* is generally indicated in all such patients too, although aspirin may partially reduce the benefits of *ACEIs* through its effect on kinins. Therefore, aspirin should be limited to patients with CAD or some patients with atrial fibrillation in the setting of CHF.

4. *Aggressive lipid therapy* has been documented to have major benefits in the setting of CAD (see also Chapter 24). Of course, *other risk factor modifications,* including *cessation of smoking,* can be critical success factors in these patients.

5. *Optimal control of hypertension* can frequently benefit patients with CHF and even lead to some reversal of left ventricular hypertrophy (LVH) and diastolic dysfunction.

6. When valvular heart disease contributes to CHF, an experienced cardiologist can be particularly helpful. Mild-to-moderate mitral regurgitation can often be secondary to left ventricular dilatation and may not be the primary problem in some patients. Timing of *valve surgery* is a difficult decision, although in general patients with symptoms of CHF related to their valve problem should be considered for surgery. Increasing skill with repair of regurgitant valves has lowered the threshold for surgical intervention in some patients as compared with replacement with prosthetic devices. *Endocarditis prophylaxis* must also always be remembered in this patient population.

7. With regard to cardiomyopathies, addressing underlying etiology may be helpful. Many patients with alcohol-induced cardiomyopathy benefit from *alcohol abstinence.* In patients with active myocarditis, selected patients may benefit from aggressive *anti-inflammatory therapy* anecdotally, although this has been difficult to demonstrate in controlled trials. For patients with end-stage heart failure, *heart transplantation* remains a potentially life-saving intervention in appropriately selected patients.

8. For patients with advanced ventricular arrhythmias, particularly those with symptoms, treatment with *implantable defibrillator* or carefully chosen *antiarrhythmic therapy* such as amiodarone may also be beneficial. *Cardiac resynchronization therapy* can also help symptoms and survival in certain subsets of patients.

MENTOR TIPS DIGEST

- Always ask yourself: (1) What is the underlying cause of the patient's CHF? and (2) What precipitated the current exacerbation?
- ACEIs, beta blockers, and spironolactone have been documented to improve mortality in patients with CHF.

Resources

American College of Cardiology Foundation, American Heart Association. Diagnosis and management of chronic heart failure in the adult [booklet].

Bristow MR, Saxon LA, Boehmer J, et al. Cardiac-resynchronization therapy with or without an implantable defibrillator in advanced chronic heart failure. New England Journal of Medicine 350:2140–2150, 2004.

Kadish A, Dyer A, Daubert JP, et al. Prophylactic defibrillator implantation in patients with nonischemic dilated cardiomyopathy. New England Journal of Medicine 350:2151–2158, 2004

Chapter Self-Test Questions

Circle the correct answer. After you have responded to the questions, check your answers in Appendix A.

1. What is the most frequently occurring proximate cause of death in persons with heart failure?

   a. Lethal arrhythmia

   b. Embolic stroke

   c. Pulmonary edema

   d. End-stage kidney disease

2. Heart failure often causes which of these electrocardiogram abnormalities?

   a. High peaked T waves

   b. Mobitz type 1 second-degree AV block

   c. Mobitz type 2 second-degree heart block

   d. Left bundle branch block

3. A 74-year-old woman has long-standing hypertension that is well controlled with nifedipine. She complains of gradual onset difficulty breathing when lying flat in bed. She notes ankle swelling in the morning. On examination, pulse is 90 and regular; blood pressure is 120/70. There are crackles only in the lung bases and a third heart sound. Electrocardiogram shows regular sinus rhythm, left ventricular

hypertrophy, and no ischemic changes. Serum electrolytes and creatinine levels are normal. What is the initial most appropriate next step?

a. Begin digoxin 0.125 mg daily, and observe over a few weeks.

b. Begin furosemide 20 mg daily, and observe over a few weeks.

c. Discontinue nifedipine, and observe over a few weeks.

d. Order transthoracic echocardiogram.

See the testbank CD for more self-test questions.

20

CHAPTER

HYPERTENSION

David B. Neely, MD

I. Overview

A. Hypertension (HTN) is common.

> Approximately 26% of adults in the United States have HTN.

B. Unfortunately, fewer than 50% of these patients have their blood pressure (BP) controlled adequately.

C. HTN is a risk factor for coronary heart disease (CHD), stroke, renal insufficiency, renal failure, and other types of vascular disease.

II. Benefits of Treatment

A. Stroke risk reduction

> A reduction of 5 mm Hg diastolic blood pressure (DBP) is associated with a 35%–40% decreased incidence of stroke.

    1. The benefits occur quickly; therefore, there is no upper age limit for treatment.

B. CHD amelioration

    1. In the last 50 years, cardiovascular mortality has decreased significantly, in part secondary to better control of HTN.

    2. The risk of myocardial infarction (MI) is reduced 20%–25% with 5 mm Hg reduction in DBP.

C. Decrease in other risks

> The risks of heart failure and renal disease are clearly reduced with lower BP; however, the major mortality benefits of BP treatment depend on the reduction of CHD and stroke.

III. Definition

A. The definition of HTN is systolic BP (SBP) greater than 140 and diastolic BP (DBP) greater than 90.

 The Joint National Committee (JNC) on Prevention, Detection, Evaluation, and Treatment of High Blood Pressure has released a new classification scheme for HTN (Table 20.1).

 Management is determined by the highest category, either systolic or diastolic.

 According to the JNC, 115/75 is the optimal BP as defined as the BP that predicts the longest life.

1. The risk of CHD doubles with each increment of 20/10 above this goal.

B. Patients should be treated to a goal less than 140/90; patients with diabetes or renal disease should be treated to a goal of less than 130/80.

IV. Etiology

A. First distinction: primary (essential) HTN versus secondary HTN.

 95% of patients with high BP have primary HTN.

B. 5% of patients with high BP may have secondary HTN.

1. The incidence of a secondary cause of HTN may be increased in:

a. Patients younger than 35 without a family history of HTN.

TABLE 20.1 BP Classification Scheme		
BP Classification	**SBP**	**DBP**
Normal	<120	<80
Prehypertension	120–139	80–89
Stage I	140–159	90–99
Stage II	>160	>100

b. Patients whose HTN has a sudden onset or is severely elevated.

c. Patients whose HTN is resistant to three medications, one of which is a diuretic.

2. Secondary causes:

a. Parenchymal renal disease

 The most common cause of secondary HTN is parenchymal renal disease.

  i. This occurs in about 3% of all patients with hypertension and is easily ruled out by a serum creatinine.

b. Renovascular HTN is next most common form

  i. Fibromuscular dysplasia is common in young women.

  ii. Atherosclerotic renovascular disease is often found in older patients with significant cardiovascular disease (CVD).

c. Primary hyperaldosteronism

  i. Classically the patient has a low potassium level (<3.5), although in many patients the potassium could be at a low normal level.

  ii. The most common cause is bilateral adrenal hyperplasia.

  iii. Primary hyperaldosteronism is treated medically.

  iv. Plasma renin activity (PRA) and plasma aldosterone activity (PAC) and the ratio of PRA to PAC can be a helpful diagnostic screening test.

d. Pheochromocytoma

  i. This is rare.

  ii. The patient classically has paroxysm of HTN, sweats, and palpitations.

  iii. However, over half of patients with pheochromocytoma present with a steady elevation of BP.

  iv. A 24-hour urine collection for metanephrines is a simple screen.

e. Cushing disease

  i. This is a rare cause of secondary HTN.

  ii. Patients classically are obese with stria.

  iii. A 24-hour urine collection for cortisol is a good screen.

f. Sleep apnea newly recognized cause of secondary HTN

  i. Patients are often obese with daytime somnolence.

V. BP Measurement

A. BP can easily fluctuate 10–20 mm Hg throughout the day; the higher the BP, the greater the fluctuation.

    1. The BP readings of the nurse, student, and attending physician may vary.

B. Accurate BP measurement is key.

    1. The patient should be seated quietly for at least 5 minutes.

    2. The patient's feet should be flat on the floor, and the arm should be supported at the level of the heart.

    3. An appropriately-sized cuff should be used.

 The most frequent mistake in BP measurement is using a cuff that is too small.

    4. Two measurements should be made after the preceding conditions are met.

VI. Evaluation

A. Initial evaluation of patient with HTN should focus on three factors

    1. Other cardiovascular risk factors that will influence the prognosis

    2. Evidence of target organ damage that will influence the urgency of treatment and the target BP

    3. Causes for secondary HTN, which are relatively rare but important to discover

B. History

    1. History is primarily focused on assessing risk for acquiring CHD

        a. Personal history of diabetes

        b. Family history of HTN, CHD, stroke, renal disease

        c. Lifestyle—exercise, cigarette smoking, alcohol, diet, illicit drugs

C. Physical examination

    1. The physical examination should focus on the heart, lungs, pulses, abdominal bruits, presence of peripheral edema, and a funduscopic examination looking for evidence of target organ damage and searching for clues to secondary causes.

D. Laboratory examination

    1. Electrolytes, blood urea nitrogen (BUN), creatinine (Cr), urinalysis

    2. Lipid panel, glucose

    3. Electrocardiogram (ECG)

VII. Patients to Treat

A. It is helpful to *consider HTN as a risk factor for CVD* rather than a disease in itself.

 The decision about BP treatment should not be determined solely by the level of BP.

    1. See Tables 20.2 and 20.3.

B. *Age:* the risks of CHD and stroke increase markedly with age. The absolute benefits of HTN treatment increase with age.

C. *Sex:* CHD risk is 2–3 times higher in men than women.

D. *Diabetes:* Diabetes triples the risk of CHD and stroke.

E. *Smoking:* Smoking doubles the risk of heart disease.

F. *Lipids:* High cholesterol is a major risk for CHD; as cholesterol rises, the need to treat blood pressure rises.

G. *Pre-existing vascular disease* in self or family increases the patient's risk of CHD.

TABLE 20.2 Factors Influencing Prognosis in Hypertension		
Risk Factors for CVDs Used for Risk Stratification	**Target Organ Damage**	**Associated Clinical Conditions**
High levels of SBP and DBP	Left ventricular hypertrophy (ECG, echocardiogram, or radiogram)	Cerebrovascular disease
Men >55 years		Ischemic stroke
Women >85 years	Proteinuria and/or slight elevation of plasma creatinine in concentration (1.2–2.0 mg/dL)	Cerebral hemorrhage
Smoking		Transient ischemic attack
Total cholesterol >65 mmol/L (250 mg/dL)		MI
Diabetes	Ultrasound or radiologic evidence of atherosclerotic plaque (carotid, iliac, and femoral arteries; aorta)	Angina
Family history of premature CVD		Coronary revascularization
	Generalized or focal narrowing of retinal arteries	Congestive heart failure (CHF)

TABLE 20.3			
Stratification of Risk to Quantify Prognosis			
	BP (mm Hg)		
Other risk factors and disease history	Grade 1 (Mild hypertension) SBP 140–159 or DBP 90–99	Grade 2 (Moderate hypertension) SBP 160–179 or DBP 100–109	Grade 3 (Severe hypertension) SBP ≥180 or DBP ≥110
No other risk factors	Low risk	Medium risk	High risk
1–2 risk factors	Medium risk	Medium risk	Very high risk
3 or more risk factors or target organ damage or diabetes	High risk	High risk	Very high risk
Associated clinical conditions (see Table 20-2	Very high risk	Very high risk	Very high risk

An otherwise healthy patient with a BP of 185/115 has a similar CV risk as a patient with diabetes and a BP of 145/95. A young patient without other risk factors with a BP of 150/95 can be managed without medicine for months, even years. A patient with a BP of 150/95 and a previous MI probably needs prompt pharmacologic treatment.

VIII. Nonpharmacologic Treatment (Table 20.4)

A. Dietary Approaches to Stop Hypertension (DASH) diet

1. This is a diet rich in fruits, vegetables, and whole grains.

2. All patients with prehypertension, stages I and II, should be prescribed the DASH diet.

 DASH diet compliance can lower BP as much as 8–14 mm Hg.

TABLE 20.4

Lifestyle Modifications to Manage HTN

Modification	Recommendation	Approximate SBP Reduction, Range
Weight reduction	Maintain normal body weight (BMI, 18.5–24.9)	5–20 mm Hg/10-kg weight loss
Adopt DASH eating plan	Consume a diet rich in fruits, vegetables, and low-fat dairy products, with a reduced content of saturated and total fat	8–14 mm Hg
Dietary sodium, reduction	Reduce dietary sodium intake to no more than 100 mEq/L (2.4 g sodium or 6 g sodium chloride)	2–8 mm Hg
Physical activity	Engage in regular aerobic physical activity such as brisk walking (at least 30 minutes per day, most days of the week)	4–9 mm Hg
Moderation of alcohol consumption	Limit consumption to no more than two drinks per day (1 oz or 30 mL ethanol [e.g., 24 oz beer, 10 oz wine, or 3 oz 90-proof whiskey]) for most men and no more than one drink per day for women and lighter-weight persons	2–4 mm Hg

B. Weight reduction
  1. A loss of only 10 kg may reduce BP 5–20 mm Hg.
  2. It is difficult for patients to lose weight; however, weight loss should be encouraged.
C. Sodium restriction
  1. Limiting salt intake to 4 g or less will reduce BP 2–8 mm Hg.
    a. This may be higher in patients who are black, obese, or elderly.
    b. There may be no benefit to salt reduction in about half of all patients.
  2. The average American consumes about 10 g of sodium per day.

D. Exercise

    1. Aerobic exercise lasting 30 minutes 3 times a week can lower blood pressure by 4–9 mm Hg.

E. Alcohol moderation

    1. Male patients should limit their alcohol intake to two drinks per day or fewer.

    2. Female patients should limit their alcohol intake to one drink per day or fewer.

    3. Limiting alcohol intake to these levels can lower BP by 2–4 mm Hg.

F. Tobacco cessation

 Smoking cigarettes is the most important modifiable risk factor to prevent CHD.

    1. Smoking cessation does not affect HTN itself very much (BP drops by only 1–2 mm Hg), but it is still very important because of the many other ways that it reduces disease risk.

IX. General Principles of Drug Treatment

A. Drug types

 Use a thiazide diuretic, beta blocker, or angiotensin-converting enzyme inhibitor (ACEI) as first-line therapy.

    1. These drugs have been shown to reduce mortality rates in large randomized studies.

    2. They are inexpensive.

B. Monotherapy

    1. Begin with low doses of the drug.

    2. If no or minimal BP lowering is not achieved, consider changing to another drug class.

 Monotherapy is effective in 70% of patients.

 Stage II HTN generally requires two BP medications.

C. Side effects
1. Doubling the initial dose will double the incidence of side effects without necessarily doubling the BP-lowering effects.

 Physicians routinely underestimate the side effects and overestimate the benefits of interventions.

 a. When physicians were asked how many of their patients had side effects from their BP medications, they indicated 10%.
 b. When patients were asked the same question, they indicated 50%.
D. Cost of drugs (Table 20.5)
E. Renin and HTN
1. Elderly and black patients tend to have low renin HTN.
 a. Diuretics (D) and dihydropyridine calcium channel blockers (C) tend to work better in low renin HTN.
2. Young and white patients tend to have high renin HTN.
 a. Beta blockers (B) and ACEIs (A) tend to work better in high renin HTN.
3. Measuring a patient's renin level has not been shown to be clinically helpful; however, the above guidelines are often helpful in initiating therapy.
 a. Use an A or B drug in young or white patients.
 b. Use a C or D drug in elderly or black patients.
F. Be aware of the major advantages and disadvantages of the major drugs (Table 20.6).

X. Medications
A. Diuretics
1. Diuretics are inexpensive, effective, and well tolerated in low doses.

TABLE 20.5 Cost of HTN Drugs	
Drug	**Cost**
Diuretics	$5/month
Beta blockers	$10/month
ACE inhibitors	$40/month
Calcium channel blockers	$70/month

TABLE 20.6 Advantages/Disadvantages of HTN Drugs

	Major Advantages/Indications	Major Disadvantages/Contraindications
Diuretics	Inexpensive Heart failure	Gout Increase incidence of diabetes
Beta blockers	Inexpensive (if generic) Angina Post-MI Heart failure Tachyarrhythmia	Asthma Chronic obstructive pulmonary disease Heart block Very physically active patients
ACEIs	Heart failure Ejection fraction <40% Post-MI Diabetic nephropathy	Pregnancy Bilateral renal artery stenosis Renal insufficiency
Angiotensin receptor blockers	Early trials suggest may be as good as ACEIs Use in patients with ACEI-induced cough	Experience much less than with ACEIs Very expensive
Calcium channel blockers	Angina Systolic HTN in the elderly or African Americans	CHF Very expensive No proven mortality benefits
Clonidine	Very effective BP lowering Inexpensive (generic) Patch—fewer side effects, more expensive	Many nuisance side effects such as sedation, dry mouth
Alpha blockers	Benign prostatic hypertrophy (BPH)	Increased heart failure in a major BP trial (ALLHAT)

Diuretics have been used in the major trials that have demonstrated a reduction in mortality and cardiovascular events.

2. They are drastically underutilized.
   a. One reason is that older studies used doses of 50–100 mg that produced many more side effects than the currently used doses of 12.5–25 mg of hydrochlorothiazide.
   b. A major reason may be the powerful influence of drug representatives and advertising. The influence of marketing in general is well documented, and the need for doctors to be mindful of this influence is well documented.
3. Hypokalemia has the following diuretic profile.
   a. Mild hypokalemia is not a problem for most patients taking a diuretic.
   b. There have been case-controlled studies demonstrating a reduction of sudden death as a result of using potassium-sparing diuretics in combination with thiazide diuretics.
   c. In patients at risk of arrhythmias or any patient with heart disease, a potassium-sparing diuretic should be considered.

B. Beta blockers
   1. Beta blockers have been used in most major trials that have demonstrated a mortality rate benefit.
   2. In addition, beta blockers have mortality rate benefits when used in patients' post-MI or CHF.
   3. They are useful for symptom control in patients with tachyarrhythmia and angina.
   4. However, in the last few years there have been concerns raised that in patients without an MI or CHF (the majority of patients with HTN), beta blockers prevent fewer cardiovascular endpoints, especially stroke, than other antihypertensive medicines. Given that two thirds of the beta-blocker studies have used atenolol, it is difficult to sort out whether this is a class effect or an atenolol effect.

C. ACEIs
   1. There have been multiple trials suggesting that ACEIs as a class may have beneficial effects on cardiovascular and renal morbidity and mortality rates that exceed their BP-lowering effects.
   2. The mechanisms of ACEI beneficial effects are often uncertain.
   3. The advantages are as follows.

a. Diabetes incidence is not increased.
b. The incidence of MI is reduced.
c. Proteinuria is reduced.
d. Mortality due to CHF is reduced.

 An ACEI should be considered for most hypertensive patients with diabetes, proteinuria, renal insufficiency, or CVD.

4. Cough is the most common side effect, occurring in up to 5% of patients.
   a. If coughing is present, changing to an angiotensin receptor blocker is the recommendation.
   b. Angioedema is a rare side effect of ACEI therapy, occurring in 0.1%–0.2% of patients.
D. All other medications, including calcium channel blockers, angiotension receptor blockers, alpha blockers, and clonidine, should be added only if the preceding agents are not tolerated due to side effects or unsuccessful in lowering BP.

XI. Refractory HTN

 The most common cause of refractory HTN is poor compliance.

A. Poor compliance can happen for understandable reasons, but it needs to be identified and improved in order to make treatment effective.
   1. Several factors may lead patients to comply poorly.
      a. *Cost:* medicines are often expensive.
      b. *Side effects:* medicines can often produce side effects.
      c. *Lack of immediate reward:* HTN medicines rarely produce any improvement in short-term well-being.
      d. *Effort:* it can be challenging to stick to dietary or exercise plans.
   2. The physician needs to ask directly but nonjudgmentally, "In a week, how many pills do you miss?"
   3. An assessment of compliance is one of the most important tasks of the physician when seeing patients with HTN.
B. After poor compliance, secondary causes of HTN should be considered.

C. Look for medication interactions.

    1. Review the patient's drug list to find potential interactions.

    2. Over-the-counter medications can be the cause.

        a. Decongestants raise BP and are a commonly used class of drugs.

        b. Nonsteroidal anti-inflammatory drugs (NSAIDs) can negate the effects of BP therapy.

D. Consider diuretic changes.

 "More diuretics" is often the answer.

    1. Renal insufficiency and high sodium intake are well-understood problems.

    2. A less well-recognized mechanism is that the kidney seems to retain sodium in response to most BP medications.

    3. Once a patient requires three different medications, the use of furosemide can be helpful. As these patients are usually not fluid-overloaded, they usually do not lose large amounts of water and potassium.

 MENTOR TIPS DIGEST

- Approximately 26% of adults in the United States have HTN.
- A reduction of 5 mm Hg DBP is associated with a 35%–40% decreased incidence of stroke.
- The risks of heart failure and renal disease are clearly reduced with lower BP; however, the major mortality benefits of BP treatment depend on the reduction of CHD and stroke.
- The JNC on Prevention, Detection, Evaluation, and Treatment of High Blood Pressure has released a new classification scheme for HTN.
- Management is determined by the highest category, either systolic or diastolic.
- According to the JNC, 115/75 is the optimal BP as defined as the BP that predicts the longest life.
- 95% of patients with high BP have primary HTN.
- The most common cause of secondary HTN is parenchymal renal disease.

- The most frequent mistake in BP measurement is using a cuff that is too small.
- The decision about BP treatment should not be determined solely by the level of BP.
- DASH diet compliance can lower BP as much as 8–14 mm Hg.
- Smoking cigarettes is the most important modifiable risk factor to prevent CHD.
- Use a thiazide diuretic, beta blocker, or ACEI as first-line therapy for HTN.
- Monotherapy is effective in 70% of patients.
- Stage II HTN generally requires two BP medications.
- Physicians routinely underestimate the side effects and overestimate the benefits of interventions.
- Diuretics have been used in the major trials that have demonstrated a reduction in mortality and cardiovascular events.
- An ACEI should be considered for most hypertensive patients with diabetes, proteinuria, renal insufficiency, or CVD.
- The most common cause of refractory HTN is poor compliance.
- With refractory HTN, "more diuretics" is often the answer.

Resources

Antihypertensive and Lipid-Lowering Treatment to Prevent Heart Attack Trial (ALLHAT). Major outcomes in high-risk hypertensive patients randomized to angiotensin-converting enzyme inhibitor or calcium channel blocker vs. diuretic. Journal of the American Medical Association 288:2981–2997, 2002.

Cialdini R. Influence, science and practice, 4th ed., Allyn and Bacon Publishers, Delaware, 2000.

Dickerson JEC, et al. Optimization of antihypertensive treatment by crossover rotation of four major classes. Lancet 353:2008–2013, 1999.

Graves JW. Management of difficult-to-control hypertension. Mayo Clinic Procedures 75:278–284, 2000.

Hansson L, et al. Effects of intensive blood-pressure lowering and low-dose aspirin in patients with hypertension: Principal results of the hypertension optimal treatment (HOT) randomised trial. Lancet 351:1755–1762, 1988,

Haynes RB, et al. Increased absenteeism from work after detection and labeling of hypertensive patients. New England Journal of Medicine 299:741–744, 1978.

No Free Lunch website: http://www.nofreelunch.org/index.htm
This Web site encourages "health care providers to practice medicine on the basis of scientific evidence rather than on the basis of pharmaceutical promotion."

Seventh Report of the Joint National Committee on Prevention, Detection, Evaluation, and Treatment of High Blood Pressure: The JNC 7 report. Journal of the American Medical Association 289:2560–2572, 2003.

Siscovick D, et al. Diuretic therapy for hypertension and the risk of primary cardiac arrest. New England Journal of Medicine 330:1852–1857, 1994.

U.S. National Heart, Lung, and Blood Institute. DASH diet booklet: http://www.nhlbi.nih.gov/health/public/heart/hbp/dash/new_dash.pdf
This booklet explains the DASH diet to patients.

U.S. National Heart, Lung, and Blood Institute. Risk assessment tool for estimating your 10-year risk of having a heart attack: http://hp2010.nhlbihin.net/atpiii/calculator.asp
Risk assessment tool (based on the Framingham Heart Study) for estimating 10-year risk of having a heart attack.

Chapter Self-Test Questions

Circle the correct answer. After you have responded to the questions, check your answers in Appendix A.

1. What is the prevalence of hypertension among adults in the United States?

   a. Less than 10%

   b. 20%–30%

   c. 50%–60%

   d. Greater than 90%

2. What is the correct classification for a BP of 125/85 according to JNC-7?

   a. Normal

   b. Pre-hypertension

    c. Stage 1 hypertension

    d. Stage 2 hypertension

3. What is the correct classification for a BP of 140/85 according to JNC-7?

    a. Normal

    b. Pre-hypertension

    c. Stage 1 hypertension

    d. Stage 2 hypertension

 See the testbank CD for more self-test questions.

21

ASTHMA

Michael J. Moore, MD

I. Definition
A. Good general definition of asthma:

> Asthma is a chronic disease of the airways that is complex and characterized by variable and recurring symptoms, airflow obstruction, bronchial hyperreactivity, and airways inflammation.

B. National Institutes of Health (NIH) working definition of asthma:
1. Asthma is a chronic inflammatory disorder of the airways in which many cells and cellular elements play a role; in particular, mast cells, eosinophils, T lymphocytes, macrophages, neutrophils, and epithelial cells.
2. In susceptible individuals, this inflammation causes recurrent episodes of wheezing, breathlessness, chest tightness, and coughing, particularly at night or in the early morning.
3. These episodes are usually associated with widespread but variable airflow obstruction that is often reversible either spontaneously or with treatment.
4. The inflammation also causes an associated increase in the existing bronchial hyperresponsiveness to a variety of stimuli.

II. Burden of Asthma: Epidemiology and Economics
A. Prevalence
1. Worldwide distribution and estimated global prevalence of 300 million patients.

> U.S. prevalence estimate is 10.9% of population.

B. Morbidity and mortality rates
  1. The World Health Organization (WHO) estimates 15 million disability-adjusted life years lost annually due to asthma.
  2. Estimated worldwide deaths: 250,000 per year.
  3. U.S. case fatality rate is 5.2 deaths per 100,000 cases.
C. Social and economic data

 Patients with asthma commonly miss school or work and suffer a decreased quality of life.

  1. Total cost (direct and indirect) of asthma-related illness was estimated at $6.2 billion in 1990.
  2. Emergency room use, hospitalization, and death comprise 43% of the economic impact.

III. Pathogenesis

 The factors involved in the development of asthma are complex, interactive, and highly dependent on the interplay between host factors (primarily genetics) and environmental exposures.

A. Host factors (genetics)
  1. Asthma has a clear heritable component with multiple genes playing a role.
  2. Genetic factors are also involved in the response to asthma therapy.
B. Environmental
  1. Allergens: indoor and outdoor allergens can cause asthma exacerbations; play important but undefined role in development of asthma
  2. Infections
     a. Some viral infections (respiratory syncytial virus [RSV], parainfluenza virus) in infancy share many features of childhood asthma.
     b. Approximately 40% of children admitted to the hospital with documented RSV will continue to wheeze or have asthma later in childhood.
     c. The "hygiene hypothesis" follows.

  i. Early childhood infections influence development of immune system along a "nonallergic" pathway

  ii. May explain observation that children at increased risk of infection (e.g., attend day care) have decreased incidence of asthma and other allergic diseases later in life.

IV. Pathophysiology

 A. Asthma is caused by a complex interaction between cells, mediators, and cytokines that result in airway inflammation.

 B. This results in important physiologic changes in airway structure and function, including airway smooth muscle contraction, hypertrophy and hyperplasia, stimulation of mucous secretion, and airway epithelial dysfunction.

 C. Infiltrating inflammatory cells produce a wide variety of mediators including histamine, platelet activating factor, and derivatives of the arachidonic cascade that can result in bronchoconstriction.

V. Natural History

 Asthma can develop at any age.

 A. Early-onset asthma

  1. Children with early-onset disease may "outgrow" their asthma in 30%–50% of cases; this asthma is more common in males than females.

  2. Risk factors for persistent asthma include severe atopy, marked bronchial hyperreactivity, and a history of difficult-to-control asthma.

  3. Lung growth appears to be normal but can be decreased in more severe disease.

 B. Adult-onset asthma

  1. Patients with adult-onset asthma, severe disease, and abnormal pulmonary function tests (PFTs) are less likely to have remission.

  2. Some patients over time develop irreversible airflow obstruction that may be related to structural changes in the airways (airway remodeling) in the setting of chronic inflammation.

VI. Diagnosis

 Asthma is a clinical diagnosis that is made based on history, physical examination, and diagnostic testing including objective measurement of lung function.

A. History

 Classic triad of symptoms: shortness of breath, wheeze, and cough with or without sputum production.

1. Cough or dyspnea can be isolated features
2. Symptoms tend to be episodic, often with acute onset; may be historically linked to exposures to known triggers and can have periods of prolonged remission
3. Cough in asthma
   a. Can predate a formal diagnosis of asthma by years and be an isolated feature of asthma, i.e., cough-variant asthma
   b. Typical triggers include cigarette smoke, cold air, laughter, deep inhalation, forced exhalation
   c. Coughing paroxysms triggered by deep breathing maneuver suggests bronchial hyperreactivity; can be useful bedside test
4. Other symptoms: chest tightness, substernal pressure, chest pain, nocturnal awakenings

B. Physical findings/examination
1. Acute asthma
   a. Wheeze
      i. Characteristic diffuse musical wheeze
      ii. Presence or intensity does not reliably predict severity of airflow obstruction
   b. Tachypnea and tachycardia (universal)
   c. Prolonged expiratory phase
   d. Hyperinflation of chest
   e. Mild hypoxemia
2. Severe asthma
   a. Wheeze
      i. Loud, high-pitched, and inspiratory and expiratory wheezing is generally associated with more severe obstruction.
      ii. Wheezing may be absent, suggesting poor air movement and impending respiratory failure.

b. Respiratory distress including the inability to speak in full sentences

c. Accessory muscle use

d. Pulsus paradoxus

e. Diaphoresis

f. Severe hypoxemia and mental status changes possibly in extreme cases

C. Objective measures of lung function

   1. Spirometry

   a. Measures forced expiratory volume in 1 second (FEV_1), forced vital capacity (FVC), and FEV_1/FVC ratio

   b. Airflow obstruction demonstrated by decreased FEV_1, decreased FEV_1/FVC ratio, and "scooping" in the expiratory flow limb of flow volume loop

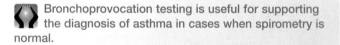 Reversible airflow obstruction is the *sine qua non* of asthma and is considered significant with a 12% improvement in FEV_1 and an absolute increase of 200 mL after administration of a short-acting beta agonist.

   2. Bronchoprovocation testing

Bronchoprovocation testing is useful for supporting the diagnosis of asthma in cases when spirometry is normal.

   a. Inducible bronchial hyperreactivity is demonstrated by a significant decrease in FEV_1 after nebulized administration of an agonist (e.g., methacholine, histamine).

   b. The test is highly sensitive but not specific for asthma.

VII. Differential Diagnosis

A. Acute viral tracheobronchitis

   1. Can result in persistent cough following typical upper respiratory infection (URI) symptoms

   2. Bronchial hyperresponsiveness persisting for up to 6 weeks

   3. May also be manifestation of mild intermittent asthma

B. Chronic obstructive pulmonary disease (COPD)

   1. Also associated with symptom triad of shortness of breath (SOB), wheeze, and cough.

   2. Can be difficult to differentiate from asthma.

C. Gastroesophageal reflux
  1. Can present with cough and chest tightness with or without classic dyspepsia
  2. Can exacerbate asthma; treatment of gastroesophageal reflux disease (GERD) can improve asthma control
D. Cardiac ischemia (chest tightness, chest pain/pressure, dyspnea)
E. Upper airway obstruction
F. Congestive heart failure
G. Vocal cord dysfunction
H. Parasitic infections *(Strongyloides)*
I. Cough secondary to drugs
J. Eosinophilic pneumonia

VIII. Management

A. Successful management of asthma
  1. Routine monitoring of symptoms and objective measures of lung function
  2. Control of asthma triggers
  3. Pharmacologic therapy
  4. Patient education
B. Goals of asthma care
  1. Avoid frequent, severe, and troublesome asthma symptoms (e.g., cough/breathlessness during night, early morning, or after physical activity).
  2. Prevent acute exacerbations that require urgent medical intervention.
  3. Maintain ability to pursue daily activities including participation in athletics without limitation due to asthma symptoms.
  4. Optimize lung function.
  5. Optimize pharmacotherapy while minimizing or avoiding side effects.
  6. Provide effective education.
C. Pharmacologic therapy

 Basic distinction: controller therapy versus reliever therapy.

  1. *Controller therapy:* chronic pharmacotherapy to prevent symptoms of asthma

2. *Reliever therapy:* short-acting pharmacotherapy used on "as-needed" (PRN) basis to treat current asthma symptoms
3. Route of administration
   a. Asthma therapy can be delivered by inhalation, orally, and intravenously.
      i. Inhalation therapy has the major benefit of delivery of drug directly to the airways, resulting in a higher local concentration with fewer systemic side effects.
4. Classes of asthma medications
   a. Anti-inflammatory agents (generally used as controller medications)
      i. Reduce airway inflammation and improve lung function, decrease bronchial hyperreactivity, decrease symptoms, reduce frequency and severity of asthma exacerbations, reduce mortality, improve quality of life
      ii. Prevent migration and activation of inflammatory cells, interfere with production of prostaglandins and leukotrienes, reduce microvascular leak, enhance action of beta-adrenergic receptors on airway smooth muscle
      iii. Corticosteroids
          (1) May be inhaled, oral, or intravenous
              (A) Inhaled corticosteroids (ICSs) are most effective medications for treatment of persistent asthma.
              (B) Examples of inhaled agents are fluticasone, beclomethasone, and flunisolide.
              (C) Oral and intravenous corticosteroids are generally used for acute asthma exacerbations.
      iv. Mast cell stabilizers
          (1) Limited role as controller therapy in adult asthma but have excellent safety profile
          (2) May be useful for some adults with mild persistent asthma or exercise-induced asthma
          (3) Cromolyn sodium and nedocromil sodium available in inhaled form
      v. Leukotriene modifying agents
          (1) Includes 5-lipoxygenase inhibitors (Zileuton) and cysteinyl leukotriene receptor blockers (Zafirlukast, Montelukast)

(2) Shown to have small and variable bronchodilator effect, reduce symptoms including cough, improve lung function, and reduce airway inflammation and asthma exacerbations

(3) May be useful in mild persistent asthma, preventing allergen-induced asthma, exercise-induced asthma, and aspirin-induced bronchospasm

> Leukotriene-modifying agents are less effective than ICSs as monotherapy and less effective than long-acting beta agonists (LABA) as add-on therapy for poorly controlled asthma.

b. Bronchodilators
  i. Short-acting
    (1) β_2-adrenergic agonists (albuterol, pirbuterol, levalbuterol)
      (A) Used as reliever therapy for acute asthma symptoms

> Regular use without concomitant use of an ICS is associated with poor asthma control and heightened bronchial hyperreactivity.

    (2) Inhaled anticholinergic agent (ipratropium)
      (A) Provides bronchodilation via decreased vagal tone of airways
      (B) Primarily used for the treatment of COPD but often combined with albuterol (Combivent/ Duoneb) for treatment of acute asthma
  ii. LABAs: (salmeterol, formoterol)
    (1) Used as asthma controller therapy and to control nocturnal asthma symptoms

> LABAs have been associated with increased risk of asthma-related death and are not appropriate for monotherapy as asthma controller therapy.

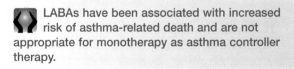

(2) Fixed-dose combination therapy of ICS and LABA (Advair) associated with increased patient compliance and assures LABA always delivered with ICS.

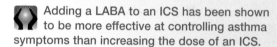 Adding a LABA to an ICS has been shown to be more effective at controlling asthma symptoms than increasing the dose of an ICS.

iii. Theophylline
(1) Bronchodilator with modest anti-inflammatory effects

 Data suggest that it is not effective as a first-line controller medication.

(2) Sustained-release formulations can be used as add-on agent to ICS, but less effective than LABA
(3) Side effects, especially in high doses, limit usefulness
  c. Immunomodulating agents
      i. Various agents have been investigated for their ability to maintain long-term asthma control or steroid-sparing effects.
      ii. These agents include methotrexate, cyclosporin A, intravenous immunoglobulin (IVIG), clarithromycin, omalizumab (anti-IgE), and others.
      iii. Omalizumab has the following profile.
          (1) Only agent approved by the U.S. Food and Drug Administration (FDA) for asthma
          (2) Recombinant DNA-derived humanized anti-IgE monoclonal antibody that prevents IgE from binding to mast cells and basophils
          (3) Indicated as adjunctive therapy in patients with allergies and severe persistent asthma that is inadequately controlled with the combination of high-dose ICS and LABA
          (4) Local side effects common; urticaria and anaphylactic reactions reported in 0.1%–0.2% of treated patients
D. Step therapy approach (Fig. 21.1)
  1. Treatment should be adjusted in a continuous cycle, determined by the patient's asthma control.

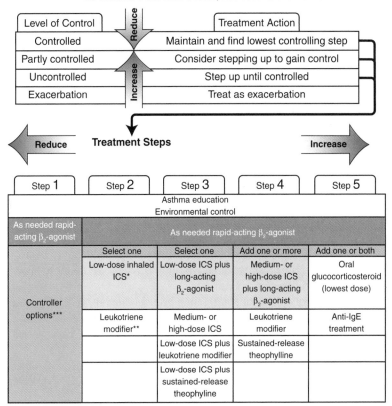

Management Approach Based on Control
for Children Older Than 5 Years, Adolescents and Adults

Level of Control	Reduce / Increase	Treatment Action
Controlled	Reduce	Maintain and find lowest controlling step
Partly controlled	Increase	Consider stepping up to gain control
Uncontrolled		Step up until controlled
Exacerbation		Treat as exacerbation

◄ Reduce   Treatment Steps   Increase ►

	Step 1	Step 2	Step 3	Step 4	Step 5
		Asthma education			
		Environmental control			
	As needed rapid-acting β_2-agonist	As needed rapid-acting β_2-agonist			
		Select one	Select one	Add one or more	Add one or both
Controller options***		Low-dose inhaled ICS*	Low-dose ICS plus long-acting β_2-agonist	Medium- or high-dose ICS plus long-acting β_2-agonist	Oral glucocorticosteroid (lowest dose)
		Leukotriene modifier**	Medium- or high-dose ICS	Leukotriene modifier	Anti-IgE treatment
			Low-dose ICS plus leukotriene modifier	Sustained-release theophylline	
			Low-dose ICS plus sustained-release theophyline		

*ICS=inhaled glucocorticosteroids
**=Receptor antagonist or synthesis inhibitors
***Preferred controller options are shown in shaded boxes

Alternative reliever treatments include inhaled anticholinergics, short-acting oral β_2-agonists, some long-acting β_2-agonists, and short-acting theophylline. Regular dosing with short- and long-acting β_2-agonist is not advised unless accompanied by regular use of an inhaled glucocorticosteroid.

FIGURE 21.1 Asthma management approach, based on level of control, ages 5 through adult. *(From Global Initiative for Asthma: GINA Report 2006: Global Strategy for Asthma Management and Prevention, Chapter 4, page 59. http://www.ginasthma.com/)*

 2. Therapy should be "stepped up" when symptoms are partly controlled or uncontrolled until control is achieved.

 3. Therapy should be "stepped down" when control is achieved for at least 3 months.

 4. Reliever therapy is used at each step for quick relief of symptoms as needed.

E. Monitoring

 1. Ongoing monitoring is essential to maintain control and to establish the lowest step and dose to minimize cost and maximize safety.

 2. Symptom assessment consists of the following.

  a. Suggested points of inquiry

   i. Frequency of short-acting bronchodilator use

   ii. Frequency of daytime symptoms

   iii. Frequency of nocturnal symptoms

   iv. Limits to physical activity or missed work/school

   v. Asthma exacerbations since last visit

  b. Well-controlled asthma: daytime symptoms no more than two times per week and nighttime symptoms no more than two times per month.

  c. Frequent use of short-acting bronchodilators, generally more than two to three puffs per day, is a marker for poorly controlled asthma.

  d. Patient perception of dyspnea/severity

   i. Patient perception of control poorly correlates with objective measures of lung function

   ii. May be linked to near-fatal or fatal asthma

   iii. Objective monitoring of lung function is essential

 3. Objective measures of lung function consists of the following.

  a. Peak expiratory flow rate (PEFR)

   i. Simple, inexpensive measure of airflow obstruction for home use

   ii. Repeated measurements used to determine relative changes and track trends in asthma control

   iii. Single measurements not accurate for airflow obstruction or useful for diagnosis of asthma

  b. Spirometry

   i. Serial measurements used to monitor asthma control

   ii. Generally limited to clinician office use

F. Control of triggers

 Identification and avoidance of asthma "triggers" are critical components of asthma management.

1. Common triggers include allergens, respiratory infections, inhaled irritants, physical activity, emotional distress, gastroesophageal reflux, and medicines (nonselective beta blockers, aspirin).

G. Asthma action plans
1. Written, customized plan for patient-initiated changes in therapy, based on individual patients' range of peak flow measurements and/or asthma symptoms

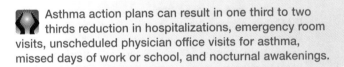 Asthma action plans can result in one third to two thirds reduction in hospitalizations, emergency room visits, unscheduled physician office visits for asthma, missed days of work or school, and nocturnal awakenings.

2. Examples can be found at www.ginasthma.com or www.nhlbi.nih.gov/guidelines/asthma.

IX. Referral to Pulmonary Specialist
A. Diagnostic uncertainty
B. Difficulty in achieving or maintaining asthma control
C. Need for Step 4 care.

 MENTOR TIPS DIGEST

- Asthma is a chronic disease of the airways that is complex and characterized by variable and recurring symptoms, airflow obstruction, bronchial hyperreactivity, and airways inflammation.
- U.S. prevalence estimate is 10.9% of population.
- Patients with asthma commonly miss school or work and suffer a decreased quality of life.
- The factors involved in the development of asthma are complex, interactive, and are highly dependent on the interplay between host factors (primarily genetics) and environmental exposures.

- Asthma can develop at any age.
- Asthma is a clinical diagnosis that is made based on history, physical examination, and diagnostic testing including objective measurement of lung function.
- Classic triad of symptoms in asthma: shortness of breath, wheeze, and cough with or without sputum production.
- Reversible airflow obstruction is the *sine qua non* of asthma and is considered significant with a 12% improvement in FEV_1 and an absolute increase of 200 mL after administration of a short-acting beta agonist.
- Bronchoprovocation testing is useful for supporting the diagnosis of asthma in cases when spirometry is normal.
- Basic distinction in pharmacologic therapy: controller therapy versus reliever therapy.
- Leukotriene-modifying agents are less effective than ICSs as monotherapy and less effective than long-acting beta agonists (LABA) as add-on therapy for poorly controlled asthma.
- Regular use of β_2-adrenergic agonists without concomitent use of an ICS is associated with poor asthma control and height-enced bronchial hyperreactivity.
- LABAs have been associated with increased risk of asthma-related death and are not appropriate for monotherapy as asthma controller therapy.
- Adding a LABA to an ICS has been shown to be more effective at controlling asthma symptoms than increasing the dose of an ICS.
- Data suggest that theophylline is not effective as a first-line controller medication.
- Identification and avoidance of asthma "triggers" are critical components of asthma management.
- Asthma action plans can result in one third to two thirds reduction in hospitalizations, emergency room visits, unscheduled physician office visits for asthma, missed days of work or school, and nocturnal awakenings.

Resources

Busse WW, Lemanske RF. Advances in immunology: Asthma. New England Journal of Medicine 344:350–362, 2001.

Global initiative for asthma: GINA report 2006: Global strategy for asthma management and prevention. Accessed 5/1/07 at http://www. ginasthma.com/

National Asthma Education and Prevention Program. Expert panel 2 report: Guidelines for the diagnosis and treatment of asthma. Accessed 5/1/07 at http://www.nhlbi.nih.gov/guidelines/asthma/ asthgdln.pdf

Wechsler ME, Lehman E, Lazarus SC, et al. Beta-adrenergic receptor polymorphisms and response to salmeterol. American Journal of Respiratory and Critical Care Medicine 173:519–526, 2006.

Weiss KB, Gergen PJ, Hodgson TA. An economic evaluation of asthma in the United States. New England Journal of Medicine 326:862–866, 1992.

Chapter Self-Test Questions

Circle the correct answer. After you have responded to the questions, check your answers in Appendix A.

1. Among Americans who have asthma, about how many die each year?

   a. 5–10/100,000

   b. 50–100/100,000

   c. 500–1000/100,000

   d. 5000–10000/100,000

2. Based on the Global Initiative for Asthma prevalence data, how many of the approximately 300 million persons who live in the United States have asthma?

   a. About 30,000

   b. About 300,000

   c. About 3,000,000

   d. Over 30,000,000

3. According to the NIH, which characterizes the primary pathophysiology of asthma?

   a. Reversible constriction of airways

   b. Irreversible constriction of airways

   c. Inflammation of airways

   d. Anxiety-medicated airways disease

 See the testbank CD for more self-test questions.

22

CHRONIC OBSTRUCTIVE PULMONARY DISEASE

Michael J. Moore, MD

I. Definition

    A. There is no universally accepted definition of chronic obstructive pulmonary disease (COPD).

    B. Most recent published consensus definition by the Global Initiative of Obstructive Lung Disease (GOLD).

> GOLD defines COPD as a disease state characterized by airflow obstruction that is no longer fully reversible, usually progressive, and associated with an abnormal inflammatory response to noxious particles or gases.

    C. Other expert panels have defined COPD as a disease state characterized by chronic airflow limitation due to chronic bronchitis and emphysema.

        1. Chronic bronchitis can be defined clinically as a chronic productive cough for at least 3 consecutive months in 2 consecutive years.

        2. Emphysema can be defined pathologically as abnormal enlargement of airspaces distal to the terminal bronchioles accompanied by destruction of their walls.

II. Epidemiology

> COPD is underdiagnosed and undertreated, and it is a major cause of morbidity and mortality globally.

A. Approximately 24 million people in the United States showing evidence of impaired lung function
B. Data from 2000 indicate COPD responsible for:
   1. 8 million outpatient visits
   2. 1.5 million emergency department visits
   3. 726,000 hospitalizations
C. Mortality

 COPD was the fourth leading cause of death in 2002 (125,500).

   1. Significantly increased rate of death from COPD among women since 1980.
   2. Among the six leading causes of death in the United States; only COPD has been increasing steadily since 1970.

III. Risk Factors
A. Cigarette smoking

 Cigarette smoking is most important risk factor, involving 85%–90% of all cases.

   1. However, only 15%–25% of smokers will be diagnosed with COPD, but a majority will develop some loss of lung function.
   2. Pipe and cigar smoking as well as passive smoking may confer risk for adult COPD.
B. Some occupations (e.g., coal miners, grain handlers, and cement and cotton workers) at increased risk, especially with concomitant exposure to tobacco smoke
C. Environmental factors (e.g., indoor use of biomass fuels, exposure to urban pollution and particulate matter)
D. Genetic factors
   1. α_1-antitrypsin deficiency responsible for <1% of COPD in United States
   2. Multiple gene polymorphisms associated with increased risk
E. Gender: males more at risk than females
F. Low socioeconomic status
G. Bronchial hyperresponsiveness: strong predictor of progressive airflow obstruction in smokers

H. Asthma: many adult nonsmokers develop fixed airflow limitation over time

I. Childhood illness: prematurity, low birth rate, frequent respiratory tract infections, symptomatic childhood asthma

J. Dietary: vitamin C and E deficiency

IV. Pathophysiology

A. Chronic exposure to noxious gases and particulate matter induce a chronic innate and adaptive inflammatory immune response.

1. Important cell mediators of inflammation include macrophages, neutrophils, CD8+ T cells, and eosinophils.

2. Other mediators of inflammation include inflammatory cytokines, chemotactic factors, growth factors, and proteases.

B. Airway inflammation leads to small airway disease and parenchymal destruction and results in airflow limitation.

C. Emphysematous destruction of lung parenchyma leads to loss of alveolar attachments and decreases the maximum expiratory flow secondary to decreased elastic recoil.

D. Other important changes include goblet cell hyperplasia, mucous gland hyperplasia, and mucus hypersecretion.

V. Natural History

COPD is characterized by a prolonged preclinical period of 20–40 years, with a marked continuous decline in lung function (Fig. 22.1).

A. Exertional dyspnea generally develops when the FEV_1 is 40%–50% of predicted.

B. Disability is common when the FEV_1 is approximately 30% of predicted.

VI. Diagnosis

The diagnosis of COPD should be considered in current or former smokers and in never-smokers with other risk factors who present with cough, sputum production, or dyspnea.

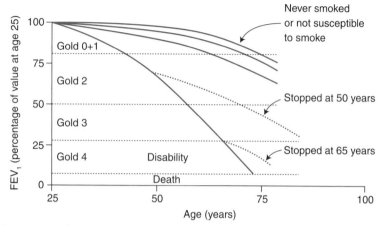

FIGURE 22.1 Rate of decline in FEV$_1$ with age. *(From Hogg JC. Pathophysiology of airflow limitation in chronic obstructive pulmonary disease. Lancet 2004; 364:709–721, Figure 1, p. 709.)*

A. Symptoms usually present in fifth decade and after smoking a pack per day for at least 20 years
  1. Chronic cough $\pm$ sputum production
  2. Dyspnea with exertion
  3. Wheezing
B. Physical examination
  1. Prolonged expiratory phase
  2. Wheeze
  3. Chest wall hyperinflation
  4. Limited diaphragmatic excursion
  5. Distant breath and heart sounds
  6. Severe signs including cyanosis, accessory muscle use, and pursed-lip breathing
C. Imaging
  1. Chest x-ray findings
    a. Low flat diaphragm
    b. Increased retrosternal airspace
    c. Pruning of arterial tree
    d. Bullae

2. Computed tomography findings
   a. Focal areas of low attenuation with "Swiss cheese" appearance
   b. Low attenuation areas small (<1 cm), round or oval, without definable walls
D. Pulmonary function testing
   1. Spirometry

 Spirometry measures expiratory airflow and is most important for diagnosis and staging.

   a. Decreased FEV_1
   b. Decreased ratio of FEV_1/FVC
   c. Flow-volume loop shows "scooping" in expiratory limb

 The FEV_1 is best correlated with morbidity and mortality.

   2. Lung volumes
      a. Total lung capacity (TLC): increased when hyperinflation is present
      b. Residual volume (RV): increased when air trapping is present
   3. Diffusing capacity (DLCO)
      a. Indirect measure of gas exchange
      b. Predicts loss of alveolar-capillary units and suggests presence of emphysema
E. Laboratory
   1. CBC: chronic hypoxemia may lead to secondary polycythemia
   2. α_1-antitrypsin levels in selected patients
   3. Highly sensitive C-reactive protein: increased regardless of smoking status; associated with increased morbidity and mortality

VII. Differential Diagnosis
A. Asthma
B. Acute bronchitis
C. Cystic fibrosis
D. Upper airway obstruction
E. Congestive heart failure

F. Sarcoidosis

G. Some pneumoconioses

VIII. Staging of COPD

A. Multiple respiratory/thoracic societies have severity staging scores

    1. All based on FEV_1

    2. Most recent from GOLD

B. GOLD stage criteria

    1. Stage 0: "at risk" group

        a. Normal spirometry

        b. Chronic symptoms (cough, sputum production)

    2. Stage I: mild COPD

        a. FEV_1/FVC <70%

        b. FEV_1 ≥80% predicted

        c. With or without chronic symptoms

    3. Stage II: moderate COPD

        a. FEV_1/FVC <70%

        b. FEV_1 between 50% and 79% predicted

          i. Stage IIa: FEV_1 between 50% and 70%

          ii. Stage IIb: FEV_1 between 30% and 49%

        c. With or without chronic symptoms

    4. Stage III: severe COPD

        a. FEV_1/FVC <70%

        b. FEV_1 ≥30% and <50% predicted

        c. With or without chronic symptoms

    5. Stage IV: very severe COPD

        a. FEV_1/FVC <70%

        b. FEV_1 <30% predicted *or*

        c. FEV_1 <50% and respiratory failure or clinical signs of right heart failure

IX. Management

A. Stable COPD

    1. Smoking cessation

 Stopping smoking can slow the loss of lung function and decrease symptoms at any point in time.

a. First-line treatments include nicotine replacement therapy and either buproprion or varenicline.

b. See smoking cessation guidelines at www.surgeongeneral.gov/tobacco/default.htm

2. Pharmacologic therapy

 All symptomatic patients warrant a trial of drug treatment.

a. Goals of pharmacologic therapy

   i. Reduce or eliminate symptoms.

   ii. Increase exercise capacity.

   iii. Decrease the number or severity of exacerbations.

   iv. Improve health status.

b. Bronchodilators

   i. Three types in common clinical use: beta-agonists, anticholinergics, and methylxanthines

   ii. Documented clinical outcomes

     (1) Short-acting bronchodilators can acutely increase exercise tolerance.

     (2) Anticholinergics given four times a day can improve health status over a 3-month period compared with placebo.

     (3) Long-acting inhaled beta-agonists improve health status, reduce symptoms, decrease rescue medication, use and increase the time between exacerbations compared with placebo.

     (4) Combination therapy has the following profile.

       (A) Short-acting agents (albuterol/ipratropium) produce a greater change in spirometry over 3 months than either agent alone.

       (B) Combination therapy with long-acting inhaled beta-agonists and ipratropium leads to fewer exacerbations than either drug alone.

       (C) Combination therapy with long-acting beta-agonists and theophylline appear to produce a greater spirometric response than either drug alone.

c. Inhaled corticosteroid (ICS)
  i. Available agents: beclomethasone, budesonide, triamcinolone, fluticasone, flunisolide
  ii. Generally used for patients with more advanced disease (usually classified as an FEV_1 <50% predicted *or* presence of frequent exacerbations).
  iii. Documented clinical outcomes
    (1) Decrease in exacerbations per year
    (2) Decreased rate of deterioration in health status
    (3) No clear evidence of effect on rate of change of FEV_1 in any severity category of COPD

d. Clinical use
  i. Intermittent symptoms (cough, wheeze, exertional dyspnea)
    (1) Short-acting inhaled beta-agonist *or*
    (2) Short-acting inhaled anticholinergic agent
  ii. Persistent symptoms (dyspnea, nocturnal symptoms)
    (1) Scheduled short-acting beta-agonist four times a day
    (2) Combination short-acting bronchodilators (albuterol/ipratropium)
    (3) Consider adding long-acting beta-agonist or long-acting anticholinergic + short-acting "reliever" agents as needed
  iii. Persistent symptoms refractory to preceding therapies
    (1) Try alternate-class bronchodilator
    (2) Combine long-acting bronchodilator and ICS
      (A) Indication for ICS includes FEV_1<50% of predicted or frequent exacerbations
      (B) Single-inhaler combination therapy with LABA and ICS (Advair) appears to have benefits greater than each agent alone
  iv. Benefit still limited or side effects
    (1) Add or substitute long-acting theophylline

e. Other therapies
  i. Systemic corticosteroids
    (1) No role in stable COPD
    (2) Important for acute exacerbations
  ii. Vaccination
    (1) Yearly influenza vaccination reported to reduce serious illness and death in COPD
    (2) Pneumococcal vaccine

3. Oxygen therapy

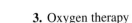 Long-term oxygen therapy (LTOT) improves survival, exercise tolerance, sleep quality, and cognitive performance.

  a. Treating hypoxemia more important versus concern for carbon dioxide (CO_2) retention
  b. Indications for supplemental oxygen
    i. $P_{A}O_2$ <55 mm Hg
    ii. SaO_2 <88%
    iii. SaO_2 ≥88% with presence of cor pulmonale
  c. Therapeutic goal SaO_2 >90% during rest, sleep, and exertion
4. Pulmonary rehabilitation
  a. Multidisciplinary program individually designed to optimize physical and social performance and preserve patient autonomy
  b. Typically includes exercise training, education, psychosocial/ behavioral intervention, nutritional therapy, outcome assessment, promotion of long-term adherence to rehabilitation recommendations
  c. Documented benefits are decreased dyspnea, improved exercise tolerance and health status, decreased health-care utilization.
5. Nutrition
  a. COPD associated with negative energy and protein balance; weight loss or being underweight associated with increased mortality risk
  b. Nutritional therapy
    i. Goal: prevention of weight loss, preservation of energy/protein balance
    ii. Most effective when combined with exercise
6. Surgery for COPD

In highly selected patients, bullectomy and lung volume reduction surgery may result in improved spirometry, lung volume, exercise capacity, dyspnea, and health-related quality of life.

  a. In highly selected patients, lung transplantation can result in improved pulmonary function, exercise capacity, and quality of life as well as possible survival.

B. Acute exacerbation

   1. Definition

      a. Change in natural course of disease, characterized by increased dyspnea, cough, and/or change in sputum quantity or quality, which requires a change in management

   2. Assessment

      a. Assess severity of symptoms, perform physical examination, and look for presence of high-risk comorbid conditions to determine need for inpatient or outpatient care.

      b. High-risk comorbid conditions include pneumonia, congestive heart failure (CHF), new cardiac arrhythmia, renal or liver failure, and history of previous exacerbations.

      c. A physical examination looks for the following.

         i. Tachypnea, tachycardia, and hyper- or hypotension

         ii. Respiratory distress indicated by inability to speak in full sentences, air movement on chest auscultation, and use of accessory muscles

      d. Pulse oximetry or arterial blood gas looks for presence of hypoxemia and/or hypercapnia.

      e. Selected patients should get chest x-ray (CXR), laboratory evaluation, electrocardiogram (EKG), and sputum culture.

   3. Outpatient treatment

      a. Patient education to ensure proper inhaler technique and use of spacer device (if not already using one)

      b. Bronchodilators

         i. Short-acting bronchodilators (albuterol/ipratropium)

         ii. Consider nebulizer

         iii. Consider LABA (if not already using)

      c. Corticosteroids

         i. Oral prednisone 30–40 mg/day × 5–10 days

         ii. Consider ICS (if not already using)

      d. Antibiotics

         i. Particularly in patients with change in quantity or quality of sputum

         ii. First-line drugs: amoxicillin, doxycycline, macrolides

   4. Inpatient

      a. Indications for hospitalization

         i. Presence of high-risk comorbidities

         ii. Failure of outpatient therapy

         iii. Marked increase in dyspnea

    iv. Inability to sleep or eat due to symptoms
    v. New or worsening hypercapnia
    vi. New or worsening hypoxemia
    vii. Change in mental status
    viii. Lack of home support
    ix. Uncertain diagnosis
b. Bronchodilators
    i. Short-acting bronchodilators (albuterol/ipratropium) with spacer or nebulizer
    ii. Increase dose and/or frequency
c. Supplemental oxygen
d. Systemic corticosteroids
    i. Oral (if tolerates) or intravenous steroids
    ii. Dose variable; trial of higher-dose steroids may be indicated depending on severity and response
e. Antibiotics
    i. Particularly in patients with change in quantity or quality of sputum
    ii. Base on local resistance patterns for *Streptococcus pneumoniae, Haemophilus influenza,* and *Moraxella catarrhalis*
f. Ventilatory support

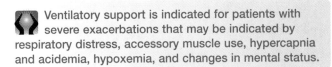

Ventilatory support is indicated for patients with severe exacerbations that may be indicated by respiratory distress, accessory muscle use, hypercapnia and acidemia, hypoxemia, and changes in mental status.

    i. Ventilatory support can be invasive or noninvasive.
    ii. Noninvasive positive-pressure ventilation (NIPPV) is first-line therapy and has been shown in multiple randomized controlled trials to decrease intubation rates, mortality, infection, and hospital length of stay

X. End-of-Life Planning
  A. Acute exacerbations of COPD can result in respiratory failure and need for mechanical ventilation.
  B. It is currently not possible to determine which patients will have greater benefit versus burden with advanced life support, i.e., need for tracheostomy and long-term ventilator assistance.

C. End-of-life planning should occur in periods of stable disease.

  1. Prepare patients for life-threatening exacerbations.

  2. Provide information regarding probable outcomes and existence of palliative care options.

  3. Enquire about patient preferences regarding end-of-life care.

  4. Help patient execute a living will and durable power of attorney for health care.

XI. Prognosis

A. FEV_1 is the most commonly used predictor of clinical outcomes.

B. Other factors associated with poor clinical outcomes include presence of prior acute exacerbations with or without respiratory failure, low body mass index (BMI), poor functional capacity, presence of hyperinflation, and current cigarette smoking.

C. BODE index consists of the following (Fig. 22.2).

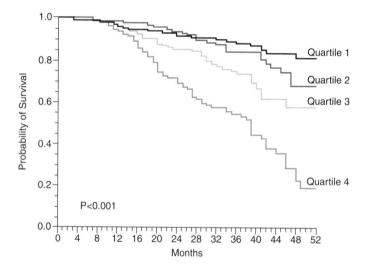

Figure 22.2 Kaplan-Meier survival curves for the four quartiles of the body mass index, degree of airflow obstruction and dyspnea, and exercise capacity index. Quartile 1 is a score of 0–2, quartile 2 is a score of 3–4, quartile 3 a score of 5–6, and quartile 4 a score of 7–10. Survival differed significantly among the four groups (p <0.001 by the log-rank test). *(From Celli BR, Cote CG, Marin JM, et al: The body-mass index, airflow obstruction, dyspnea, and exercise capacity index in chronic obstructive pulmonary disease. New England Journal of Medicine 2004; 350(10):1005–1012, Figure 1A, p. 1010.)*

1. Validated multidimensional index developed to predict death in individual patients
2. Four components
   a. Body mass index (B)
   b. Airflow obstruction (O)
   c. modified Medical Research Council (MMRC) dyspnea score (D)
   d. Exercise capacity (E)
3. 10-point scale, with higher numbers predictive of death

XII. Referral to Pulmonary Specialist

A. Referral to specialist care: confirm diagnosis, perform additional investigations, optimize and initiate treatment, exclude other illnesses
B. Possible indications for referral
   1. Disease onset at age <40 years
   2. Frequent exacerbations (two or more per year) despite adequate treatment
   3. Rapidly progressive course of disease
   4. Severe COPD (FEV_1 <50% predicted) despite optimal treatment
   5. Need for oxygen therapy
   6. Onset of comorbid illness (osteoporosis, heart failure, bronchiectasis, lung cancer)

MENTOR TIPS DIGEST

- GOLD defines COPD as a disease state characterized by airflow obstruction that is no longer fully reversible, usually progressive, and associated with an abnormal inflammatory response to noxious particles or gases.
- COPD is underdiagnosed and undertreated, and it is a major cause of morbidity and mortality globally.
- COPD was the fourth leading cause of death in 2002 (125,500).
- Cigarette smoking is the most important risk factor for COPD, involving 85%–90% of all cases.
- COPD is characterized by a prolonged preclinical period of 20–40 years with a marked continuous decline in lung function.
- The diagnosis of COPD should be considered in current or former smokers and in nonsmokers with other risk factors who present with cough, sputum production, or dyspnea.

- Spirometry measures expiratory airflow and is most important for diagnosis and staging.
- The FEV_1 is best correlated with morbidity and mortality.
- Stopping smoking can slow the loss of lung function and decrease symptoms at any point in time.
- All symptomatic patients warrant a trial of drug treatment.
- Long-term oxygen therapy (LTOT) improves survival, exercise tolerance, sleep quality, and cognitive performance.
- In highly selected patients, bullectomy and lung volume reduction surgery may result in improved spirometry, lung volume, exercise capacity, dyspnea, and health-related quality of life.
- Ventilatory support is indicated for patients with severe exacerbations that may be indicated by respiratory distress, accessory muscle use, hypercapnia and acidemia, hypoxemia, and changes in mental status.

Resources

American Thoracic Society. Standards for the diagnosis and care of patients with chronic obstructive pulmonary disease. American Journal of Respiratory and Critical Care Medicine 152:S77–S121, 1995.

Celli BR, Cote CG, Marin JM, et al. The body-mass index, airflow obstruction, dyspnea, and exercise capacity index in chronic obstructive pulmonary disease. New England Journal of Medicine 350:1005–1012, 2004

Chapman KR, Mannino DM, Soriano JB, et al. Epidemiology and costs of chronic obstructive pulmonary disease. European Respiratory Journal 2006; 27:188–207

Mannino DM, Homa DM, Akinbami LJ, et al. Chronic obstructive pulmonary disease surveillance—United States, 1971–2000. MMWR Surveillance Summary 51:1–16, 2002.

Pauwels RA, Buist AS, Calverley PM, et al. Global strategy for the diagnosis, management and prevention of chronic obstructive pulmonary disease. NHLBI/WHO global initiative for chronic lung disease (GOLD) workshop summary. American Journal of Respiratory Critical Care Medicine 163:1256–1276, 2001.

Rabe KF, Beghé B, Luppi F, et al. Update in chronic obstructive pulmonary disease 2006. American Journal of Respiratory Critical Care Medicine 175:1222–1232, 2007.

Sutherland ER, Cherniack RM. Current concepts: Management of chronic obstructive pulmonary disease. New England Journal of Medicine 350:2689–2697, 2004.

Chapter Self-Test Questions

Circle the correct answer. After you have responded to the questions, check your answers in Appendix A.

1. Which description is characteristic of COPD?

    a. Airways obstruction that improves 20% with albuterol

    b. Airways obstruction that is not fully reversible with albuterol

    c. Restrictive lung disease due to chronic tobacco exposure

    d. Alveolar infiltration with inflammatory cells

2. Which is minimal manifestation in order to make a diagnosis of COPD?

    a. Daily cough for more than 6 months

    b. Daily sputum-producing cough for more than 6 months

    c. Productive cough for at least 3 months in 2 consecutive years

    d. Productive daily cough for at least 3 months

3. Concerning the relationship between cigarette smoking and COPD, which of the following statements is correct?

    a. Most persons who smoke pipe tobacco will develop COPD.

    b. Most persons who smoke cigarettes will develop COPD.

    c. Among persons with COPD, 15%–25% have been cigarette smokers.

    d. Among cigarette smokers, 15%–25% will develop COPD (85%–90% of COPD patients had been smokers).

See the testbank CD for more self-test questions.

23

DIABETES

Jeffrey S. Royce, MD, and Martin S. Lipsky, MD

I. Introduction

A. Diabetes is a group of metabolic disorders characterized by hyperglycemia caused by two types of anomalies.

    1. Defects in insulin secretion

    2. Insulin resistance

II. Epidemiology

A. Diabetes is one of the most common diseases seen in a primary care setting.

    1. In the United States, 21 million people have diabetes (7% of the population).

    2. Diabetes accounts for one-sixth of all health-care expenditures.

III. Classification and Diagnosis

A. Classification

    1. Type 1 diabetes

        a. Results from beta-cell destruction

        b. An absolute insulin deficiency

        c. Requires insulin to avoid ketoacidosis

    2. Type 2 diabetes

        a. Formerly known as non–insulin-dependent diabetes mellitus

        b. Accounts for 90% of all cases of diabetes

        c. Caused by insulin resistance and a progressive secretory defect of insulin

    3. Other specific types

        a. Genetic defects

        b. Endocrinopathies such as Cushing disease

c. Pancreatic disease
d. Chemical- /drug-induced, e.g., thiazides and corticosteroids
4. Gestational diabetes mellitus
B. Diagnosis (Table 23.1)
  1. Plasma glucose
    a. The criteria for diagnosing diabetes in adults include a single plasma glucose level greater than or equal to 200 mg/dL accompanied by classic symptoms such as polyuria, polydipsia, or an unexplained weight loss.
    b. Additional criteria include fasting blood glucose of at least 126 mg/dL on two occasions or a 2-hour postprandial glucose of 200 mg/dL or higher.
    c. Blood glucose meters are not always accurate, and a finger-stick testing result should be verified with a plasma glucose level.

 Measuring the fasting plasma glucose (FPG) is the most common means of testing for diabetes.

    d. The benefits of using the FPG include ease of testing, patient acceptability, and low cost when compared with a glucose tolerance test.

 Oral glucose tolerance testing is used primarily to screen for diabetes during pregnancy.

TABLE 23.1	
Diagnostic Criteria for Diabetes	
Glucose Level Type	**Values**
Fasting blood glucose	≥126 on two or more separate occasions
Random blood glucose	≥200 mg/dL with polyuria, polydipsia, and polyphagia
2-hour postprandial glucose	≥200 mg/dL

2. Glycosylated hemoglobin

   a. Although a glycosylated hemoglobin (Hgb_{A1c}) is not part of the diagnostic criteria, it is an essential component for measuring overall glucose control.

   b. Hgb_{A1c} is formed when glucose is bound non-enzymatically to the hemoglobin molecule and reflects the average level of glucose over the preceding 120 days.

   c. The Hgb_{A1c} provides an objective index that correlates with the risk of diabetic complications.

   d. If a patient is self-monitoring blood sugar levels at home, the Hgb_{A1c} can validate the accuracy.

   e. Although the optimal frequency is not certain, experts recommend two assays per year in stable type 2 diabetes.

   f. Testing three or four times per year may be indicated when adjusting therapy.

IV. Complications

  A. Patients with diabetes often develop long-term complications in addition to the symptoms related to elevated blood sugars.

 Maintaining glucose control as close to normal as possible reduces the risk of diabetic complications.

  1. The Diabetes Control and Complication Trial (DCCT) firmly established the benefit of good control in type 1 diabetics for reducing the risk of microvascular (such as retinopathy or neuropathy) complications. However, the DCCT did not establish that good glycemic control reduced macrovascular complications (atherosclerotic disease).

  2. The United Kingdom Prospective Diabetes Study (UKPDS) demonstrated that maintaining near normal glucose levels in type 2 diabetics also reduces microvascular complications.

The American Diabetes Association (ADA) recommends trying to achieve an Hgb_{A1c} of <7%. Levels above 8% suggest the need to reexamine treatment, either by reemphasizing the adherence to current therapy or by changing management.

B. Macrovascular complications
 1. Atherosclerotic disease, commonly referred to as macrovascular disease, accounts for approximately 75% of all excess mortality in patients with type 2 diabetes mellitus.
 2. Most of the excess mortality rate is due to cardiovascular disease and to complications from cerebral vascular or peripheral vascular disease.
 3. In addition to maintaining good glycemic control, it is critically important to address other cardiovascular risk factors such as smoking, hypertension, and hyperlipidemia.
 4. The Seventh Report of the Joint National Committee on Prevention, Detection, Evaluation, and Treatment of High Blood Pressure (JNC-VII) recommends a blood pressure of less than 130/80 mm Hg for patients with diabetes.

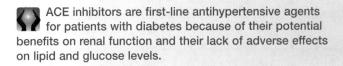

ACE inhibitors are first-line antihypertensive agents for patients with diabetes because of their potential benefits on renal function and their lack of adverse effects on lipid and glucose levels.

 5. Many patients with type 2 diabetes have hyperlipidemia. Because of the high prevalence of coronary artery disease with diabetes, the National Cholesterol Education Panel (NCEP) recommends annual screening for diabetic patients and initiating pharmacologic treatment at low-density lipoprotein (LDL) levels of 130 mg/dL or higher, with an LDL target of 100 mg/dL or lower.
 6. The ADA also recommends prophylactic aspirin use for patients age 50 or older or those with cardiovascular risk factors.
 7. Type 2 diabetes is often associated with a cluster of risk factors known as the metabolic syndrome or insulin-resistance syndrome, characterized by hyperinsulinemia and insulin resistance.
 a. The metabolic syndrome is characterized by central obesity, dyslipidemia, impaired fibrinolysis, and hypertension, each of which is a risk factor for macrovascular disease.
C. Microvascular complications
 1. Retinopathy is one of earliest signs of microvascular disease
 a. The ADA recommends annual dilated eye examinations for patients with diabetes.

     b. Any evidence of retinopathy merits an evaluation by an ophthalmologist as timely appropriate laser therapy may be effective in preserving vision.

     c. Diabetes accounts for about 12% of all new cases of adult blindness.

2. Nephropathy

 Nephropathy is one of the most common diabetic complications.

     a. The ADA recommends screening for microalbuminuria to detect early nephropathy. Microalbuminuria is defined as the presence of 30–300 mg of urinary protein excreted over 24 hours (more than 300 mg is considered macroalbuminuria).

     b. Microalbuminuria is most commonly measured using a spot urine to determine the albumin:creatinine ratio. This measurement correlates very well with a 24-hour urine collection.

     c. The presence of microalbuminuria should signal the clinician to do a careful retinal examination because retinopathy may also be a marker for cardiovascular disease.

Intensifying glycemic control, reducing blood pressure to less than 130/80 mm Hg, and reducing protein intake are all strategies that may slow the progression of nephropathy.

     d. Angiotensin-converting enzyme (ACE) inhibitors have been shown to have renal protective effects independent of their antihypertensive effects. For patients who cannot take ACE inhibitors, angiotensin-II receptor blockers (ARBs) are an alternative.

     e. Diabetic nephropathy accounts for about a third of all patients with end-stage renal disease.

3. Neuropathy

     a. Diabetic autonomic neuropathy can cause bladder and bowel dysfunction, impotence, orthostatic hypotension, and diarrhea.

     b. Patients with diabetes may also experience serious sensory neuropathy.

     c. The presence of a neuropathy and vascular insufficiency makes the diabetic patient prone to foot problems.

Painful neuropathies may respond to tricyclic antidepressants, gabapentin (Neurontin), pregabalin (Lyrica),
or duloxetine (Cymbalta).

V. Management

A. Diet (Table 23.2) and exercise

    1. Overview

 Diet and exercise are the cornerstones of therapy for
type 2 diabetes.

       a. Of patients with type 2 diabetes, 80%–90% are overweight,
making weight loss a common and important goal.

       b. Often a modest loss of 10–20 pounds may be sufficient to
improve glycemic control.

       c. Reducing fat intake is also important because of the risk of
developing vascular disease and dyslipidemia.

    2. Exercise

       a. The ADA recommends that individuals with diabetes try to
achieve 30–45 minutes of moderate exercise at least three
times per week.

       b. Before starting an exercise program, patients with diabetes
merit a thorough evaluation, including an assessment for
macrovascular and microvascular complications that might
be aggravated by physical activity.

TABLE 23.2	Nutritional Recommendations for Diabetes
Nutritional Component	**Recommendations**
Protein	10%–20% of calories; lower in patients with nephropathy
Fat	≤30% of caloric intake, ≤10% from saturated fats
Carbohydrates	60%–70% of caloric intake
Fiber	25–30 g/day dietary fiber
Alcohol	≤2 oz per day for men, ≤1 oz for women

c. Many experts recommend that individuals undergo EKG stress testing before embarking on a vigorous exercise program.

    d. Patients with peripheral neuropathy need to avoid exercise regimens that might damage their feet, and individuals with retinopathy should avoid exercises that require straining.

B. Pharmacologic treatment with oral agents

  1. Overview

    a. Diet and exercise are often insufficient to achieve glycemic control. Pharmacologic therapy should be considered when glycemic goals are not met by diet and exercise alone within 3 months.

    b. In addition to insulin, five classes of oral agents are available for treating type 2 diabetes. All these medications need the presence of endogenous or exogenous insulin to be effective.

  2. Biguanide

    a. The only biguanide on the market in the United States is glucophage (Metformin).

    b. It acts by inhibiting hepatic gluconeogenesis and by increasing glucose uptake in the peripheral tissues.

    c. Metformin when used alone does not cause hypoglycemia but can potentiate hypoglycemia when used in conjunction with insulin or sulfonylureas.

    d. The most common side effects of Metformin are gastrointestinal (GI) (e.g., diarrhea, nausea, or dyspepsia).

    e. These are generally mild and often resolve spontaneously within 1–2 weeks.

    f. A rare ($<1:100,000$) but potentially fatal complication is lactic acidosis.

    g. Avoiding the use of Metformin in patients with renal dysfunction (creatinine >1.5 mg/dL in men; >1.4 mg/dL in women), congestive heart failure, acute or chronic acidosis, and hepatic dysfunction reduces the risk of lactic acidosis.

    h. Metformin is similar in effectiveness to sulfonylureas and reduces fasting blood sugar by 30–60 mg/dL and the Hgb_{A1C} by 1.5%.

> Because Metformin tends not to increase weight and has a modest beneficial effect on lipid levels, some experts view it as a first choice for monotherapy in obese individuals with type 2 diabetes.

3. Sulfonylureas

  a. Sulfonylureas enhance insulin release from pancreatic beta cells.

  b. All sulfonylureas have the same mechanism of action and differ only in their pharmacokinetic properties.

  c. Contraindications include allergy, pregnancy, and significant renal dysfunction.

  d. The most common serious side effect of these medications is hypoglycemia.

  e. Therapy should begin with the lowest dose and titrated slowly upward until glycemic control is achieved.

  f. About 50%–70% of patients with diabetes can be initially controlled solely with a sulfonylurea.

  g. As beta-cell function deteriorates, an additional 5%–10% per year of patients formerly controlled on sulfonylureas will lose glycemic control.

> Typically, patients with significant residual beta-cell function respond best to sulfonylureas. These individuals have usually had diabetes for fewer than 5 years and tend to be lean.

  h. Sulfonylureas generally improve fasting blood sugars by 30–60 mg/dL and Hgb_{A1C} by 1.5%.

4. Thiazolidinediones (TZD)

  a. These medications (rosiglitazone, pioglitazone) work by increasing the sensitivity to insulin in the skeletal muscle, liver, and adipose tissue.

  b. They are used in combination with insulin and the other oral medications.

  c. The Hgb_{A1C} is lowered approximately 0.5%–1.4% by these agents.

  d. The most common side effects are weight gain and fluid retention. For rosiglitazone, recent safety data from controlled clinical trials revealed a potentially significant increase in the risk of heart attack and heart-related deaths.

5. Alpha-glucosidase inhibitors

  a. Alpha glucosidase is an enzyme that hydrolyzes disaccharides. Inhibiting it limits the rate of carbohydrate absorption, reducing postprandial elevation of glucose.

    b. The major side effects are flatulence, diarrhea, and abdominal pain.

    c. It has a smaller effect on fasting blood sugar than the other oral agents and lowers Hgb$_{A1C}$ approximately 0.5%.

  6. Dipeptidyl peptidase-4 (DPP-4) inhibitor

    a. Currently sitagliptin is the only FDA-approved DPP-4 inhibitor.

    b. DPP-4 is an enzyme that inactivates the incretins glucagon-like peptide-1 (GLP-1) and glucose-dependent insulin-releasing polypeptide (GIP).

    c. GLP-1 is excreted by small-intestine L cells.

      i. Stimulates glucose-dependent insulin receptor from pancreatic beta cells

      ii. Suppresses postprandial glucagon secretion from pancreatic 2 cells

      iii. Slows gastric emptying

    d. Currently DPP-4 inhibitors are used as an adjuvant therapy with Metformin and the TZDs.

    e. Glycosylated Hgb$_{A1C}$ is lowered by a modest 0.6%–0.8%.

    f. There is no weight gain caused by DPP-4 inhibitors.

 The DPP-4 inhibitors are eliminated renally; thus, dose adjustment in moderate renal disease is necessary.

C. Parental medications administered subcutaneously

  1. Incretin mimetic (exenatide) mimics action of GLP-1

    a. Lowers postprandial glucose

    b. Used in type 2 diabetics in combination with sulfonylureas and Metformin.

    c. Appears to lower Hgb$_{A1C}$ by 0.5%–1%

    d. Is associated with weight loss

    e. High frequency of GI side effects

    f. Administered twice daily before a meal

  2. Amylin agonist (pramlintide)

    a. Pramlintide is a synthetic analogue of the beta-cell hormone amylin.

    b. Its mechanism of action is suppression of glucagon secretion, slowing of gastric emptying, induction of satiety, and reduction of food intake.

      c. It is used with insulin for the treatment of type 1 or type 2 diabetes.

      d. Pramlintide is administered subcutaneously before meals.

      e. The Hgb_{A1C} reduction is in the 0.5%–0.7% range.

      f. GI side effects such as nausea predominate.

      g. Weight loss is associated with this medication.

  3. Insulin

      a. Insulin is the oldest treatment of diabetes.

      b. Eventually almost 50% of type 2 diabetics require it.

      c. Unlike other medications, there is no maximum dosage of insulin.

      d. Characteristics of insulin preparations vary in terms of onset of action and duration of action.

      e. Patients on insulin are best managed in conjunction with self-monitoring at home using a glucometer.

D. Combination therapy

  1. Type 2 diabetes is a progressive disease. Monotherapy may be ineffective at the outset or may become ineffective with disease progression.

  2. Combination therapy with two or more agents that work by different mechanisms may reduce the blood sugar to an acceptable level.

  3. A biguanide combined with a sulfonylurea is the most widely studied combination.

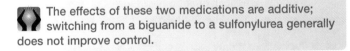 The effects of these two medications are additive; switching from a biguanide to a sulfonylurea generally does not improve control.

  4. The benefit of using insulin with oral agents over insulin alone has yet to be clearly demonstrated, but insulin and a sulfonylurea, insulin and a biguanide, or insulin and a thiazolidinedione are commonly combined.

MENTOR TIPS DIGEST

- Measuring the fasting plasma glucose (FPG) is the most common means of testing for diabetes.
- Oral glucose tolerance testing is used primarily to screen for diabetes during pregnancy.
- Maintaining glucose control as close to normal as possible reduces the risk of diabetic complications.
- The ADA recommends trying to achieve an Hgb_{A1c} of <7%. Levels above 8% suggest the need to reexamine treatment, either by reemphasizing the adherence to current therapy or by changing management.
- ACE inhibitors are first-line antihypertensive agents for patients with diabetes because of their potential benefits on renal function and their lack of adverse effects on lipid and glucose levels.
- Nephropathy is one of the most common diabetic complications.
- Intensifying glycemic control, reducing blood pressure to less than 130/80 mm Hg, and reducing protein intake are all strategies that may slow the progression of nephropathy.
- Painful neuropathies may respond to tricyclic antidepressants, gabapentin (Neurontin), pregabalin (Lyrica), or duloxetine (Cymbalta).
- Diet and exercise are the cornerstones of therapy for type 2 diabetes.
- Because Metformin tends not to increase weight and has a modest beneficial effect on lipid levels, some experts view it as a first choice for monotherapy in obese individuals with type 2 diabetes.
- Typically, patients with significant residual beta-cell function respond best to sulfonylureas. These individuals usually have had diabetes for less than 5 years and tend to be lean.
- The DPP-4 inhibitors are eliminated renally; thus, dose adjustment in moderate renal disease is necessary.
- The effects of biguanides and sulfonylureas are additive; switching from a biguanide to a sulfonylurea generally does not improve control.

Resources

American Diabetes Association. Clinical practice recommendations 2007. Diabetes Care 23:S1–S65, 2007.

This position paper provides guidelines for care in terms of treatment goals, monitoring patients, and prevention strategies. It reflects a combination of evidence from the medical literature and expert opinion.

American Diabetes Association. http://www.diabetes.org/ada/facts.asp

This Web site is an excellent resource for information about diabetes and complications, epidemiology, demographics, and management in special populations.

DCCT Research Group. The effect of intensive diabetes management on long-term complications in insulin-dependent diabetes mellitus. New England Journal of Medicine 329:977–86, 1993.

A landmark study that provided evidence that tight control for patients with type 1 diabetes reduced complications.

Nathan D, et al. Management of hyperglycemia in type 2 diabetes: A consensus algorithm for the initiation and adjustment of therapy. Diabetes Care 29:1963–1972, 2006.

Chapter Self-Test Questions

Circle the correct answer. After you have responded to the questions, check your answers in Appendix A.

1. What is the most common cause of diabetes mellitus in the United States?

   a. Autoimmune beta-cell destruction with absolute insulin deficiency

   b. Progressive beta-cell insulin secretory failure associated with insulin resistance

   c. Pancreatic disease with beta-cell destruction

   d. Glucocorticoid-induced hyperglycemia

2. A 53-year-old man has polyuria, polydipsia, and 5-pound weight loss for a month. His body mass index is 31. Past medical history and physical examination are otherwise unremarkable. Which of the following test results would confirm your clinical suspicion of diabetes?

   a. Non-fasting plasma glucose 215 mg/dL

   b. Single-fasting plasma glucose 185 mg/dL

   c. 2-hour postprandial plasma glucose 185 mg/dL

   d. Hgb_{A1c} 8.1%

3. A 53-year-old man has polyuria, polydipsia, and 5-pound weight loss for a month. His body mass index is 31. Past medical history and physical examination are otherwise unremarkable. You have confirmed the diagnosis of type-2 diabetes by appropriate testing. What should be initial therapy in order to achieve Hgb_{A1c} <7.0%?

   a. Glyburide 1.25–2.5 mg daily

   b. Metformin 1000 mg daily

   c. Insulin glargine 10–20 units every morning

   d. Initiate calorie-restricted diet and vigorous exercise at least three times weekly

See the testbank CD for more self-test questions.

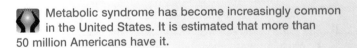

24

CHAPTER

HYPERLIPIDEMIA

Gary J. Martin, MD

I. Pathophysiology and Epidemiology

A. Hyperlipidemia has many causes and in most patients is multifactorial. The basic causes are related to liver metabolism, genetic traits, and diet. In some patients the genetic tendencies are strong enough to be apparent, and the patient has a familial hyperlipidemia. Most patients have either pure hypercholesterolemia or a mixed pattern with increased triglycerides also.

B. Metabolic syndrome is a fairly common presentation with low high-density lipoprotein (HDL) and elevated triglycerides as well as often an elevated blood sugar, blood pressure, and excess abdominal fat. It is associated with inflammatory and prothrombotic markers. Table 24.1 has the most widely accepted criteria in the United States.

> Metabolic syndrome has become increasingly common in the United States. It is estimated that more than 50 million Americans have it.

II. Signs and Symptoms

A. Patients with hyperlipidemia should always have their history explored for signs of hypothyroidism, nephrotic syndrome, and such target organ damage as coronary artery disease, peripheral vascular disease, and cerebral vascular disease.

B. Clues may be found on physical examination, including checking the Achilles tendon for thickening, the skin for xanthelasma, and the cornea for premature arcus senilis.

TABLE 24.1

Definition of Metabolic Syndrome

The American Heart Association (AHA) and the U.S. National Heart, Lung, and Blood Institute (NHLBI) recommend that the metabolic syndrome be identified as the presence of three or more of these components:

Components	Values
Elevated waist circumference	Men: Equal to or greater than 40 inches (102 cm) Women: Equal to or greater than 35 inches (88 cm)
Elevated triglycerides	Equal to or greater than 150 mg/dL
Reduced HDL cholesterol	Men: Less than 40 mg/dL Women: Less than 50 mg/dL
Elevated blood pressure	Equal to or greater than 130/85 mm Hg
Elevated fasting glucose	Equal to or greater than 100 mg/dL

III. History and Physical Examination

A. Key parts of the history include:

1. A history of diabetes

2. Coronary artery disease (angina, prior myocardial infarction)

3. Peripheral vascular disease (claudication or transient ischemic attacks)

4. Drugs that may adversely affect lipids, including progestins, anabolic steroids, corticosteroids, and anti-retrovirals

B. Key parts of the physical examination include:

1. Waist circumference, as it may provide additional information beyond body mass index.

2. Carotid and femoral bruits, as possible signs of atherosclerosis

IV. Differential Diagnosis

A. Liver disease, hypothyroidism, and nephrotic syndrome should be ruled out initially in patients with hyperlipidemia because the secondary causes are often quite treatable and might need attention independently.

 Mild hypothyroidism can contribute to significant elevation of lipids, and treatment can improve cholesterol levels.

V. Laboratory Testing

   A. Thyroid-stimulating hormone (TSH), basic chemical panel, and a hepatic panel including an albumin test are appropriate tests.

   B. Fasting lipids are the gold standard, although there is increasing evidence that measuring triglycerides postprandial may have even more predictive value for atherosclerosis. Testing urine for proteinuria is also a useful screen for nephrotic syndrome.

VI. Management

   A. Management is divided into primary prevention for patients with no apparent end-organ damage and secondary prevention for patients with known coronary or peripheral vascular disease.

   B. Diet is the mainstay of treatment and is appropriate for all patients and adequate for many.

   C. American Heart Association has a recommended diet based on many epidemic studies. This diet is low in fat and cholesterol.

      1. The Mediterranean diet has been tested in randomized trials and has been shown to reduce recurrent myocardial infarctions in patients with a previous infarct. This is a diet that is high in grains and low in meat and that uses olive oil.

   D. Many patients need medication for their cholesterol to get to a low-density lipoprotein (LDL) goal. Table 24.2 lists the risk factors that should be weighed in this decision.

   E. For primary prevention patients, an LDL goal is generally <160 (Table 24.3).

   F. For most patients with coronary or peripheral vascular disease, or diabetes that is now being used as a proxy for atherosclerosis, the goal is an LDL <100. Recent data suggest that patients with acute coronary syndromes and even stable coronary disease may be better off with an LDL of 50–70 mg/dL. At these levels, patients have fewer recurrent events and possibly more regression of plaque.

   G. Most information is available for the statins, particularly atorvastatin, pravastatin, and simvastatin.

      1. Pravastatin, lovastatin, and simvastatin are available as generic drugs. Many statins average about $100/month for patients.

      2. Two national chains offer pravastatin and lovastatin for $4/month.

   H. Statins vary in their potency and dose-response curve, providing a 30%–50% reduction in LDL. The most potent statins are atorvastatin and rosuvastatin.

TABLE 24.2

Major Risk Factors (Exclusive of LDL Cholesterol) That Modify LDL Goals*

Risk Factor	Details
Cigarette smoking	Counsel on means of cessation
Hypertension	BP ≥140/90 mm Hg or on antihypertensive medication
Low HDL cholesterol	<40 mg/dL†
Family history of premature coronary heart disease (CHD)	CHD in male first-degree relative <55 years CHD in female first-degree relative <65 years
Age	Men ≥ 45 years Women ≥55 years*

*In ATP III, diabetes is regarded as a CHD risk equivalent.

†HDL cholesterol ≥60 mg/dL counts as a "negative" risk factor; its presence removes one risk factor from the total count.

Adapted from U.S. National Institutes of Health. Third Report of the National Cholesterol Education Program (NCEP) Expert Panel on Detection, Evaluation, and Treatment of High Blood Cholesterol in Adults (Adult Treatment Panel) Executive Summary. May 2001; NIH Publication Number 01-3670.

TABLE 24.3

Treatment Goals Based on Patient Risk

Risk Category	LDL Goal	LDL Level to Initiate Therapeutic Lifestyle Change	LDL Level to Consider Drug Therapy
CHD or CHD risk equivalents (10-year risk >20%)	<100 mg/dL	≤ 100 mg/dL	≥130 mg/dL (100–129 mg/dL: drug optional)* 10-year risk at 10%–20%: ≥130 mg/dL
2+ risk factors (10-year risk ≤ 20%)	<130 mg/dL	≥ 130 mg/dL	10-year risk <10%: ≥160 mg/dL

Treatment Goals Based on Patient Risk (continued)			
Risk Category	LDL Goal	LDL Level to Initiate Therapeutic Lifestyle Change	LDL Level to Consider Drug Therapy
0–1 risk factor†	<160 mg/dL	≥160 mg/dL	≥190 mg/dL (160–189 mg/dL: LDL-lowering drug optional)

*Some authorities recommend use of LDL-lowering drugs in this category if an LDL cholesterol <100 mg/dL cannot be achieved by therapeutic lifestyle changes. Others prefer use of drugs that primarily modify triglycerides and HDL, e.g., nicotinic acid or fibrate. Clinical judgment may also call for deferring drug therapy in this subcategory.

†Almost all people with 0–1 risk factor have a 10-year risk <10%; this 10-year risk assessment in people with 0–1 risk factor is necessary.

Adapted from U.S. National Institutes of Health. Third Report of the National Cholesterol Education Program (NCEP) Expert Panel on Detection, Evaluation, and Treatment of High Blood Cholesterol in Adults (Adult Treatment Panel) Executive Summary. May 2001; NIH Publication Number 01-3670.

I. Fibrates are used for patients who have low HDLs and elevated tryglycerides, i.e., triglycerides greater than at least 200 mg/dL. There is much less information documenting benefits for fibrates, but some studies suggest fewer recurrent myocardial infarctions in patients treated with these drugs.

J. Niacin is an inexpensive alternative. It does have relatively modest LDL-lowering effects but can raise HDL significantly.

K. The following are important facts about statins.

Statins for the most part are well-tolerated drugs, but rare cases of rhabdomyolysis occur (<1%). More frequently, cases of myalgias are seen with normal or mild creatinine phosphokinase (CPK) elevations.

1. Mild liver function abnormalities (transaminase elevations) can also be seen in up to 2% of patients. However, these are rarely clinically significant.

2. Combination treatment is generally reserved for patients with known atherosclerosis that is otherwise poorly controlled.

Fibrates and niacin may be combined with statins; however, they may increase the risk of rhabdomyolysis.

3. The best monitoring for rhabdomyolysis is an "activated" patient who understands what the symptoms may be and knows to stop the drug and contact the physician the same day diffuse unexplained muscle aches occur.

4. Periodic CPK monitoring, although sometimes done, is not particularly helpful unless used to evaluate symptoms of myalgia

5. One needs to be sensitive that many additional medications can elevate statin levels and thereby precipitate rhabdomyolysis. This includes fairly common drugs such as antifungals and macrolides and even grapefruit juice.

L. Bile sequestrant agents, such as cholestyramine, colesevelam, and cholestipol, are also used in some patients who do not reach a goal with a statin or who cannot tolerate a statin. These drugs are limited by the fact that they also absorb other medications and need to be separated by a number of hours from other doses. They can worsen hypertriglyceridemia.

M. Ezetimibe has had the most impressive impact as an adjunct therapy with statins. This drug has been documented to be safe in terms of drug interactions with statins and can provide an additional 25% reduction in LDL levels. It may also be an option for patients who cannot tolerate statins. Unfortunately, ezetimibe has not been studied in any clinical outcome trials, but several are in progress.

MENTOR TIPS DIGEST

- Metabolic syndrome has become increasingly common in the United States. It is estimated that more than 50 million Americans have it.
- Mild hypothyroidism can contribute to significant elevation of lipids, and treatment can improve cholesterol levels.
- Statins for the most part are very well tolerated drugs, but rare cases of rhabdomyolysis occur (<1%). More frequently, cases of myalgias are seen with normal or mild CPK elevations.

Resources

Blankenhorn DM, et al. Beneficial effects of combined colestipol-niacin therapy on coronary atherosclerosis and coronary venous bypass grafts. Journal of the American Medical Association 257:3233–3240, 1987 *The first report of regression of coronary atherosclerosis in subjects intensively treated with lipid-lowering medications.*

Cannon CP, Braunwald E, McCabe CH, et al. Comparison of intensive and moderate lipid lowering with statins after acute coronary syndromes. New England Journal of Medicine 350:15, 2004. *This study from 2004 supported getting to LDL levels of approximately 60–80 mg/dL.*

Downs JR, Clearfield M, Weiss S, et al. Primary prevention of acute coronary events with lovastatin in men and women with average cholesterol levels: Results of AFCAPS/TexCAPS. Journal of the American Medical Association 279:1615–1622, 1998.

Forrester JS, et al. Lipid lowering versus revascularization: An idea whose time (for testing) has come. Circulation 96:1360–1362, 1997

Haffner SM, Lehto S, Ronnemaa T, et al. Mortality from coronary heart disease in subjects with type 2 diabetes and in nondiabetic subjects with and without prior myocardial infarction. New England Journal of Medicine 339:229–234, 1998.

La Rosa JC, Grundy SM, Waters DD, et al. Intensive lipid lowering with atorvastatin in patients with stable coronary disease. New England Journal of Medicine 352: 1425–1435, 2005.

MRC/BHF Heart Protection study Collaborative Group. MRC/BHF heart protection study of cholesterol lowering with simvastatin in 20,536 high-risk individuals: A randomized placebo-controlled trial. Lancet 360:7–22, 2002.

National Institute of Health. Third report of the national cholesterol education program expert panel on detection, evaluation, and treatment of high blood cholesterol in adults (adult treatment panel) executive summary. May 2001; NIH Publication Number 01-3670.

Nissen SE, Tuzcu EM, Schoenhagen P, et al. Effect of intensive compared with moderate lipid-lowering therapy on progression of coronary atherosclerosis. JAMA 2004; 291:1071–1080. *This is another study from 2004 that supported getting to LDL levels of approximately 60–80.*

Nissen SE; Nicholls SJ; Sipahi I, et al. Effect of very high-intensity statin therapy on regression of coronary atherosclerosis: The ASTEROID trial. Journal of the American Medical Association 295:1556–1565, 2006.

Pasternak RC, Smith SC, Bairey-Merz CN, et al. ACC/AHA/NHLBI clinical advisory on the use and safety of statins. Circulation 106:1024–1028, 2002.

Pitt B, Waters D, Brown WV, et al. Aggressive lipid-lowering therapy compared with angioplasty in stable coronary artery disease. New England Journal of Medicine 341:70–76, 1999.

Lipid lowering actually led to lower event rate than PCI in low-risk patients.

Rubins HB, Robins SJ, Colins D, et al. Gemfibrozil for the secondary prevention of coronary heart disease in men with low levels of high-density lipoprotein cholesterol: Veterans Affairs high-density lipoprotein cholesterol intervention trial study group. New England Journal of Medicine 341:410–418, 1999.

Sacks FM. High-intensity statin treatment for coronary heart disease. Journal of the American Medical Association 291:1132–1134, 2004.

Scandinavian Simvastatin Survival Study Group. Randomized trial of cholesterol lowering in 4444 patients with coronary heart disease: The Scandinavian simvastatin survival study. Lancet 344:1383–1389, 1994.

Simvastatin results in decreased CHD incidence and mortality and a 30% decrease in all-cause mortality. Coronary artery disease patients LDL 187→122 with simvastatin: mortality 12% versus 8% (5.4 yr F/U).

Shepherd J, et al. Prevention of coronary heart disease with pravastatin in men with hypercholesterolemia. New England Journal of Medicine 333:1301–1307, 1995.

Primary prevention ("west of Scotland study") LDL 192→140. Approximately 10% versus 6% major event rate over 6 years.

Singh RB, Dubnov G, Niaz MA, et al. Effect of an Indo-Mediterranean diet on progression of coronary artery disease in high risk patients (Indo-Mediterranean diet heart study): A randomized single-blind trial. Lancet 360:1455–1461, 2002.

Smith SC, Allen J, Blair SN, et al. AHA/ACC guidelines for secondary prevention for patients with coronary and other atherosclerotic vascular disease: 2006 Update. Journal of the American College of Cardiology 47:2130–2139, 2006.

Most recent guidelines that advocate for LDL <70, beta blockers (BB), angiotensin-converting enzyme inhibitor (ACEI), exercise, BMI <25, blood pressure (BP) control <130–140/80–90, ASA, and quitting smoking.

Chapter Self-Test Questions

Circle the correct answer. After you have responded to the questions, check your answers in Appendix A.

1. What is a physical finding that suggests hyperlipidemia?

   a. Subcutaneous cholesterol-filled nodules

   b. Flare-shaped red deposits in retina

   c. Periarticular swelling of the distal phalangeal joints of hands

   d. Third heart sound

2. What ocular physical finding suggests hyperlipidemia?

   a. Cloudiness in lens

   b. Brown deposit around periphery of cornea seen with slit-lamp

   c. White-gray deposit around periphery of cornea

   d. Blue sclerae

3. A 64-year-old woman has been under your care for years. Several screening total cholesterol measurements had been 180–200 mg/dL. Now random total cholesterol is 286 mg/dL. Which test is most appropriate?

   a. Serum Apo-B

   b. Serum direct LDL

   c. ACTH

   d. TSH

See the testbank CD for more self-test questions.

25

OBESITY

Robert F. Kushner, MD

I. Pathophysiology

A. Etiology

 The etiology of obesity is multifactorial.

1. Obesity is brought about by an interaction between predisposing genetic and metabolic factors and a rapidly changing environment.
2. Interactive influences include social, behavioral, physiologic, metabolic, cellular, and molecular factors.
3. By definition, obesity is a disease of energy imbalance, in which energy$_{in}$ exceeds energy$_{out}$. The resultant accretion of body fat and, to a lesser extent, lean body mass, is a function of time (months or years) $\times$ surplus energy (kcalories). This concept is consistent with the First Law of Thermodynamics, or the Law of Conservation of Energy.
4. There is a positive energy balance produced whenever energy intake is increased, energy output is lowered, or both occur.
5. Energy balance is critical. A daily calorie mismatch of only $+1\%$ would theoretically lead to a gain of approximately 2.5 pounds of fat per year.
6. Heredity clearly plays a role in human obesity. The evidence for a genetic basis for obesity comes from several areas of investigation, including animal models, human inherited disorders (e.g., Prader-Willi syndrome), adoption studies, human twin studies, family metabolic studies, and human intervention studies.

B. Pathology

 Obesity is a pervasive and insidious disorder affecting nine organ systems and over 40 conditions and diseases.

1. Obesity-related comorbidities
    a. Endocrine: type 2 diabetes, dyslipidemia, metabolic syndrome, polycystic ovarian syndrome (PCOS)
    b. Cardiovascular: hypertension, congestive heart failure (CHF), atrial fibrillation, left ventricular hypertrophy (LVH)
    c. Respiratory: reduced lung compliance, asthma, obstructive sleep apnea (OSA), obesity hypoventilation syndrome
    d. Gastrointestinal: gallstones, gastroesophageal reflux disease (GERD), nonalcoholic fatty liver disease (NAFLD)
    e. Genitourinary: urinary incontinence, hypogonadism (male), complications of pregnancy, uterine cancer, obesity-related nephropathy
    f. Integument: carbuncles and furuncles, intertrigo, stretch marks, venous stasis pigmentation
    g. Musculoskeletal: arthralgias and arthritis, Blount disease (childhood)
    h. Psychological: reduced quality of life, depression, poor self-esteem and body image
2. Pathophysiology

 The pathophysiology of obesity is multifactorial.

    a. It is the result of changes in diet, physical inactivity, hemodynamics, weightbearing mechanics, and metabolic and endocrine abnormalities.
    b. Alterations in function are often insidious, progressing from subclinical physiologic changes to reduction in quality of life and symptomatic disease states.
    c. New insights include the following.

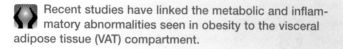

Recent studies have linked the metabolic and inflammatory abnormalities seen in obesity to the visceral adipose tissue (VAT) compartment.

    i. The VAT adipocytes and adipose connective tissue secrete products called adipokines. These bioactive peptides act locally and distally through autocrine, paracrine, and endocrine effects.

    ii. Secreted factors include the energy balance-regulating hormone leptin, cytokines such as interleukin (IL)-6 and tumor necrosis factor (TNF)-alpha, prothrombotic agents such as plasminogen activator inhibitor 1 (PAI-1), and a component of the blood-pressure regulating system: angiotensinogen.

    iii. In obesity, increased production of most adipokines affects multiple functions such as appetite and energy balance, immunity, insulin sensitivity, angiogenesis, blood pressure, lipid metabolism, and hemostasis. For example, IL-6 leads to hypertriglyceridemia by stimulating lipolysis and hepatic triglyceride secretion; TNF-alpha directly decreases insulin sensitivity and increases lipolysis in adipocytes.

II. Epidemiology

A. The prevalence of obesity is increasing to epidemic proportions in the United States.

About two-thirds of American adults are overweight, and about one-third is obese.

About one-third of American children and adolescents (age 6–19 years) is overweight or obese.

1. An analysis based on the 1999–2000 data from the National Health and Nutrition Examination Survey (NHANES) estimated the adult numbers at 64.5% (overweight) and 30.5% (obese); 31% of children and adolescents were overweight or obese.

2. Differences in prevalence exist in many segments of the population, particularly among blacks and Mexican Americans. Of adult African American women, 50% are obese, and 40% of Hispanic women are obese, compared with 30% of white women. Mexican American men have a higher prevalence of overweight and obesity (75%) than non-Hispanic white men (67%) and non-Hispanic black men (61%).

B. Obesity is now considered a global health problem. The World Health Organization (WHO) has concluded that "overweight and obesity are now so common that they are replacing the more traditional public health concerns such as undernutrition and infectious diseases as some of the most significant contributors to ill health."

III. Prevention

A. Maintaining a healthy body weight by balancing dietary calories with physical activity is recommended by all professional guidelines including the 2005 USDA Dietary Guidelines for Healthy Americans.

 Clinicians should provide behavioral counseling on preventing weight gain as part of preventive counseling.

IV. Signs and Symptoms

A. Obese patients at very high absolute risk who trigger the need for intense risk-factor modification and management include those with the following pathology.

1. Established coronary heart disease

2. Presence of other atherosclerotic diseases such as peripheral arterial disease, abdominal aortic aneurysm, or symptomatic carotid artery disease

3. Type 2 diabetes

4. Sleep apnea

B. Additional triggers for treatment include development of any other obesity-related comorbid condition listed earlier.

 The number and severity of organ-specific comorbid conditions usually rise with increasing levels of obesity.

V. History and Physical Examination

A. A comprehensive history that addresses issues and concerns specific to obesity should be taken.

1. Chronological history of weight gain; age at onset, description of weight gain (and loss), and inciting events

2. Response to previous weight-loss attempts

3. Effect of excess body weight on health; important to elicit patients' own perceptions regarding how overweight affects them physically, psychologically, and socially

4. Expectations from a weight management program

5. A thorough medication history to uncover possible drug-induced weight gain and medications interfering with weight loss (such as antipsychotics, antidepressants, mood stabilizers, antidiabetic agents, and steroids)

6. Determination of fitness level; cardiorespiratory fitness (measured by maximal treadmill exercise test) is important predictor of all-cause mortality independent of body mass index (BMI) and body composition

B. For the physical examination, the following insights apply.

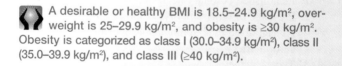 Assessment of risk status due to overweight or obesity is based on the patient's BMI, waist circumference, and the existence of comorbid conditions.

1. BMI is calculated as weight (kg)/height (m)^2, or as weight (pounds)/height (inches)^2 × 703.

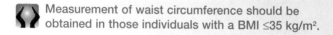 A desirable or healthy BMI is 18.5–24.9 kg/m^2, overweight is 25–29.9 kg/m^2, and obesity is ≥30 kg/m^2. Obesity is categorized as class I (30.0–34.9 kg/m^2), class II (35.0–39.9 kg/m^2), and class III (≥40 kg/m^2).

Measurement of waist circumference should be obtained in those individuals with a BMI ≤35 kg/m^2.

a. Abdominal fat is clinically defined as a waist circumference ≥102 cm (≥40 inches) in men and ≥88 cm (≥35 inches) in women according to the APT III report. Lower waist circumference thresholds exist for Asian populations.

> An increased waist circumference has been found to be predictive of the risk of having hypertension, diabetes, dyslipidemia, and the metabolic syndrome compared with those who have normal waist circumference.

   2. Special attention needs to be given to measurement of blood pressure.

   a. A bladder cuff that is not the appropriate width for the patient's arm circumference will cause a systematic error in blood pressure measurement. The error in blood pressure measurement is larger when the cuff is too small relative to the patient's arm circumference than when it is too large—a situation commonly encountered among the obese.

   b. It has been demonstrated that the most frequent error in measuring blood pressure is "mis-cuffing," with undercuffing large arms accounting for 84%.

VI. Differential Diagnosis

A. In the majority of patients, obesity is the result of environmental exposure to increased caloric intake and reduced energy expenditure associated with a poorly defined genetic vulnerability.

   1. Single-gene disorders are uncommon and include the syndromes of Prader-Willi, Bardet-Biedl, Cohen, and Alström, along with deficiencies in the leptin and MC4 receptors.

B. Laboratory tests consist of the following.

   1. There is no single laboratory test or diagnostic evaluation that is indicated for all patients with obesity. The specific evaluation performed should be based on presentation of symptoms, risk factors, and index of suspicion; however, many screening guidelines recommend a fasting lipid panel and blood glucose measurement at presentation.

   2. Other tests to consider include the liver function tests alanine aminotransferase (ALT) and aspartate aminotransferase (AST) (for NAFLD), thyroid-stimulating hormone (TSH) (for hypothyroidism), and a polysomnogram for patients presenting with symptoms consistent with obstructive sleep apnea.

VII. Management

A. Lifestyle modification

 Lifestyle management incorporates the three essential components of obesity care: dietary therapy, physical activity, and behavior therapy.

1. Obesity is a disease of energy imbalance; patients must learn how and when energy consumed (diet), how and when energy expended (physical activity), and how to incorporate this information into daily life (behavior therapy)
2. Diet

 The diet needs to produce a calorie deficit of 500–1000 kcal/day, resulting in a weight loss of 1–2 lb/week.

   a. This is usually consistent with a diet containing 1000–1200 kcal/day for most women and 1200–1600 kcal/day for men.
   b. The diet may be instituted using a broad range of acceptable macronutrient levels consisting of 45%–65% of total calories from carbohydrates, 20%–35% of total calories from fat, and 10%–35% of total calories from protein.
3. Physical activity
   a. In addition to increasing calorie expenditure, physical activity is beneficial for improved cardiorespiratory fitness, cardiovascular disease and cancer risk reduction, and improved mood and self-esteem.
   b. The minimum public health recommendation for physical activity is 30 minutes of moderate intensity physical activity on most, preferably all, days of the week (150 minutes per week).
   c. For long-term weight loss, higher amounts of exercise (e.g., 200–300 minutes per week or ≥2000 kcal/week) are needed.
4. Behavior therapy
   a. The most commonly used approaches include motivational interviewing, transtheoretical model and stages of change, and cognitive behavioral therapy (CBT).
   b. CBT incorporates various strategies intended to help change and reinforce new dietary and physical activity be-

haviors. Strategies include self-monitoring techniques (e.g., journaling, weighing and measuring food and activity), stress management, stimulus control, social support, problem solving, and cognitive restructuring, i.e., helping patients develop more positive and realistic thoughts about themselves.

> When recommending any behavioral lifestyle change, have the patient identify what, when, where, and how the behavioral change will be performed.

   c. Have the patient and yourself keep a record of the anticipated behavioral change, and monitor progress at the next office visit.

   d. Combined interventions of diet, physical activity, and behavior therapy provide the most successful therapy for weight loss and weight maintenance.

B. Pharmacotherapy

> Adjuvant pharmacologic treatments should be considered for patients with a BMI ≥ 30 kg/m^2 or with a BMI ≥ 27 kg/m^2 who also have concomitant obesity-related risk factors or diseases and for whom dietary and physical activity therapies have not been successful.

  1. Centrally acting anorexiant medications

    a. Sibutramine (Meridia) functions as a serotonin and norepinephrine reuptake inhibitor (SNRI).

      i. Sibutramine produces a dose-dependent weight loss (available doses are 5-, 10-, and 15-mg capsules), with an average loss of about 5%–9% of initial body weight at 12 months.

      ii. The most commonly reported adverse events are headache, dry mouth, insomnia, and constipation. A dose-related increase in blood pressure and heart rate may require discontinuation of the medication. A dose of 10–15 mg/day causes an average increase in systolic and diastolic blood pressure of 2–4 mm Hg and an increase in heart rate of 4–6 beats/min.

    b. Phentermine is a centrally acting anorectic drug and a derivative of amphetamine.

       i. The development of drug tolerance, a characteristic feature of amphetamine and other drugs in this class, is commonly reported by patients after a few weeks or months.

       ii. Because phentermine was originally approved for short-term use only, there are no published studies of phentermine monotherapy beyond 9 months.

       iii. There are several trade brands of phentermine. Initial dose is typically 15 mg/day, with maximum dose at 30 mg/day.

       iv. Side effects include those associated with central nervous system stimulation, such as elevation of blood pressure, increased heart rate, palpitations, insomnia, and dry mouth.

2. Peripherally acting medication

    a. Orlistat (Xenical) is a potent, slowly reversible inhibitor of pancreatic, gastric, and carboxyl ester lipases and phospholipase A_2, which are required for the hydrolysis of dietary fat in the gastrointestinal tract into fatty acids and monoacylglycerols. Orlistat (Alli) was approved as a 60-mg over-the-counter medication in February 2007.

       i. Taken at a therapeutic dose of 120 mg three times a day, orlistat blocks the digestion and absorption of about 30% of dietary fat.

       ii. Orlistat produces a weight loss of about 9%–10% compared with a 4%–6% weight loss in the placebo-treated groups.

       iii. Gastrointestinal tract adverse effects occur in at least 10% of orlistat-treated patients. Effects include oily spotting, flatus with discharge, fecal urgency, fatty/oily stool, oily evacuation, and increased defecation.

C. Surgical (bariatric) treatment

> Bariatric surgery should be considered for patients with severe obesity (BMI >40 kg/m^2) or those with moderate obesity (BMI >35 kg/m^2) associated with a serious medical condition.

1. Weight loss surgeries are in one of two categories: restrictive and restrictive malabsorptive.

a. Restrictive surgeries limit the amount of food the stomach can hold and slow the rate of gastric emptying. Laparoscopic adjustable silicone gastric banding (LASGB) is an example.

b. Restrictive malabsorptive bypass procedures combine the elements of gastric restriction and selective malabsorption. The Roux-en-Y gastric bypass (RYGB) is an example.

2. These procedures are generally effective in producing an average weight loss of approximately 30%–35% of total body weight that is maintained in nearly 60% of patients at 5 years.

Bariatric surgery is the most effective weight loss therapy for patients with clinically severe obesity.

3. The restrictive-malabsorptive procedures produce a predictable increased risk for micronutrient deficiencies of vitamin B_{12}, iron, folate, calcium, and vitamin D, based on surgical anatomical changes. The patients require lifelong supplementation with these micronutrients and should be managed by a team of specialists including a registered dietitian.

MENTOR TIPS DIGEST

- The etiology of obesity is multifactorial.
- Obesity is a pervasive and insidious disorder affecting nine organ systems and over 40 conditions and diseases.
- The pathophysiology of obesity is multifactorial.
- Recent studies have linked the metabolic and inflammatory abnormalities seen in obesity to the visceral adipose tissue (VAT) compartment.
- About two-thirds of American adults are overweight, and about one-third is obese.
- About one-third of American children and adolescents (age 6–19 years) is overweight or obese.
- Clinicians should provide behavioral counseling on preventing weight gain as part of preventive counseling.
- The number and severity of organ-specific comorbid conditions usually rise with increasing levels of obesity.

- Assessment of risk status due to overweight or obesity is based on the patient's BMI, waist circumference, and the existence of comorbid conditions.
- A desirable or healthy BMI is 18.5–24.9 kg/m^2, overweight is 25–29.9 kg/m^2, and obesity is ≥ kg/m^2. Obesity is categorized as class I (30.0–34.9 kg/m^2), class II (35.0–39.9 kg/m^2), and class III (≥40 kg/m^2).
- Measurement of waist circumference should be obtained in those individuals with a BMI ≤35 kg/m^2.
- An increased waist circumference has been found to be predictive of the risk of having hypertension, diabetes, dyslipidemia, and the metabolic syndrome compared with those who have normal waist circumference.
- Lifestyle management incorporates the three essential components of obesity care: dietary therapy, physical activity, and behavior therapy.
- The diet needs to produce a calorie deficit of 500–1000 kcal/day, resulting in a weight loss of 1–2 lb/week.
- When recommending any behavioral lifestyle change, have the patient identify what, when, where, and how the behavioral change will be performed.
- Adjuvant pharmacologic treatments should be considered for patients with a BMI ≥30 kg/m^2 or with a BMI ≥27 kg/m^2 who also have concomitant obesity-related risk factors or diseases and for whom dietary and physical activity therapies have not been successful.
- Bariatric surgery should be considered for patients with severe obesity (BMI >40 kg/m^2) or those with moderate obesity (BMI >35 kg/m^2) associated with a serious medical condition.
- Bariatric surgery is the most effective weight loss therapy for patients with clinically severe obesity.

Resources

Buchwald H, et al. Bariatric surgery: A systematic review and meta-analysis. Journal of the American Medical Association 292:1724, 2004.

Haslam DW, James WPT. Obesity. Lancet 366:1197, 2005.

Jakacic JM, et al: Appropriate intervention strategies for weight loss and prevention of weight regain for adults. Medicine and Science in Sports and Exercise 33:2145, 2001.

Kushner RF. Roadmaps for clinical practice: Case studies in disease prevention and health promotion—assessment and management of adult obesity: A primer for physicians. www.ama-assn.org/ama/pub/category/10931.html

McTigue KM, et al: Screening and interventions for obesity in adults: Summary of the evidence for the U.S. Preventive Services Task Force. Annals of Internal Medicine 139:933, 2003.

National Heart, Lung, and Blood Institute (NHLBI) and North American Association for the Study of Obesity (NAASO). Practical guide to identification, evaluation, and treatment of overweight and obesity in adults. Bethesda, MD: National Institutes of Health, NIH Pub. 00-4084, Oct. 2000.

National Heart, Lung, and Blood Institute (NHLBI). Clinical guidelines on the identification, evaluation, and treatment of overweight and obesity in adults. The evidence report. Obesity Research 6:51S, 1998.

Padwal R, Li SK, Lau DCW. Long-term pharmacotherapy for overweight and obesity: A systematic review and meta-analysis of randomized controlled trials. International Journal of Obesity 27:1437, 2003.

U.S. Preventive Services Task Force. Screening for obesity in adults: Recommendations and rationale. Annals of Internal Medicine 139:930, 2003.

Yanovski S, Yanovski JA: Obesity. New England Journal of Medicine 346:591, 2002.

Chapter Self-Test Questions

Circle the correct answer. After you have responded to the questions, check your answers in Appendix A.

1. There is an association between obesity and which of the following?

a. Type 1 diabetes mellitus

b. Diabetes insipidus

    c. Polycystic ovarian syndrome

    d. Interstitial pulmonary fibrosis

2. There is an association between obesity and which cardiovascular disease?

    a. Hypertrophic cardiomyopathy

    b. Pulmonic stenosis

    c. Rheumatic valvular disease

    d. Myocardial infarction

3. A 60-year-old woman who was previously healthy presented with hematemesis. Subsequent testing demonstrated esophageal varices and hepatic cirrhosis. She admits to one to two glasses of wine in an average week and denies binge drinking. She denies taking any prescription or over-the-counter medicine. After her condition has been stabilized, her physical examination is notable for BMI 33 and normal ophthalmological, lung, and cardiovascular systems. Serum AST = 68 IU/L, ALT = 86 IU/L. TSH and iron results are normal. What is the most likely cause of cirrhosis in this patient?

    a. Obesity

    b. Chronic alcoholism despite her denial

    c. Chronic acetaminophen use despite her denial

    d. Hepatic atherosclerosis

 See the testbank CD for more self-test questions.

DIAGNOSIS AND MANAGEMENT OF AGE-RELATED CONDITIONS

26

WELL-CHILD VISIT

Janice A. Litza, MD, and Adam D. Rosenfeld, DO

I. Fundamentals of Well-Child Examination

A. The purpose of the examination is to assess the overall well-being of the child and child-family unit and to provide guidance how the family can stimulate the physical and mental growth of the child. Most of the time the child is well, and physicians provide reassurance to the parents. Visit schedules are set according to major age groups and comprise the following.

1. *Newborn:* within 1–2 weeks of birth
2. *Infant:* at 2, 4, 6, 9, and 12 months

3. *Toddler:* at 12, 15, and 18 months; 2 and 3 years old
4. *Preschool:* annual visits beginning at 3 years old
5. *Elementary school age:* annual visits 5 through 10 years old
6. *Middle school age:* annual visits 10 through 13 years old
7. *Teenager:* annual visits 13 through 18 years old

B. Each examination should include a review of the medical history and assess family dynamics.
1. Any parental and child concerns that begin at school age and allow opportunity to interact and build trust with the child
2. Review of *interval medical problems* (active, chronic, resolved)
3. Urgent-care history versus well-child examination history

> Many young children just starting in day care or school have numerous colds with frequent urgent-care examinations and need to be monitored for more serious underlying issues. Urgent-care examinations do not substitute for well-child examinations.

4. Review of *medications* and supplements, including vitamins and over-the-counter medications that can cause serious injury to children if not used correctly.
5. *Birth history*

> Birth history and key highlights should be documented in past medical history for review and assessed in any new patient.

   a. Birth history should include:
      i. Prenatal course
      ii. Labor and delivery method (cesarean section, normal spontaneous vaginal delivery [NSVD], instrument-assisted delivery)
      iii. Gestational age (full term/preterm)
      iv. Birth weight
      v. Apgar scores (low numbers indicate there may have been problems at birth, which parents were not aware of or forgot after a couple of years, at a time when development may be lagging as a first indication of birth trauma)
      vi. Bonding: postpartum depression, substance use, sibling rivalry

6. *Family history:* can be very dynamic and must be updated every examination; includes family history of genetic abnormalities

7. *Immunization history:* for timing, appropriateness, and assessment of any reactions or refusal of any immunizations
8. *Social history* and *home environment:* parent involvement with child including marital status, who lives in the home, other adults who spend time interacting with child (grandparents, aunts, uncles, step-family, siblings, day care, babysitters), day-care/babysitter/school information, passive exposure to smoking, lead potential in very old houses, peeling paint, fire and carbon monoxide alarms present and working, neighborhood safety
C. Examine physical characteristics for possible disease, developmental assessment, appropriate growth, and abuse concerns.
  1. Development divided into milestones in a few key areas; important to review these milestones to ensure child progressing and that appropriate anticipatory guidance according to the child's developmental stage being provided
   a. Motor
   b. Cognitive
   c. Language
   d. Social and emotional
  2. Observation: parent-child interactions, appropriate behavior toward physician, activity with toys and items in examination room
  3. Build trust: playfully including child in discussion early on or using a book to build trust (critical for ease of physical examination)

> As with any other patient, examining in the easiest and least invasive areas first and finishing with the most invasive or uncomfortable is key (may vary).

D. All well-child examinations have anticipatory guidance packed into them. It is best done while taking history and performing the examination. Otherwise, parents and children will not remember a "checklist" of what to do and what not to do. Use any opportunity to reinforce positive parental and child behaviors, and frame a few key other areas around safety and normal development of the child.
E. One mechanism for remembering general areas for well-child examination is the mnemonic SNASI (safety, nutrition, activity, socialization, immunizations). Document a few key points of discussion so that following examinations can build on what was discussed previously.

The SNASI areas of anticipatory guidance are safety, nutrition, activity, socialization, and immunizations.

F. Immunizations are often the dreaded part of well-child examination for parents and children. See full immunization schedule, and use Centers for Disease Control as updated source for immunizations. The schedule can be downloaded into a hand-held device. Review possible immunization reactions.

II. Age-Specific Examination Guidelines

A. Newborn and infant examinations

1. In the first year of life, major transitions are made along all of the developmental milestones, and much opportunity exists to educate parents on nurturing their child and keeping the child safe. Most parental concerns center around nutrition, elimination, and socialization. Most critical times for changes in family dynamics and home environment and child's well-being depend on the well-being and functioning of the caregivers. Leading causes of death in this age group are suffocation, motor vehicle accidents, and homicide.

B. 2-month examination

1. Common parental concerns: nutrition: starting solids (not yet), breastfeeding, spitting up; parent(s) returning to work; crying responsiveness—let cry or pick up (pick up); assessment of social/home environment: caregivers other than parents; focus on attention to growth curve and deviations from normal pattern; developmental milestones include *motor*—lifts head in prone, eyes follow past midline and fix on objects, pulls to sit with head lag; *social*—smiles responsively, consoled by being held; and *language*—listens and responds when speaker is quiet, coos

2. Anticipatory guidance

   a. *Safety:*
   i. Incorrect use of child safety seats accounting for many deaths at this age

 Stress car-seat safety: rear-facing in middle of back seat (can turn car seat around when baby is 20 pounds).

   ii. Fall protection: infant beginning to roll and move
   iii. Choking hazard: remove objects smaller than 1 inch or with small parts; no ribbons or string to attach pacifier to child

ⁱᵛ· Sleeping safety

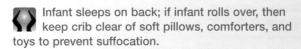 Infant sleeps on back; if infant rolls over, then keep crib clear of soft pillows, comforters, and toys to prevent suffocation.

ᵛ· Burn caution: infant begins to grab for things, including cups that may contain hot liquid

b. *Nutrition:*

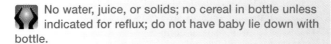 No water, juice, or solids; no cereal in bottle unless indicated for reflux; do not have baby lie down with bottle.

ⁱ· Stools: normal stooling pattern; will push with bowel movements; less frequent with formula-fed infants; stool usually yellow and liquid in exclusively breast-fed infants; stress the wide range of normal bowel habits in infants; constipation—stool is small-caliber and hard; cries with bowel movement; anal fissures present

c. *Activity:*

ⁱ· Encourage "tummy time" while awake; infant sleeps most of night except for one or two feedings. Parents have been so compliant with placing their children on their backs to prevent sudden infant death syndrome (SIDS), they fail to place the child on its stomach when awake, which leads to developmental delays in upper body and neck strength.

d. *Social:*

ⁱ· Cuddling/holding and talking encourages bonding and does not spoil the baby.

ⁱⁱ· Respond to crying promptly to provide reassurance to infant. Crying will decrease in time as infant knows needs will be met quickly. Maximum hours of crying per day occur at 6 weeks and coincide with incidence of shaken baby syndrome.

Prevent shaken baby syndrome by advising parents and caregivers that, when they become frustrated, it is safest to place child gently in a safe place and walk away to call for help or take a break until they are calm.

iii. Assess signs of postpartum depression that may affect bonding negatively.

    e. *Immunizations:*

      i. Inactivated polio vaccine (IPV); hepatitis B (Hep B) No. 2; pneumococcal; *Haemophilus influenzae* type b (Hib); diphtheria, tetanus, and pertussis (DTaP); rotavirus

C. 4-month examination

  1. Development

    a. *Motor:* pulls to sit without head lag, holds rattle, lets go of objects, rolls over, bears some weight on legs

    b. *Social:* regards strangers with interest, laughs and smiles, initiates social contact

    c. *Cognitive:* stares at own hand, crumples paper happily

    d. *Language:* recognizes sounds such as parents' voices

  2. Anticipatory guidance

    a. *Safety:* rear-facing car seat, small object caution, child more mobile and can get under furniture, keep cords from window blinds and appliances high and wrapped up

    b. *Nutrition:*

 Child can begin solids with rice cereal mixed with milk in bowl with spoon.

      i. First tooth may show up; Tylenol and chew toys best for discomfort (can have fever with teething)

    c. *Activity:* floor time important; cannot spoil child by responding to basic needs when crying; lie down to sleep when drowsy, not asleep to develop routine; child sleeps all night; parents may want to start childproofing house

    d. *Social:* child enjoys people and being talked to, music, cuddling

    e. *Immunizations:* DTaP No. 2, IPV No. 2, pneumococcal No. 2, Hib No. 2, rotavirus No. 2; Hep B may be extra dose in combination vaccine, but not required

D. 6-month examination

  1. Development

    a. *Motor:* raking grasp with fingers, passes cube from hand to hand, will grab book with two hands and put in mouth, pulls to sit with head forward, turns head to localize sounds

    b. *Cognitive:* looks for fallen objects, more attentive to surroundings

    c. *Language:* babbles, smiles at other babies and familiar things in books

2. Anticipatory guidance
  a. *Safety:* outlets need covers; poisonous substances, including medications, locked away; car seat may be facing front in back seat if child heavier than 20 lbs; child starting to crawl and pull up on furniture; keep stairs blocked, secure furniture, and put objects higher on shelves or away
  b. *Nutrition:*
    i. Introduce new solid every 3 days to assess for intolerance allergies

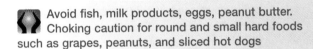 Avoid fish, milk products, eggs, peanut butter. Choking caution for round and small hard foods such as grapes, peanuts, and sliced hot dogs

    ii. Meats at 7–8 months; allow child to feed self with hands and begin to use spoon; introduce cup
    iii. Brush or clean teeth with washcloth (fluoride if needed)
  c. *Activity:* child should be sitting up; crawling begins; enjoys books and listening to reading
  d. *Socialization:* begin routine for bedtime and anticipate beginning of separation anxiety
  e. *Immunizations:* DTaP No. 3, IPV No. 3, Hep B No. 3, pneumococcal No. 3, Hib No. 3, rotavirus No. 3, consider flu shot if in season
E. 9-month examination
  1. Development/examination
    a. *Motor:* thumb-finger or pincer grasp, grabs items efficiently, crawls, pulls to stand, sits without support
    b. *Cognitive:* inspects object, puts things in mouth, bangs cubes, looks for hidden object
    c. *Language:* babbles, begins "mama/dada" sounds
    d. *Social:* plays "peek-a-boo" and "pat-a-cake"; shy with strangers
  2. Anticipatory guidance
    a. *Safety:* keep in car seat at all times; electrical outlet and cord cautions; can strangle self with cords

 Do not leave child alone in bath, near toilet, or pool.

    b. *Nutrition:* child should eat meals with family; supplement with milk in cup and occasional bottle; transition continues to cup; some decrease in appetite is normal; assure adequate growth on pediatric growth charts; brush teeth, no bottle or cup in bed to avoid dental caries; minimal juice

    c. *Activity:* continue to establish bedtime routine; child more mobile so needs constant supervision, enjoys simple games

    d. *Socialization:* stranger anxiety; separation anxiety; use books for language development; talks frequently throughout the day

    e. *Immunizations:* usually none unless needed for catch-up; flu shot second dose during flu season (4 weeks after first dose)

  3. Toddler years: ages 1 to 3 years. child is more mobile, fearlessly curious, independent with increasing language skills; most parental concerns center around speech development and discipline; conflict frequent between toddlers and parents over picky eating, bedtime, and toileting; leading safety issues and causes of death include motor vehicle accidents, drowning, burns

F. 12-month examination

  1. Development

    a. *Motor/examination:* intoe-ing, either as a result of femoral anteversion, tibial torsion, or metatarsus adductus is common; normal bruising of shins with active children; first steps; stands alone

    b. *Cognitive:* looks for hidden objects

    c. *Language:* first words in addition to "mama/dada" and jargoning

    d. *Social:* consolable; explores present environment under parental observation

 Red flag: if no pointing, babbling, other gestures by 12 months: consider autistic spectrum disorder.

  2. Anticipatory guidance

    a. *Safety:* street safety, electrical cord, water safety—no buckets of water; small pools; bath time alone; burns—keep bath water at 100 degrees and water thermostat at 120 degrees; choking—small objects and food caution; lower crib mattress; child requires constant supervision

    b. *Nutrition:*

 Phase out bottle by using for water only; everything else in cup.

    c. *Activity:* enjoys outside playground; gauge activities to temperament and plan for transition to quieter activities; naps two or three times a day

    d. *Socialization:* positive reinforcement; books along with familiar objects; will want same book read repeatedly

    e. *Immunizations:* MMR No. 1, varicella No. 1, Hib No. 4, pneumococcal No. 4, annual flu shot

        i. Lead and Hgb/hematocrit screens for high-risk populations

G. 15- and 18-month examinations

  1. Development/examination

    a. *Motor:* walks well, scribbles spontaneously, rolls ball, by 18 months can walk up steps and backward, stacks two cubes

    b. *Cognitive:* uses objects correctly in play; can point to body parts; works wind-up toys and on-off buttons

    c. *Language:* follows single-step command without gesture; has at least one word; by 18 months should have six words, not echolalic, and indicates desired objects with index finger

    d. *Social:* "reads" parents' expressions; uses "feeling" words (sad, happy, scared)

 Red flag: if no single words by 16 months: consider autism spectrum disorder.

  2. Anticipatory guidance

    a. *Safety:* car seat, water/electrical safety, poisons

    b. *Nutrition:* variety of healthy foods offered at meals; fruits/vegetables that are favorite at most meals

    c. *Activity:* more advanced toys such as riding cars; naps once or twice per day; enjoys books and points to objects

 No television recommended under 2 years old.

    d. *Socialization:* substitution of activities and praise for discipline; limited choices reduce power struggles

    e. *Immunizations:* DTaP No. 4, annual flu shot

H. 2-year examination

  1. Development

    a. *Motor:* walks backward and up and down steps independently; copies a circle by 30 months, kicks ball

    b. *Social:* may be clingy (normal); dresses self mostly, with supervision

    c. *Cognitive:* can substitute one thing for another in play; combines play actions (rocks doll and puts to bed) by 30 months; wants same books over and over

    d. *Language:* two-word phrases, vocabulary of 20 words, points to at least one body part, names several body parts by 30 months, follows two-prepositional commands with block (behind, under, next to, in)

 Red flag: if no two-word spontaneous phrases by 24 months of age: consider autism spectrum disorder.

Red flag: loss of previously learned language or social skills at any age: consider autism spectrum disorder.

  2. Anticipatory guidance

    a. *Safety:* discipline—pick "battles" carefully to minimize power struggles; respond directly and in timely manner to undesired behavior; may still distract or substitute activity unless unsafe, then need to clarify why activity unsafe

    b. *Nutrition:* all types of solid foods with an abundance of foods containing calcium

    c. *Activity:*

 Toilet training: do not rush the toddler! Positive reinforcement is the key.

    d. *Socialization:* parents should ask questions and interact with books and relate stories to child's life

    e. *Immunizations:* review and annual flu shot; lead and hematocrit screenings for high-risk population

I. Preschool-age (3- to 5-year-old) examinations

  1. Child fine-tuning early skills in all areas of development; speech development most critical and often area of concern for parents; age for toilet training if not already accomplished.

  2. Development

    a. *Motor:*

      i. 3-year-old: jumps with both feet off floor, stacks tower, mature crayon grasp, holds book without help

      ii. 4-year-old: balances on one foot for 4–5 seconds, copies the "equal sign =," makes three-part or more person, turns book pages one at a time

     iii. 5-year-old: balances on one foot for 5–10 seconds, copies square and triangle

  b. *Social:*

       i. 3-year-old: separates more easily from caregivers; on average, diapers dry all night; sits for 5-minute story or longer

      ii. 4-year-old: understands taking turns; uses words, not hitting; retells familiar story; makes up "tall tale"

     iii. 5-year-old: plays well with group of children; dresses with little help

  c. *Cognitive:*

       i. 3-year-old: plays out familiar events and changes outcomes; duplicates simple actions

      ii. 4-year-old: talks for doll and assigns roll to other children in play; pretends to read and write

     iii. 5-year-old: plays out imaginary scripts (e.g., space voyage); understands simple concepts: "If I cut an apple in half, how many pieces will I have?" "What do you do to make water boil?" "Candy and ice cream are both good to ____?"

  d. *Language:*

       i. 3-year-old: forms three- or four-word sentences; speech easily understood; gives full name; knows "cold," "tired," "hungry"; likes rhymes and nonsense words

      ii. 4-year-old: forms sentences with mostly correct grammar; asks questions

     iii. 5-year-old: correct use of "me" and "I"; uses past tense and plurals

3. Anticipatory guidance

  a. *Safety:* water safety, seat belts

  b. *Nutrition:* bedwetting common and accidents still occur and can escalate as a response to stress or change in home environment (e.g., new sibling) but generally resolves by 12 years; picky eating—parents advised to continue to offer healthy choices and can be creative to offer fruits with dinner if needed versus giving in to junk food

  c. *Activity:* encourage imaginative and interactive play; books important for beginning letter recognition and writing

Television time should be less than 2 hours per day.

    d. *Socialization:* should be interacting with other children; parallel play lessens; preschool introduces routine, structure; will listen to reading up to 10–20 minutes; parents should ask "What will happen next?" and encourage story telling

    e. *Immunizations:* At 4 or 5 years, child needs booster shots for MMR, IPV, DtaP, and varicella; annual flu shot

J. Elementary-age (5- to 10-year-old) examinations

  1. Development

    a. *Motor:* walks backward heel to toe; begins sports/dance; copies diamond shape

    b. *Social:* plays rule-based games; has "best" friend; parents assess school performance and possible learning disabilities, ADHD.

    c. *Cognitive:*

      i. 6-year-old: Asks, e.g., how are peaches and plums alike? why do we wear shoes?; able to repeat 4-digit strings and calculate simple math

      ii. 7-year-old: repeats five digits forward and three digits backward; asks, e.g., how are a cat and a mouse alike? how are a penny and a nickel alike?; knows left and right; able to write and calculate simple math

      iii. 8-year-old: asks how similar things are alike and different (fish/boat, dime/nickel, book/video) and calculates more advanced math

      iv. 9–10-year-old: repeats four digits in reverse; gives names of the days of the week in reverse order; knows month order; simple recall of three objects; can tell time in minutes and hours

    d. *Language:*

      i. 6-year-old: fluency, names four or five things to eat or wear in 20 seconds; knows names of most letters and recognizes a few words; reads books aloud, early chapter books

      ii. 7-year-old: can read simple paragraph story and tell what happened in summary; spells three-letter words

      iii. 8-year-old: more spelling and comprehension of stories

  2. Anticipatory guidance

    a. *Safety:* protective gear, seat belts, water safety

    b. *Nutrition:*

Healthy food and beverage choices encouraged—limit "junk."

   c. *Activity:* television time maximum of 2 hours and includes all television/computer activity; organized sports

   d. *Socialization:* bullying assessment, school activities

   e. *Immunizations:* reviewed, annual flu shot

K. Preteen or middle-school-age (10- to 13-year-old) examinations

  1. Development

    a. *Motor/examination:* puberty changes begin; review Tanner staging; screen for obesity; menses (may not begin until 15 years old); acne

    b. *Cognitive:* assess school performance and for any learning difficulties

  2. Anticipatory guidance

    a. *Safety:* drowning risk, protective gear with sports

    b. *Nutrition:* tends to fall into junk-food habits, skips meals; needs healthy encouragement; preventive health screening considered especially for cholesterol and diabetes if overweight; increase calcium intake

 Eating disorders may begin to appear more clearly in this age group.

    c. *Activity:* begins to focus on a few sports and extracurricular activities in which excels

    d. *Socialization:* bullying: identify who might be object of bullying as well as teens who are bullying; provide counseling for intervention

 Discuss influence of drugs, alcohol, and sex. Easiest to ask when parent not in room. Begin in the context of their friends, and then assess their own feelings to peer pressure and if/how they respond. Discuss Internet safety.

    e. *Immunizations:* HPV series, annual flu shot

L. Teen (13- to 18-year-old) examinations

  1. Development at this age is physical, with puberty changes; address common concerns such as acne, menses, body's sexual responses, hormonal fluctuations that lead to emotional changes; struggles for independence yet needs the limit-setting and support of parents for protection from external influences; may struggle with body image, self-esteem, and peer pressure despite external appearances of confidence, school success, athletic ability, and social acceptance; fears should be assessed and normalized; parenting should have real-life consequences with responsibilities, goal setting, rules/limits, and rewards; calmness and consistency are critical for parents—engaging other adults in school, church, family for reinforcement is helpful.

2. Development
   a. *Motor/examination:* physical maturity and puberty; Tanner staging; sports physical examination separate from normal well-child and includes hernia and musculoskeletal examination
   b. *Cognitive:* School performance and career goals
3. Anticipatory guidance
   a. *Safety:* driving safety; high-risk behavior at various levels with sense of invincibility; leading cause of deaths in this group are motor vehicle accidents, drowning, suicide, and homicide; explore Internet safety and predator awareness; discuss sexual activity and diseases
   b. *Nutrition:* discuss junk food versus healthy habits for life-time, eating disorders, body image; consider screening for diabetes and cholesterol
   c. *Activity:* encourage activity of any kind to get teens away from television, Internet, gaming systems that are not physically interactive
   d. *Socialization:* assess for peer pressure, depression, coping mechanisms for stress, self-esteem issues for all teens and pressure for performance from parents and coaches; cutting, tattooing, piercing health hazards
   e. *Immunizations:* HPV, DTaP, meningococcal, annual flu shot

 MENTOR TIPS DIGEST

General Tips
- Many young children just starting in day care or school have numerous colds with frequent urgent-care examinations and need to be monitored for more serious underlying issues. Urgent-care examinations do not substitute for well-child examinations.

- Birth history and key highlights should be documented in past medical history for review and assessed in any new patient.
- As with any other patient, examining in the easiest and least invasive areas first and finishing with the most invasive or uncomfortable is key (may vary).
- The SNASI areas of anticipatory guidance are safety, nutrition, activity, socialization, and immunizations.

2-Month Examination
- Stress car-seat safety: rear-facing in middle of back seat (can turn car seat around when baby is 20 pounds).
- Infant sleeps on back; if infant rolls over, then keep crib clear of soft pillows, comforters, and toys to prevent suffocation.
- No water, juice, or solids; no cereal in bottle unless indicated for reflux; do not have baby lie down with bottle.
- Prevent shaken baby syndrome by advising parents and caregivers that, when they become frustrated, it is safest to place child gently in a safe place and walk away to call for help or take a break until they are calm.

4-Month Examination
- Child can begin solids with rice cereal mixed with milk in bowl with spoon.

6-Month Examination
- Avoid fish, milk products, eggs, peanut butter. Choking caution for round and small hard foods such as grapes, peanuts, and sliced hot dogs

9-Month Examination
- Do not leave child alone in bath, near toilet, or pool.

12-Month Examination
- Red flag: if no pointing, babbling, other gestures by 12 months: consider autistic spectrum disorder.
- Phase out bottle by using for water only; everything else in cup.

15- and 18-Month Examinations
- Red flag: if no single words by 16 months: consider autism spectrum disorder.
- No television recommended under 2 years old.

2-Year Examination
- Red flag: No two-word spontaneous phrases by 24 months of age: consider autism spectrum disorder.

- Red flag: Loss of previously learned language or social skills at any age: consider autism spectrum disorder.
- Toilet training: do not rush the toddler! Positive reinforcement is the key.

Preschool-Age (3- to 5-Year-Old) Examinations
- Television time should be less than 2 hours per day.

Elementary-Age (5- to 10-Year-Old) Examinations
- Healthy food and beverage choices encouraged—limit "junk."

Preteen or Middle-School-Age (10- to 13-Year-Old) Examinations
- Eating disorders may begin to appear more clearly in this age group.
- Discuss influence of drugs, alcohol, and sex. Easiest to ask when parent not in room. Begin in the context of their friends, and then assess their own feelings to peer pressure and if/how they respond. Discuss Internet safety.

Resources

American Academy of Family Physicians. www.aafp.org
  Specific articles on newborn examination and sports physical through AAFP journal articles.
American Academy of Family Physicians' Family Doctor. www.familydoctor.org
  Teen and parent information on a variety of anticipatory guidance topics.
Reach Out and Read (ROR). www.reachoutandread.org
  Developmental milestones and parent/patient handouts on language development and book use.
U.S. Centers for Disease Control and Prevention (CDC). www.cdc.gov
  Many tools available, including immunization chart, off-cycle timing.

Chapter Self-Test Questions

Circle the correct answer. After you have responded to the questions, check your answers in Appendix A.

1. A mother of a 9-month-old boy brings him in for an urgent examination for a respiratory infection. Chart review shows only urgent-care examinations. When you recommend that she bring him for a well-child examination, she asks why she cannot have the child's immunizations from the nurse to save on fees? What is an appropriate response?

a. Your practice policy requires well-child examinations yearly.

b. A concern about potential litigation requires well-child examinations.

c. You need to observe the child's activity and socialization development.

d. You need to assess for child abuse.

2. Which of the following is among the three most common mortality causes in the first year for a child in the United States?

a. Suffocation

b. Intussusception

c. Volvulus

d. Retinoblastoma

3. A 5-year-old child has a positive test screening for lead. Subsequent blood lead is high. Which of these environmental conditions would likely be responsible for this finding?

a. Both parents smoke cigarettes in the home.

b. The family lives in a high-rise apartment building in a smoggy city.

c. The family lives in a 100-year-old home undergoing extensive renovation.

d. The tap water in a suburban area has a municipal well for water supply.

See the testbank CD for more self-test questions.

27

FEVER IN CHILDREN

Karin G. Patterson, DO, and Sandra A. Pagan, MD, MPA

I. Definition
   A. No universally recognized definition of fever
   B. Consensus: fever is rectal temperature higher than 100.4°F (38°C)
   C. If temperature higher than 106°F: much higher risk of bacterial infection
   D. Fever of unknown origin (FUO): illness lasting more than 3 weeks with a temperature higher than 101°F and an uncertain diagnosis after a 1-week investigation in the hospital
   E. Fever without localizing signs (FWLS): brief febrile illness for which there are no localizing findings

II. Epidemiology
   A. Fever in children is common.

> Most children undergo evaluation for a febrile illness before age 3 years.

> Almost a third of pediatric outpatient visits are for fever.

III. Pathophysiology
   A. Generation of fever in response to hypothalamic stimuli, such as:
      1. Cutaneous vasoconstriction
      2. Skin temperature falls
      3. Cold receptors in the skin sense this as cold
   B. Defervescence: body temperature falls in response to:
      1. Cutaneous vasodilation
      2. Drenching sweats; typically terminate an episode of fever

C. Fever detrimental if:
  1. Convulsion risk

 In children, high fevers should be suppressed to prevent convulsions.

  2. Extreme hyperthermia (>108°F); may cause:
    a. Direct cellular damage (especially to vascular endothelium, brain, muscle, and heart; frequently associated with disseminated intravascular coagulation (DIC)
    b. Metabolic derangements (hypoxia, acidosis, hyperkalemia), which may further contribute to coma, seizures, arrhythmias, or hypotension.
  3. Body temperatures of 113°F uniformly lethal

IV. Differential Diagnosis
  A. Infectious

 Majority of fevers in children are due to an infectious cause.

  1. Viral (majority of infections): most are nonspecific, self-limiting illnesses
    a. Upper respiratory infection (croup, bronchiolitis, etc.); pharyngitis; otitis media; sinusitis; gastroenteritis; exanthem
  2. Bacterial
    a. Urinary tract infection (UTI); meningitis; pneumonia; sinusitis; cellulitis; otitis media; pelvic inflammatory disease; osteomyelitis

 UTI is the main source of bacterial infection among febrile infants and young children.

  B. Neoplasms
    1. Lymphoma, leukemia, renal cell carcinoma, atrial myxoma, metastases to bone or liver
  C. Collagen-vascular and other multisystem disease
    1. Juvenile rheumatoid arthritis (JRA), systemic lupus erythematosus (SLE), polyarteritis nodosa, Wegener granulomatosis, mixed connective tissue disease, sarcoidosis

D. Other

1. Appendicitis, noninfectious granulomatous diseases, inflammatory bowel disease, drug fever (especially to antibiotics), factitious fever, miscellaneous uncommon diseases (familial Mediterranean fever, Whipple disease), undiagnosed

V. History and Physical Examination

A. Should reveal diagnostic clues so that laboratory and study results may be used selectively

B. Assess host for vulnerability (immunocompromised) and for exposure (travel, drugs, sick contacts) (Table 27.1).

TABLE 27.1	Fever in Children: History and Physical Examination Clues		
System	**History: Assess for Localizing Symptoms**	**Physical: Assess for Focal Signs**	**Potential Diagnoses**
Vital Signs	Temperatures reported Heart racing Breathing history Urine output	Fever Tachycardia Tachypnea Hypotension Hypoxia	Need to incorporate vitals with other findings; important in determining "toxicity" of patients and hydration status
Head, ears, eyes, nose, throat	Headache Ear pain or drainage Eye pain or discharge Rhinorrhea Sinus tenderness Sore throat Toothache	Anterior oral ulcers Pharyngeal vesicles Tonsillary hypertrophy Pharyngeal erythema or exudates Tooth/gum abnormalities Salivary gland tenderness Strawberry tongue	Herpes simplex virus (HSV) gingivostomatitis Coxsackievirus Pharyngitis Dental abscess Kawasaki disease Mononucleosis Otitis media Sinusitis

Fever in Children: History and Physical Examination Clues (Continued)

System	History: Assess for Localizing Symptoms	Physical: Assess for Focal Signs	Potential Diagnoses
		Petechiae at junction of hard and soft palate Tympanic membrane with erythema or effusion, may be bulging Sinus tenderness with percussion, +transillumination	
Neck	Neck pain or stiffness Neck swelling or mass	Nuchal rigidity (Kernig Brudzinski signs) Lymphadenopathy Thyroid tenderness	Meningitis Pharyngitis, mononucleosis Thyroiditis
Respiratory	Cough Dyspnea Wheeze	Quality of cough Nasal flaring, retractions Rhonchi, rales, wheeze	Croup Bronchiolitis (+/− respiratory syncytial virus [RSV]) Pneumonia (bacterial or viral)
Cardiovascular	Dyspnea Chest pain	Murmur (?new) Pulses, capillary refill	Endocarditis Dehydration
Gastrointestinal	Vomiting Diarrhea	Organomegaly, masses	Gastroenteritis Appendicitis

(continued on page 380)

TABLE 27.1	Fever in Children: History and Physical Examination Clues (Continued)		
System	History: Assess for Localizing Symptoms	Physical: Assess for Focal Signs	Potential Diagnoses
	Abdominal pain	Tenderness, guarding, rebound Hernia	Strangulated, incarcerated hernia
Genitourinary	Dysuria Hematuria Flank pain Vaginal discharge Pelvic pain Testicular pain	CVA tenderness Female: cervical motion tenderness, abnormal discharge, adnexal tenderness Male: testicular pain, mass or color changes	Urinary tract infection Pyelonephritis Pelvic inflammatory disease Testicular torsion
Neurologic	Confusion Seizures	Focal deficits Alteration in consciousness (confusion, delirium, stupor)	Meningitis Encephalitis
Dermatologic	Rash Change in consistency Pruritis Painful lesions	Petechiae Pustular lesions Cellulitis Exanthem Erythema chronicum migrans Turgor	Meningococcemia Rocky Mountain spotted fever Gonococcemia *Staphylococcus* infection Viral Lyme disease Dehydration
Musculoskeletal	Joint or bone pain Trauma	Range of motion of joints involved Swelling or effusion of joints Strength, symmetry Bony deformities	Septic arthritis Osteomyelitis

VI. Diagnostic Evaluation

A. Overview

1. A thorough history and physical will typically uncover the obvious source of infection (e.g. otitis media, gastroenteritis, upper respiratory infection). However, 20% of febrile children have no apparent source of infection after history and physical examination.

 A small percentage of children with fever will have an occult serious bacterial infection (SBI), including bacteremia, urinary tract infection, occult pneumonia, or meningitis.

B. Diagnostic approach by age

 All temperatures should be taken rectally.

1. Neonates (0–28 days):
   a. 10%–20% of well-appearing neonates with a temperature 100.4°F (38°C) or higher have a serious bacterial infection.

    Clinical impression is not reliable in this age group.

    Rectal temperature 100.4°F(38°C) or higher requires a full septic workup.

   b. Workup includes hospitalization, blood culture, urine culture, lumbar puncture, and empiric antibiotics (Table 27.2) pending culture results.
2. Young infant (1–3 months):
   a. 7%–10% of young infants with temperature 100.4°F (38°C) or higher have SBI

   Clinical impression is not reliable in this age group.

   The diagnostic and clinical criteria in Table 27.3 are used to identify febrile young infants at low risk for SBI.

TABLE 27.2 Common Pediatric Infectious Sources of Fever*

Infection	Diagnostic Evaluation	Pathogens	Treatment
Gastroen-teritis	Basic metabolic panel → electrolyte imbalances Bloody diarrhea → stool culture, fecal leukocytes (*Campylobacter, Shigella, Yersinia,* or toxic strains of *Escherichia coli*) Winter → *Rotavirus* test of stool Stool culture for ova, parasites, *C. difficile* (if prolonged) Blood culture if clinical suspicion	Community-acquired: Viruses, *E. coli* *Salmonella* *Shigella* *Yersinia* *Campylobacter* Nosocomial: *C. difficile* (antibiotics use, immunocompromised, hospitalized)	Supportive **<6 mo, bacteremia, toxic or immunocompromised:** cefotaxime or ceftriaxone Ceftriaxone or oral cefixime **Bacteremia, extraintestinal infection, immunocompromised:** trimethoprim/ sulfamethoxazole (TMP/ SMX), aminoglycoside, cefotaxime, tetracycline (>8 y) Azithromycin or erythromycin Metronidazole

Common Pediatric Infectious Sources of Fever* (continued)

Infection	Diagnostic Evaluation	Pathogens	Treatment
Meningitis	Blood culture Lumbar puncture Urinalysis and urine culture	**Neonate:** Group B streptococci, *Enterobacter* (esp. *E. coli*), *Listeria* spp.	Ampicillin + cefotaxime (alternative: ampicillin + gentamycin)
		1–3 mo: GBS, *Streptococcus pneumoniae, Haemophilus influenzae, Neisseria meningitidis, Enterobacter* spp.	Ampicillin + cefotaxime
		>3 mo: *S. pneumoniae, N. meningitidis, H. influenzae,* neonatal pathogens	Cefotaxime or ceftriaxone (+ vancomycin for *S. pneumoniae* resistance)
Pneumonia	Chest radiograph: • Focal infiltrate → bacterial Bilateral diffuse infiltrates → atypical or viral Culture for influenza, RSV, or other viruses Blood culture if clinical suspicion	**Neonate:** *E. coli,* GBS, *Staphylococcus aureus, Listeria monocytogenes, Chlamydia trachomatis*	Ampicillin + gentamycin *or* ampicillin + cefotaxime
			Febrile → IV ceftriaxone or cefotaxime
		3 wk–4 mo: *S. pneumoniae, C. trachomatis,* virus	Erythromycin (alternative: oral azithromycin)
		6 wk–4yr: Lobar: *S. pneumoniae*	PO: amoxicillin (or clindamycin) IV: ceftriaxone or cefotaxime

(continued on page 384)

TABLE 27.2	Common Pediatric Infectious Sources of Fever* (Continued)		
Infection	Diagnostic Evaluation	Pathogens	Treatment
		Atypical: *Bordetella pertussis*	Macrolide (erythromycin, azithromycin, or clarithromycin)
		RSV	Supportive care: hydration +/− albuterol nebulizer +/− oxygen
		Influenza	In 36 h: > 1 yr, influenza A/B → oseltamivir >1 yr, influenza A → amantadine
		≥4 yr: Lobar: *S. pneumoniae*	PO: amoxicillin (or erythromycin) IV: ceftriaxone or cefotaxime + PO/IV macrolide
		Atypical: *Mycoplasma pneumoniae, Chlamydia pneumoniae*	Clarithromycin or azithromycin
		Influenza	Zanamir or oseltamivir (if onset of symptoms in 36 h)

Common Pediatric Infectious Sources of Fever* (continued)

Infection	Diagnostic Evaluation	Pathogens	Treatment
Pharyngitis	Monospot Rapid streptococcus → streptococcus culture if negative and high suspicion	Group A streptococci, group C and G streptococci Viral, mononucleosis	PO: penicillin VK IM: benzathine penicillin G × 1 Supportive
Urinary tract infection	Urinalysis and culture → elevated white blood cell count, nitrites, leukocyte esterase, bacteria, positive Gram stain	**Uncomplicated:** *E. coli, Proteus* spp., *Staphylococcus saprophyticus,* enterococci	PO: TMP/SMX IV: cefotaxime OR amp and gent
	CVA tenderness → computer tomography (CT) abdomen/ pelvis → pyelonephritis Blood culture (if clinical suspicion)	**Complicated** (immunocompromised/urinary tract): above + *Pseudomonas* spp.	Ampicillin + gentamycin, Zosyn, or Timentin

---

*CBC often helpful in most cases: WBC >15,000: increased risk of occult bacteremia

Left shift—increase in immature form of neutrophils (bands, myelocytes, metamyelocytes) or increased neutrophils → bacterial

Elevated lymphocytes → viral

Elevated eosinophils → parasitic, malignancy, allergic

*First follow management as recommended by age group

TABLE 27.3	
Fever at 1–3 Months: Low-Risk Criteria	
Diagnostic	**Clinical**
White blood cell (WBC) count 5000–15,000 and <1500 bands	Previously healthy
Normal urinalysis (<5 WBC/HPF on Gram-stain smear)	Nontoxic-appearing (negative for weak cry, irritability, inconsolability, poor perfusion, poor tone, decreased activity, lethargy, hypoventilation, hyperventilation)
When diarrhea present: <5 WBC/HPF in stool	No focal bacterial infection on examination (excluding otitis media)
When respiratory symptoms present: normal chest radiograph	No increased work of breathing

b. Deciding workup plan
  i. Most important:

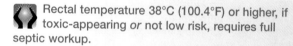

Rectal temperature 38°C (100.4°F) or higher, if toxic-appearing *or* not low risk, requires full septic workup.

   (1) Includes blood and urine culture, lumbar puncture, parenteral antibiotics (see Table 27.2).
  ii. Otherwise:
   (1) Rectal temperature 38°C (100.4°F) or higher, if nontoxic-appearing *and* low risk:
      (A) Blood and urine culture alone; follow outpatient within 24 hours *or*
      (B) Blood culture, urine culture, lumbar puncture, single dose of ceftriaxone 50 mg/kg IM in hospital; follow outpatient within 24 hours
3. Older infant or toddler (3–36 months):
  a. Fewer than 2% of well-appearing in age group with temperature higher than 39°C (102.2°F) manifest bacteremia

Clinical impression is reliable in this age group. Most have localizing sources of infection.

b. Deciding workup plan
  i. Toxic-appearing

Admit to the hospital for full septic workup.

  ii. Nontoxic appearing *and* temperature 39°C (102.2°F) or higher
    (1) Blood culture regardless of WBC count
    (2) Urine culture for males younger than 6 months or females younger than 2 years
    (3) Chest x-ray if respiratory symptoms involved
    (4) Stool culture, if blood and mucus in stool or 5 WBC/HPF or more in stool
    (5) Empiric antibiotics (after cultures) if temperature 39°C (102.2°F) or higher or if temperature 39°C or higher and WBC count 15,000 or more
    (6) Follow-up in 24–48 hours
  iii. Nontoxic-appearing *and* temperature lower than 39°C (102.2°F), follow clinically
  4. Children 3 years and older: an apparent source of infection usually present on history and physical examination; target diagnostic evaluation to findings

VII. Management
  A. Viral infection (most common): supportive care (e.g., hydration, antipyretics, supplemental oxygen, albuterol)

 Refer to Table 27.2 for most common infections, diagnoses, pathogens, and management.

  B. Management by age if no apparent source of infection (all temperatures taken **rectally**)

1. Neonates (0–28 days):
   a. Rectal temperature ≥ 38°C (100.4°F): hospitalization, blood culture, urine culture, lumbar puncture, and empiric antibiotics pending culture results

    Suggested empiric antibiotics are ampicillin and gentamicin *or* ampicillin and cefotaxime.

    Common pathogens are group B streptococcus, *E. coli,* other gram-negative rods and, less commonly, *Listeria monocytogenes.*

2. Young infant (1–3 months):
   a. Temperature higher than 38°C (100.4°F)
      i. Toxic-appearing *or* not low risk: admit for full sepsis workup
      ii. Nontoxic-appearing *and* low risk: may or may not give empiric antibiotics in hospital (ceftriaxone 50 mg/kg IM × 1); follow outpatient within 24 hours
3. Older infant or toddler (3–36 months):
   a. *S. pneumoniae* primary suspect

    In this age group, *S. pneumoniae* cause 90% of cases of occult bacteremia.

   b. Less common causes *N. meningitides, Salmonella,* and *H. influenza.*
   c. Toxic-appearing: admit to the hospital for full septic workup
   d. Nontoxic-appearing *and* temperature 39°C (102.2°F) or higher: diagnostics as preceding and empiric antibiotics (ceftriaxone 50 mg/kg IM × 1) regardless of WBC count; follow up in 24–48 hours
   e. Nontoxic-appearing *and* temperature 39°C (102.2°F) or lower: follow clinically and return in 48 hours if child febrile
4. Children 3 years and older: an apparent source of infection is usually present on history and physical examination (see Table 27.1)

MENTOR TIPS DIGEST

General Tips

- Most children undergo evaluation for a febrile illness before age 3 years.
- Almost a third of pediatric outpatient visits are for fever.
- In children, high fevers should be suppressed to prevent convulsions.
- Majority of fevers in children are due to an infectious cause.
- UTI is the main source of bacterial infection among febrile infants and young children.
- A small percentage of children with fever will have an occult serious bacterial infection (SBI), including bacteremia, urinary tract infection, occult pneumonia, or meningitis.
- All temperatures should be taken rectally.

Diagnosis in Neonates

- Clinical impression is not reliable in this age group.
- Rectal temperature higher than or 100.4°F (38°C) requires a full septic workup.

Diagnosis in Young Infants

- Clinical impression is not reliable in this age group.
- The diagnostic and clinical criteria in Table 27.3 are used to identify febrile young infants at low risk for SBI.
- Rectal temperature 38°C (100.4°F) or higher, if toxic-appearing *or* not low risk, requires full septic workup.

Diagnosis in Older Infant or Toddler

- Clinical impression is reliable in this age group. Most have localizing sources of infection.
- Admit to the hospital for full septic workup.

Management

- Refer to Table 27.2 for most common infections, diagnoses, pathogens, and management.
- In neonates, suggested empiric antibiotics are ampicillin and gentamicin *or* ampicillin and cefotaxime.
- In neonates, common pathogens are group B streptococcus, *E. coli,* other gram-negative rods and, less commonly, *Listeria monocytogenes*.
- In older infants or toddlers, *S. pneumoniae* cause 90% of cases of occult bacteremia.

Resources

Ahmed, S. et al. Evaluation and treatment of urinary tract infections in children. American Family Physician 57, 1998.

Alpern ER, Alessandrini EA, Bell LM, et al. Occult bacteremia from a pediatric emergency department: Current prevalence, time to detection, and outcome. Pediatrics 106:505–511, 2000.

Baraff LJ. Management of fever without source in infants and children. Annals of Emergency Medicine 36:602–614, 2000.

Baraff LJ, Bass JW, Fleisher GR, et al. Practice guideline for the management of infants and children to 36 months of age with fever without source. Pediatrics 92:1–12, 1993

Baskin MN. The prevalence of serious bacterial infections by age in febrile infants during the first 3 months of life. Pediatric Annals 22:462–466, 1993.

Chiu CH, Lin TY, Bullard MJ. Identification of febrile neonates unlikely to have bacterial infections. Pediatric Infectious Disease Journal 16:59–63, 1997.

Jaskiewicz JA, McCarthy CA, Richardson AC, et al. Febrile infants at low risk for serious bacterial infection: An appraisal of the Rochester criteria and implications for management. Pediatrics 94:390–396, 1994.

Krauss BS, Harakal T, Fleisher GR. The spectrum and frequency of illness presenting to a pediatric emergency department. Pediatric Emergency Care 7:67–71, 1991.

Lee GM, Harper MB. Risk of bacteremia for febrile young children in the post-*Haemophilus influenzae* type B era. Archives of Pediatric Adolescent Medicine 152:624–628, 1998.

Lutfiyya, N, et al. Diagnosis and treatment of community-acquired pneumonia. American Family Physician 73, 2006.

See the testbank CD for self-test questions.

OTITIS MEDIA IN CHILDREN

Elizabeth Nguyen Kirchoff, DO, Christopher Varona, DO, and Joseph P. Gibes, MD

I. Infectious Versus Noninfectious Otitis Media
A. Otitis media (OM) can be divided into two categories:
   1. *Infectious:* suppurative or acute otitis media (AOM)—presence of symptoms of acute illness and signs of tympanic membrane (TM) under positive pressure (full or bulging)
   2. *Noninfectious:* nonsuppurative secretory OM, or otitis media with effusion (OME)

II. Anatomy and Function
A. Middle ear anatomy
   1. Delineated laterally by tympanic membrane (TM)
   2. TM attached to middle ears bones: ossicles
   3. Ossicles consist of malleus (most lateral, attached to TM), incus, and stapes
   4. Medial wall of middle ear consists largely of promontory of cochlea
   5. Within medial wall are round window and oval window (stapes footplate)
   6. Anterior wall contains petrous carotid artery, eustachian tube, semicanal of the tensor tympani muscle
B. Middle ear function
   1. To increase efficiency of sound energy transfer from surrounding air-filled environment to fluid-filled inner ear
   2. Sound pressure waves conducted from TM through ossicles to oval window (connected to the vestibule of inner ear)

   3. Two mechanisms of amplifying sound wave energy
      a. Difference in surface area of TM to stapes footplate
         (pressure = force/area)
      b. Difference in length of long process of malleus and incus
         provides mechanical lever that increases energy

III. Pathophysiology of AOM

 Usually AOM is preceded by an upper respiratory
infection (URI).

   A. Inflammation and secretions from URI cause occlusion of the
      eustachian tubes.
   B. Middle ear mucosa continues to absorb air as usual; air is not
      replaced because of occlusion of the eustachian tubes.

 Negative pressure created in the middle ear causes
serous fluid buildup.

 Serous fluid provides medium for bacterial or viral
growth.

   C. URI provides source of bacteria or viruses.

IV. Microbiology

 Most common bacteria are *Streptococcus pneumoniae*,
untypeable *Haemophilus*, influenza, and *Moraxella* spp.

   A. Other less common causes are *Mycoplasma* spp. and viruses.

V. Risk Factors

 Top three risk factors are: day care (predisposes to URI);
bottle feeding; and cigarette smoking in the house.

A. Other risk factors are:
1. Increased number of siblings in the house
2. Male gender
3. Cleft palate
4. Immunodeficiencies
    a. IgG subclass deficiencies
    b. AIDS
    c. Complement deficiencies
    d. Immunosuppression secondary to medications

VI. Epidemiology

A. Frequency
1. 50% of children have one episode prior to first birthday.
2. 80% of children have one episode prior to third birthday.

B. Age
1. Most common in children 6 months to 3 years; may be due to immunologic factors (lack of antibodies) and low angle of eustachian tubes in relation to nasopharynx
2. May occur in all age groups

C. Sex—males slightly more affected than females; unknown cause

D. Race
1. White Americans and Hispanics more susceptible than African Americans
2. Native Americans and Inuit Indians at higher risk

VII. Examining the Ear

A. Otoscope—can use regular otoscope and/or pneumatic

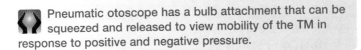

Pneumatic otoscope has a bulb attachment that can be squeezed and released to view mobility of the TM in response to positive and negative pressure.

1. Should have a properly sized speculum to permit seal in external auditory canal
2. Bright otoscopic illumination critical to adequately visualize TM
3. May require cerumen removal before examination (cerumen can limit visualization)
4. Particular attention should be paid to position and mobility of TM

VIII. Diagnosis

> A diagnosis of AOM must fulfill the following requirements: history of acute onset of signs and symptoms, presence of middle ear effusion (MEE), and signs and symptoms of middle ear inflammation.

A. Elements of preceding requirements
1. Recent or abrupt onset of signs and symptoms of middle ear inflammation and MEE
   a. Otalgia (pain, or pulling of ear in infant)
   b. Irritability in infant or toddler
   c. Otorrhea (drainage in ear)
   d. Fever
2. MEE—commonly confirmed by pneumatic otoscopy (must use a properly sized speculum to permit a seal in the external auditory canal); can be found in both AOM and OME
   a. Fullness or bulging of TM—highest predictive value for presence of MEE
   b. Air fluid level behind TM
   c. Limited or no mobility of TM—additional evidence of fluid in middle ear
   d. Otorrhea
3. Signs or symptoms of middle ear inflammation
   a. Distinct erythema of TM—must be distinguished from other elements that may cause redness of TM—crying, cerumen removal, fevers
   b. Distinct otalgia (discomfort) that interferes with regular activity or sleep
B. Typical TM findings
1. Color
   a. Normal is pearly gray
   b. Can have erythema from inflammation; must differentiate from redness caused by crying, fevers, or irritation from cerumen removal
   c. Abnormal whiteness; can be from scarring or fluid in middle ear

2. Contour
   a. Normal is slightly concave
   b. In AOM—can be full or bulging
   c. In OME—usually retracted or in neutral position
3. Translucence
   a. Normal is translucent
   b. Opacity commonly from underlying MEE
      i. Can sometimes reflect scarring
4. Structural changes
   a. Scarring
   b. Perforation
   c. Retraction pockets
5. Mobility

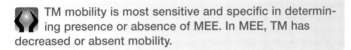 TM mobility is most sensitive and specific in determining presence or absence of MEE. In MEE, TM has decreased or absent mobility.

 Mobility is seen using pneumatic otoscopy.

C. Other tests that may assist with diagnosis of MEE
   1. Tympanometry
      a. Simple, rapid, atraumatic test
      b. Gives objective evidence of presence or absence of MEE
      c. Gives information about TM compliance in electroacoustic terms: basically equivalent to mobility of TM as visualized via pneumatic otoscopy
      d. Can be helpful in office with patients who are difficult to examine
      e. Can be used to confirm/refine/clarify otoscopic findings
      f. Can predict probability of MEE but cannot distinguish OME from AOM
   2. Acoustic reflectometry
      a. Small, portable; gives readings rapidly
      b. Estimates condition of middle ear by assessing response of TM to sound stimulus
      c. More limited than tympanometry
      d. Can predict probability of MEE but cannot distinguish OME from AOM

IX. Management

A. Definitions

 Severe illness is defined here as moderate to severe otalgia or temperature higher than 102°F (39°C) in past 24 hours.

 Nonsevere illness is defined here as mild otalgia and temperature lower than 102°F.

B. AOM

1. Antibiotic treatment

 For nonsevere illness, high-dose amoxicillin (80–90 mg/kg/day) is used.

a. Severe illness or amoxicillin failure: high-dose amoxicillin/ clavulanate (80–90 mg/kg/day of amoxicillin component)

b. Nonanaphylactic penicillin (PCN) allergy: cefdinir (14 mg/kg/day in one or two doses), cefpodoxime (10 mg/kg/day, once daily), cefuroxime (30 mg/kg/day in two divided doses)

c. Severe PCN allergy: azithromycin (multiple regimens available: one 30mg/kg dose; or 10 mg/kg every day for 3 days; or 10 mg/kg on first day, followed by 5 mg/kg daily on second through fifth days) or clarithromycin (7.5 mg/kg twice daily)

d. Unable to tolerate oral: ceftriaxone 50 mg/kg IM once

e. Other options: erythromycin-sulfisoxazole (50 mg/kg/day of erythromycin) or sulfamethoxazole-trimethoprim (10 mg/kg/ day of trimethoprim)

f. Alternative therapy for PCN-allergic patient being treated for infection known or presumed to be caused by PCN-resistant *S. pneumoniae:* clindamycin (30–40 mg/kg/day in three divided doses)

2. Observation: period of watchful waiting with close clinical follow-up; Association of American Physicians (AAP) and American Academy of Family Physicians (AAFP) guidelines

a. Acceptable for children 6 months to 2 years old with nonsevere symptoms (see below) *and* uncertain diagnosis

    b. Acceptable for older children with nonsevere symptoms, regardless of certainty of diagnosis

 Observation is an appropriate option only when follow-up can be ensured and antibacterial agents started if symptoms persist or worsen.

    c. Strategies for monitoring children being managed with initial observation include parent-initiated visit and/or phone contact for worsening condition or no improvement at 48–72 hours, a scheduled follow-up appointment in 48–72 hours, routine follow-up phone contact, or use of a safety-net antibiotic prescription to be filled if illness does not improve in 48–72 hours

3. Pain management: for all children with pain whether or not antibiotics are prescribed

    a. Acetaminophen: 10–15 mg/kg every 4–6 hours

    b. Ibuprofen: 5–10 mg/kg every 6–8 hours

C. OME

 In OME, antibiotics, steroids, antihistamines/decongestants, and mucolytics afford no long-term benefit.

1. Surgery for persistent OME should be reserved for children with significant hearing loss, persistent symptoms, risk factors for developmental difficulties, or structural damage to the tympanic membrane or middle ear.

2. Antibiotics, with or without steroids, can be considered if the parents or caregivers are strongly opposed to surgery.

MENTOR TIPS DIGEST

• Usually AOM is preceded by a URI.
• Negative pressure created in the middle ear causes serous fluid buildup.
• Serous fluid provides medium for bacterial or viral growth.

- Most common bacteria are *S. pneumococcus,* untypeable *Haemophilus,* influenza, and *Moraxella.*
- Top three risk factors are: day care (predisposes to URI); bottle feeding; and cigarette smoking in the house.
- Pneumatic otoscope has a bulb attachment that can be squeezed and released to view mobility of the TM in response to positive and negative pressure.
- A diagnosis of AOM must fulfill the following requirements: history of acute onset of signs and symptoms, presence of middle ear effusion (MEE), and signs and symptoms of middle ear inflammation.
- TM mobility is most sensitive and specific in determining presence or absence of MEE. In MEE, TM has decreased or absent mobility.
- Mobility is seen using pneumatic otoscopy.
- Severe illness is defined here as moderate to severe otalgia or temperature higher than 102°F (39°C) in past 24 hours.
- Nonsevere illness is defined here as mild otalgia and temperature lower than 102°F.
- For nonsevere illness, high-dose amoxicillin (80–90 mg/kg/day) is used.
- Observation is an appropriate option only when follow-up can be ensured and antibacterial agents started if symptoms persist or worsen.
- In OME, antibiotics, steroids, antihistamines/decongestants, and mucolytics afford no long-term benefit.

Resources

Paradise, JL. Otitis media. In Behrman RE, et al (eds): Nelson Textbook of Pediatrics, 17th ed. WB Saunders, 2004.

Pichichero, ME. Acute otitis media: Improving diagnostic accuracy. American Family Physician 61:1990–1992, 2000.

Subcommittee on Management of Acute Otitis Media. Diagnosis and management of acute otitis media: Clinical practice guideline. Pediatrics 113: 1451–1465, 2004.

Chapter Self-Test Questions

Circle the correct answer. After you have responded to the questions, check your answers in Appendix A.

1. What is the usual cause of suppurative acute otitis media?

   a. Exacerbation of chronic bacterial otitis media

   b. Complication of antecedent viral upper respiratory infection

   c. Tympanic membrane trauma from cotton-tip swab

   d. Primary bacterial infection acquired from another person

2. How does bottle-feeding an infant affect risk of acquiring suppurative acute otitis media?

   a. No risk difference

   b. Increased risk compared with breastfed infants

   c. Decreased risk compared with breastfed infants

   d. Increased risk if bottle nipples are not sterile

3. During which of these ranges are children most at risk of acute otitis media?

   a. Younger than 6 months of age

   b. 6 months to 3 years of age

   c. 7–10 years of age

   d. Older than 10 years of age

See the testbank CD for more self-test questions.

29

GERIATRIC CONDITIONS

Gary J. Martin, MD, Martin S. Lipsky, MD, and Herbert Sier, MD

I. Overview

A. The aging of the population is a situation that physicians need to consider.

1. Most specialties will be caring for older patients.

2. Some of these tactics have been garnered from geriatric evaluation services. Many randomized trials have documented these approaches.

3. Box 29.1 lists issues that are routinely evaluated in geriatric evaluation programs. In addition to an appropriate history and physical, special assessments of home safety, cognition, advance directives, and social support are helpful.

BOX 29.1

Geriatric Programs: Issues for Evaluation

Thorough history, physical examination, and:
- Activities of daily living (e.g., bathroom, bathing, eating)
- Instrumental activities of daily living (e.g., shopping, checkbook)
- Mobility
- Advance directives
- Medications
- Social network/resources
- Cognition
- Affect
- Nutrition
- Environmental safety
- Alcohol use/abuse

B. Issues that are particularly helpful to address in the management of older patients are listed in Box 29.2. In general, optimizing the care for any chronic condition such as congestive heart failure and diabetes can often improve the overall functioning of the elderly patient.

1. Addressing issues such as vision, dental conditions, and hearing can often be neglected in routine practice and yet may be a major determinant of how a patient functions.
2. Medications have a tendency to be added and added, particularly for older patients. A careful reevaluation of everything a patient is taking and dosages from all providers (and on their own) needs to be done periodically.

 In the frail elderly, addressing home safety, social support, functional capacity, and special senses can have a high yield.

BOX 29.2
Geriatric Programs: Management Strategies

Address chronic conditions.
Identify the following:
- Sensory and cognitive impairments
- Dental conditions
- Polypharmacy
- Substance abuse—especially excessive alcohol intake
- Pain
- Depression
- Incontinence
- Social isolation
- Environmental hazards
- Caregiver stress

Advise patient about and help patient take steps toward the following:
- Health maintenance/vaccinations
- Nutrition
- Exercise
- Smoking cessation
- Advance directives

II. Assessment

A. As part of the functional assessment of an older patient, a number of areas can be addressed quickly.

1. Vision can be tested with a Jaeger card.

2. Hearing can be checked by whispering an easily asked question in each ear.

3. A brief range-of-motion test of the arms and legs can be performed.

4. Careful observation of a patient getting out of a chair and walking can be very enlightening. Patients who have difficulty walking should have a full neurologic and musculoskeletal evaluation and may benefit from physical therapy.

5. Basic questions include the following.

   a. "Do you often feel sad or depressed?"

   b. "Are you able to get out of bed yourself?"

   c. "Can you dress yourself?"

   d. "Can you make your own meals?"

   e. "Can you do your own shopping?"

   f. "Do you have trouble with stairs inside or outside of your home?"

   g. "Who would be able to help you in case of an illness or emergency?"

   h. "Are you losing weight?"

   i. "Have you fallen in the last year?"

   j. "Are you having any problems with your memory?"

6. Depending on the answers to the preceding questions, further evaluation may be warranted.

7. Inquire about urinary incontinence. For example, "Do you ever lose your urine and get wet?" Incontinence can lead to the institutionalization of a patient. Appropriate treatment may allow a patient to remain home.

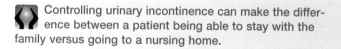

Controlling urinary incontinence can make the difference between a patient being able to stay with the family versus going to a nursing home.

B. The following syndromes are particularly relevant to older patients.

1. **Dementia** increases in frequency with age. It approaches 10%–20% in patients over 80 years of age.

    a. If there is any suspicion in an older patient, a full Mini-Mental Status Examination is recommended.

    b. There are several potentially reversible causes of dementia that can be pursued, including medications, metabolic abnormalities, and depression.

    c. Nonreversible causes of dementia include Alzheimer disease, vascular dementia, and Lewy body dementia.

    d. Treatment with drugs such as donepezil may be warranted in some patients, although the overall impact of these drugs is relatively modest.

2. Depression can present as dementia, and the two can be hard to separate at times in older patients.

    a. The Geriatric Depression Scale can be helpful in the initial evaluation of a patient suspected of depression (see Lachs, et al, 1990).

    b. If there is uncertainty, at times a therapeutic trial may be warranted or an evaluation by a psychiatrist familiar with geriatric evaluation.

3. Incontinence has the following profile.

    a. Incontinence can be divided into categories.

        i. *Stress incontinence,* which is leakage associated with intra-abdominal pressure such as coughing, laughing, or bending

        ii. *Urge incontinence,* which is usually associated with a precipitant urge to void

        iii. *Overflow incontinence,* which can be due to mechanical factors such as an enlarged prostate or less commonly to a contractile bladder

        iv. *Functional incontinence,* which is inability or unwillingness to get to a toilet or toilet substitute; can be due to a cognitive or physical functional impairment and, occasionally, a psychological factor such as depression, anger, or hostility

    b. After initial evaluation for incontinence, depending on the physician's knowledge and skills, it is usually helpful to address any potentially reversible conditions that contribute to urinary incontinence. If this is unsuccessful, then urologic consultation is generally warranted.

    c. Examples of some of the more readily treatable conditions include urinary tract infection, atrophic vaginitis, hyperglycemia, hypercalcemia, and fluid overload related to venous insufficiency with edema or congestive heart failure.

d. Drugs and side effects may contribute, such as short-acting diuretics. If the timing of these can be adjusted, this can also be helpful. As well, some patients may not realize that BID (twice a day) does not necessarily mean before bedtime for the second dose, that it may be appropriate for the second dose to be as early as 3:00 p.m. Many blood pressure medications and psychotropic drugs and other anticholinergics may be factors contributing to urinary problems.

e. For urge and stress urine incontinence, behavioral therapies are the first management strategies. Examples include bladder training and pelvic muscle exercise.

4. Iatrogenesis can be a significant issue.

a. Avoid hospitalizations whenever possible.

b. Forgoing surgery if surgical indications are marginal can avoid a downhill spiral for some patients.

> Ask whether any test or procedure will truly change the management of the patient in the context of the patient's overall condition and life expectancy.

c. Inappropriate prescribing of medications can be avoided by avoiding treating side effects of one medication with another.

d. Remember appropriate dosing in patients whose renal function is lower than their creatinine level as this may suggest age-related loss of muscle mass.

e. For hospitalized frail elderly patients, avoid sedative hypnotics, benzodiazepine, and medications with anticholinergic properties if possible.

5. Falls and gait disturbances have the following profile.

a. Falls and gait disturbances may need to be addressed, based on the patient's history or functional status assessment, including visual impairment; drug side effects causing orthostasis or vestibular disturbances; peripheral neuropathy; musculoskeletal diseases such as arthritis; foot disorders; central nervous system disease; and sedating medications including anxiolytics, sedatives, anticholinergics, and antidepressants.

b. Addressing these contributing factors as well as aggressive physical therapy to improve a patient's balance and walking can be very beneficial. Even small improvements in strength and balance can make the difference between falling and not falling. Use of assistive devices and footwear can be very helpful.

III. Other Important Concepts

A. Involving the aid of dentists, otologists, and ophthalmologists rather than depending on the patient to utilize these services is a necessary part of primary care.

B. Elder abuse and neglect are issues that must be addressed and in general reported to the appropriate state agency when identified.

C. Remember the nonspecific presentations of disease in the elderly. For example, myocardial infarction can present as sudden profound fatigue, and major infections can present with just a decline in functional status without a noticeable fever.

 MENTOR TIPS DIGEST

- In the frail elderly, addressing home safety, social support, functional capacity, and special senses can have a high yield.
- Controlling urinary incontinence can make the difference between a patient being able to stay with the family versus going to a nursing home.
- Ask whether any test or procedure will truly change the management of the patient in the context of the patient's overall condition and life expectancy.

Resources

American Geriatrics Society (AGS). Core competency. www.americangeriatrics.org/education/competency.html
Overview of what a panel of experts believes every medical student should know about geriatric issues.

Geldmacher DS, ed. Dementia update: Overview from the first annual dementia congress. Journal of the American Geriatric Society 51: S281–326, 2003.

Grossman H, Bergmann C, Parker S. Dementia: A brief overview. Mount Sinai Journal of Medicine 73:985–992, 2006.

Inouye SK. Delirium in older persons. New England Journal of Medicine 354:1157–1165, 2006.

Kane RL, Ouslander JG, Abrass IB, eds. Functional assessment. In Essentials of Clinical Geriatrics, 5th ed. New York, McGraw Hill, 2004, pp. 49–56.

Lachs MS, Feinstein AR, Cooney LM, et al. A simple procedure for general screening for functional disability in elderly patients. Annals of Internal Medicine 112:699–706, 1990.
An excellent overview of how to incorporate a comprehensive evaluation efficiently into an office visit. Includes the Mini-Mental State Examination and Geriatric Depression Scale.

Landefeld CS, Palmer RM, Kresevic DM, et al. A randomized trial of care in a hospital medical unit especially designed to improve the functional outcomes of acutely ill patients. New England Journal of Medicine 332:1338–1344, 1995.

Morley JE. Urinary incontinence and the community dwelling elder: A practical approach to diagnosis and management for the primary care geriatrician. Clinical Geriatric Medicine 20: 427–435, 2004.

Pogo Web site for medical students. www.POGO.org

Rubenstein LZ, Josephson KR, Wieland GD, et al. Effectiveness of a geriatric evaluation unit: A randomized trial. New England Journal of Medicine 311:1664–1670, 1984.

Tinetti ME. Preventing falls in elderly persons. New England Journal of Medicine 348:42–49, 2003.

Chapter Self-Test Questions

Circle the correct answer. After you have responded to the questions, check your answers in Appendix A.

1. In contrast to routine medical care of adults, geriatric assessments also include attention to which of these additional concerns?

    a. Tobacco use

    b. Living conditions, including stairs, floor coverings, and bathing facilities

    c. Screening for common malignancies

    d. Over-the-counter medication use

2. In periodic health assessment of elderly persons who deny visual complaints, what is the most appropriate way to evaluate visual acuity?

    a. Funduscopic examination

    b. Assess cranial nerves III, IV, and VI

   c. Jaeger or Snellen test

   d. Referral to ophthalmologist

3. Medical treatment can reverse which of these cognitive illnesses?

   a. Depression

   b. Alzheimer disease

   c. Lewy body disease

   d. Multiple vascular infarcts

See the testbank CD for more self-test questions.

five

WOMEN'S HEALTH

30

BENIGN BREAST DISEASE

Aparna Priyanath, MD

I. Introduction

A. Benign breast disease encompasses a heterogeneous group of disorders and conditions.

B. In the United States, approximately 16% of primary care office visits involved breast symptoms.

C. The clinical history is paramount in formulating a diagnosis in breast disease.

    1. Age

    2. Menopausal status

    3. Symptoms' relation to the menstrual cycle

    4. Quality and duration of pain

    5. Location of the symptoms

D. The diagnostic workup should include a thorough physical examination, breast imaging with mammography or ultrasound if necessary, and possibly a fine-needle aspiration or biopsy.

Women seeking an evaluation of breast symptoms often experience a great deal of anxiety. Therefore, it is often helpful to explain to the patient that the majority of benign breast diseases arise from cyclical changes within the ducts and lobules that occur throughout reproductive life.

 The palpation of a breast lump at any age warrants a workup.

Figure 30.1 is an algorithm for the evaluation of a palpable breast mass.

II. Fibrocystic Disease

A. Fibrocystic disease is a generalized term that has been used to describe benign, palpable thickening or nodularity in the breast tissue, which is usually associated with pain.

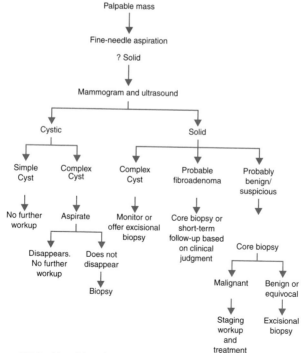

FIGURE 30.1 **Algorithm for the evaluation of a palpable breast mass.**

B. Variations in the texture of the breast may cause thickening or nodularity that is sometimes difficult to distinguish from a true mass.

> Areas of nodularity or thickening should be compared with the corresponding area of the other breast, as symmetrical changes are rarely pathologic. Often these changes fluctuate with the menstrual cycle.

C. A persistent asymmetrical area of breast tissue thickening or nodularity that is suspicious for a breast mass should prompt further evaluation.

D. The term "disease" is a misnomer as the majority of breast changes described by the term are physiologic.

E. The etiology of the changes referred to as fibrocystic disease is unknown, and clear risk factors have not been identified.

F. A clinically useful strategy, which is supported by the College of American Pathologists, classifies benign breast disease into strictly defined histologic groups (Table 30.1)

   1. Nonproliferative lesions

   2. Proliferative lesions without atypia

   3. Atypical hyperplasia, each associated with a different risk for developing subsequent cancer

> In the National Surgical Adjuvant Breast and Bowel Project P-1 Study, tamoxifen was found to reduce the 5-year risk of invasive breast cancer by 86% in women with a history of atypical hyperplasia. Recent results from the Study of Tamoxifen and Raloxifene showed similar benefits with raloxifene; however, there has not been United States Food and Drug Administration approval for this indication.

G. Thus, in women with a previous history of a benign breast biopsy, it is important to obtain histologic diagnosis and consider chemoprevention for those at higher risk of developing cancer.

H. Treatment is generally directed at the symptoms of mastalgia (see later). Although the avoidance of substances that contain methylxanthine, such as coffee, tea, cola, and chocolate, has been recommended by clinicians, there is no definite evidence that it offers a therapeutic benefit.

III. Breast Pain

   A. Breast pain, or mastalgia, is a common complaint in the primary care setting.

TABLE 30.1	Relative Risk (RR) of Breast Cancer Based on Benign Breast Disease Histological Categories (Nonproliferative Type)		
Nonproliferative	**Proliferative Without Atypia**	**Atypical Hyperplasia**	
Epithelial-related calcifications	Intraductal papilloma, sclerosing adenosis, moderate hyperplasias of the usual type	Atypical ductal or lobular hyperplasias	
RR = 1.0	RR = 1.3 (0.8–2.2)	RR = 4.3 (1.7–11.0)	

B. Mastalgia is more common in premenopausal than postmenopausal women and is rarely associated with breast cancer.

C. It is useful to consider the classification of breast pain based on its relationship to the menstrual period:

  1. Cyclic mastalgia—related to the onset of the menstrual period

   a. More common in younger women (younger than 35 years) and is often relieved after the menstrual period

   b. Usually bilateral, diffuse, and described as heaviness or soreness that radiates to the axilla or arm

   c. Usually begins 1–4 days prior to menses; however, in women who experience moderate-to-severe mastalgia, the duration can extend 5–14 days pre-menses

  2. Noncyclic mastalgia

   a. Most common in women in the 4th decade

   b. Unilateral, localized, and described as sharp or burning in quality

D. In cases of severe mastalgia, nodularity may be associated with the pain; however, the extent of mastalgia does not correlate with the amount of nodularity.

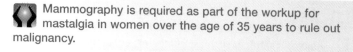

Mammography is required as part of the workup for mastalgia in women over the age of 35 years to rule out malignancy.

E. Treatment choices consist of the following.

  1. Nonsteroidal anti-inflammatory drugs (NSAIDs) are the first-line treatment of breast pain.

2. If NSAIDs fail, a trial of evening primrose oil or vitamin E may relieve breast pain, with little or no side effects.

IV. Breast Cysts

A. Cysts are a common cause of a dominant breast mass and are often difficult on physical examination to distinguish from a solid mass.

B. Ultrasound examination is used to distinguish between a cystic versus a solid lesion.

C. Cysts may fluctuate with the menstrual cycle and occur most frequently in perimenopausal women in their 40s.

D. In premenopausal women, fine-needle aspiration of the cyst should be performed. If the mass disappears and is nonbloody, no further evaluation is required. If the fluid is bloody or the palpable abnormality persists or recurs after multiple aspirations in a short time interval, a biopsy is required.

E. Cytologic examination of cystic fluid for malignancy provides little value.

V. Fibroadenomas

 Fibroadenomas are benign tumors occurring most frequently in women between the ages of 20 and 50 years.

A. Histologically, fibroadenomas display a considerable amount of morphologic variability and consist of a mixture of proliferated fibrous stroma and increased epithelial ductal structures.

B. These tumors are usually asymptomatic and are often found by either breast self-examination or incidentally during the clinical breast examination.

C. Fibroadenomas typically present as solitary masses but may be multiple in about 10%–15% of cases.

D. Classically, these tumors are smooth, nontender, discrete, and freely moveable.

1. They are usually 1–2 cm when detected and do not often increase in size beyond 2–3 cm.

2. A diagnosis based on clinical examination alone is accurate only 50%–73% of the time.

E. Ultrasound examination is disappointing as there is significant overlap in the ultrasonographic appearance of benign and malignant masses.

1. Because of the inadequacy of the examination and ultrasound alone in the diagnosis of fibroadenoma, many investigators advocate triple assessment with clinical examination, ultrasound, and aspiration with cytology.

 If the diagnosis of fibroadenoma cannot be established with certainty, excisional biopsy is the procedure of choice.

VI. Nipple Discharge

 Most nipple discharge is benign in origin.

A. Galactorrhea
   1. Milk or milk-like discharge from the breast
   2. Usually bilateral, spontaneous, or intermittent
   3. May be due to chronic breast stimulation
   4. Common drugs implicated include:
      a. Oral contraceptives
      b. Dopamine antagonists (methyldopa, phenothiazine)
   5. Laboratory evaluation should include:
      a. Pregnancy test
      b. Prolactin level
      c. Thyroid studies
B. Features associated with an increased risk of cancer include:
   1. Unilateral discharge
   2. Spontaneous appearance
   3. Bloody or guaiac-positive
   4. Association with a mass
   5. Patient older than 40 years
C. Physical examination
   1. Elicit discharge by massaging breast from periphery to center or applying warm compresses.
   2. Identify breast masses or lymphadenopathy.
   3. Determine skin color changes, nipple position, erythema, ulceration, or retraction of skin.

4. Observe the number of ducts involved.
   a. Flow from one duct is concerning for intraductal papilloma or intraductal breast carcinoma.
   b. Bilateral or multiductal discharge should be evaluated for endocrinological causes.
D. Diagnostic evaluation
   1. Guaiac tests
   2. Mammography
   3. Ductography or ductoscopy

MENTOR TIPS DIGEST

- Women seeking an evaluation of breast symptoms often experience a great deal of anxiety. Therefore, it is often helpful to explain to the patient that the majority of benign breast diseases arise from cyclical changes within the ducts and lobules that occur throughout reproductive life.
- The palpation of a breast lump at any age warrants a workup.
- Figure 30.1 is an algorithm for the evaluation of a palpable breast mass.
- Areas of nodularity or thickening should be compared with the corresponding area of the other breast, as symmetrical changes are rarely pathologic. Often these changes fluctuate with the menstrual cycle.
- In the National Surgical Adjuvant Breast and Bowel Project P-1 Study, tamoxifen was found to reduce the 5-year risk of invasive breast cancer by 86% in women with a history of atypical hyperplasia. Recent results from the Study of Tamoxifen and Raloxifene showed similar benefits with raloxifene; however, there has not been United States Food and Drug Administration approval for this indication.
- Mammography is required as part of the workup for mastalgia in women over the age of 35 years to rule out malignancy.
- Fibroadenomas are benign tumors occurring most frequently in women between the ages of 20 and 50 years.
- If the diagnosis of fibroadenoma cannot be established with certainty, excisional biopsy is the procedure of choice.
- Most nipple discharge is benign in origin.

Resources

Barton MB, Elmore JG, Fletcher SW. Breast symptoms among women enrolled in a health maintenance organization: Frequency, evaluation, and outcome. Annals of Internal Medicine 130:651–657, 1999.

Dupont WD, Parl FF, Hartman WH, et al. Breast cancer risk associated with proliferative breast disease and atypical hyperplasia. Cancer 71:1258, 1993.

Fisher B, Constantino JP, Wickerham DL, et al. Tamoxifen for prevention of breast cancer: Report of the National Surgical Adjuvant Breast and Bowel Project P-1 Study. Journal of the National Cancer Institute 90:1371–1388, 1998.

Hansen N, Morrow M. Breast disease. Medical Clinics of North America 82: 203–222, 1998.

Harris J, Lippman ME, Morrow M, et al. Diseases of the Breast, 2nd ed. Philadelphia, Lippincott Williams & Wilkins, 2000.

Vogel VG, Costantino JP, Wickerham DL, et al. Effects of tamoxifen vs raloxifene on the risk of developing invasive breast cancer and other disease outcomes: the NSABP Study of Tamoxifen and Raloxifene (STAR) P-2 Trial. Journal of the American Medical Association 295:2727–2741, 2006.

Chapter Self-Test Questions

Circle the correct answer. After you have responded to the questions, check your answers in Appendix A.

1. A 24-year-old woman found a lump in her right breast 2 days ago. The lump is mildly tender on palpation. She has no family history of breast cancer. Menarche was at age 13. Menses are regular; last menstrual period began 24 days ago. On examination, you feel a 2-cm tender firm nodule in the upper outer quadrant. The axillary examination result is negative. What is the next appropriate medical response?

   a. Reassurance that this is not malignant

   b. Reassurance that this is common; return for breast examination in 2 weeks

   c. Reassurance that this is common; return for breast examination in 3 months

   d. Diagnostic mammogram and ultrasound imaging

2. A 24-year-old woman found a lump in her right breast 2 weeks ago. The lump is mildly tender on palpation. She has no family history of breast cancer. Menarche was at age 13. Menses are regular; last menstrual period began 10 days ago. On examination 2 weeks ago, you felt a 2-cm tender firm nodule in the upper outer quadrant. The axillary examination result was negative. Examination now is unchanged. What is the next appropriate medical response?

   a. Diagnostic mammogram and ultrasound imaging

   b. Fine-needle aspiration of nodule

   c. Excisional or core biopsy of nodule

   d. Magnetic resonance image of right breast

3. A 35-year-old woman is your regular patient. While out of town, she felt a breast lump and consulted a physician. She reports that she promptly underwent needle aspiration of the mass and that the mass disappeared. She observed that the aspirated fluid was yellow and translucent. The other physician told her that nothing further would be necessary. She is a healthy mother of children ages 8 and 10 years. Menses are regular. She uses a diaphragm for contraception. On examination, you are unable to palpate any abnormality. What is the most appropriate response in answer to what intervention is necessary next?

   a. Tamoxifen 10 mg twice daily for 5 years

   b. Obtain previously aspirated fluid sample for cytologic examination

   c. Bilateral screening mammogram

   d. Reassurance and observation only

See the testbank CD for more self-test questions.

31

Preconception Care

Aarati D. Didwania, MD

I. Preconception Evaluation

A. **Complete medical history** should be taken, with particular attention paid to the presence of the following:
   1. Known medication allergies, particularly antibiotics
   2. Autoimmune disorders
   3. A history of blood transfusions and date at which each transfusion was received
   4. Breast disorders including history of biopsies and pathologies
   5. Cardiovascular conditions
   6. Domestic violence or other safety concerns at home or work
   7. Endocrine disorders
   8. Family history of any known hereditable disorders
   9. Gastrointestinal disease
   10. Hematologic disorders
   11. Kidney disease
   12. A list of all medications the patient is taking
       a. Prescription
       b. Over-the-counter
       c. Herbal or vitamin supplements
   13. Neurologic disorders
   14. Psychiatric disease
   15. Pulmonary disorders
   16. Substance abuse
   17. Surgical procedures

B. **Medications** can present teratogenic risk to the fetus. The list of medications in Box 31.1 includes common teratogens that need to be changed prior to conception. There is a risk/benefit ratio to consider when changing or discontinuing medications. If the

BOX 31.1
Common Teratogenic Medications

ACE inhibitors
Anticholinergic drugs
Antithyroid
Carbamazepine
Cyclophosphamide
Danazol
Hypoglycemic drugs
Lithium
Methotrexate
Misoprostol
Nonsteroidal anti-inflammatory drugs
Phenytoin
Psychoactive drugs
Systemic retinoids
Tetracycline
Thalidomide
Valproic acid
Warfarin

disease process cannot be controlled with a change in regimen, a decision may be needed on which risk to the fetus is greater—the risk posed by the medication or the risk posed by uncontrolled disease in the mother. This is a decision that should be made by a high-risk obstetrician.

 Consider the relative risks and benefits of each medication change.

   C. **Advanced maternal age,** defined as older than 35 years at the time of delivery, can affect pregnancy outcomes.
   1. Maternal age older than 35 years at time of delivery is associated with:
      a. Decrease in fecundity (ability to become pregnant) with advancing age
         i. 50% for women age 19–26 years
         ii. 40% for women age 27–34 years
         iii. 30% for women age 35–39 years

As a woman gets older, conception gets harder.

   b. Increased risk of spontaneous abortion due to decline in oocyte quality
   c. Increased risk of aneuploidy
   d. Coexisting medical conditions that can increase the risk of complications; risks further amplified in even older women; conditions such as hypertension and diabetes should be optimized
2. A medical assessment of women over the age of 35 years should include:
   a. Infertility evaluation if conception difficulty

 Do an infertility evaluation after 6 months if the woman is unable to become pregnant.

   b. Prenatal diagnosis via:
      i. Amniocentesis or chorionic villus sampling (CVS)
      ii. Maternal serum testing/nuchal translucency evaluation
   c. Diabetes screening
D. Substance use can affect pregnancy and fetal outcomes.

 Eliminate alcohol or tobacco for women who are planning to conceive. Suggest minimal caffeine use as well.

1. Tobacco use is associated with an increased risk of the following.
   a. Miscarriage
   b. Prematurity
   c. Low birth weight
2. Alcohol use can adversely affect pregnancy outcomes.
   a. Moderate intake is associated with subtle growth retardation and neurobehavioral effects.
   b. Fetal alcohol syndrome is associated with excessive alcohol use.
3. Caffeine content varies between products.

 More than 250 mg of caffeine per day is associated with a decrease in fertility.

More than 500 mg of caffeine per day is associated with an increase in spontaneous abortion.

E. A thorough physical examination should be performed and include the following.

1. Complete breast examination: symmetry, nipple morphology, palpable change in breast tissue, axillary adenopathy, skin changes
2. Cardiovascular examination including pulse, blood pressure, and rhythm assessment
3. Dental evaluation by a trained professional

 Dental disease is associated with a higher rate of premature birth and spontaneous abortion.

4. Pelvic examination with sexually transmitted illness (STI) screen
5. Thyroid evaluation for size and nodules

F. Laboratory evaluation should include the following.

1. Complete blood count (CBC) to assess for anemia
2. Rubella titer
3. Varicella titer
4. Hepatitis B surface antigen
5. HIV
6. Plasma glucose for patients at high-risk for diabetes

II. Specific Preconception Counseling

A. Optimizing maternal medical conditions
B. Promoting smoking cessation
C. Encouraging alcohol abstinence
D. Medication adjustment and assessment of disease process effects with a change in medication regimen

 Pseudoephedrine has the best safety record during pregnancy and is preferred over other decongestants.

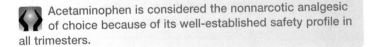 Acetaminophen is considered the nonnarcotic analgesic of choice because of its well-established safety profile in all trimesters.

    1. All medications are assigned a United States Food and Drug Association (FDA) pregnancy risk factor category. These categories are defined in Table 31.1.

E. Genetic counseling for those with heritable disorders

F. Nutritional evaluation and recommendations should include:

    1. Vitamins

 Recommend a multivitamin supplement with 400 mcg of folate to prevent neural tube defects.

    2. Vegetarian diet assessment for presence of essential amino acids and iron

    3. Avoidance of shark, swordfish, king mackerel, tuna steaks, or tilefish because of methylmercury exposure

    4. Recommend limiting caffeine consumption to less than 250 mg/day

G. Maintenance of regular exercise

 Advise women not to alter their regular exercise regimen.

H. Perform social service assessment for those at risk for domestic violence

I. Provide immunizations as needed

TABLE 31.1	FDA Pregnancy Risk Categories
Risk Category	**Profile**
A	Safety established using human studies
B	Presumed safe (animal studies)
C	Uncertain safety; animal studies show an adverse effect, no human studies
D	Unsafe; evidence of human fetal risk that may in certain clinical circumstances (i.e. life-threatening) be justifiable
X	Highly unsafe; risk of use outweighs any possible benefit

1. Influenza during flu season
2. Measles, mumps, rubella, tetanus, diphtheria, poliomyelitis, varicella

 Live viruses should be administered 1 month prior to conception.

    a. Varicella for those without previous clinical disease and negative titers
3. Hepatitis B for those at high risk

 MENTOR TIPS DIGEST

- Consider the relative risks and benefits of each medication change.
- As a woman gets older, conception gets harder.
- Do an infertility evaluation after 6 months if the woman is unable to become pregnant.
- Eliminate alcohol or tobacco for women who are planning to conceive. Suggest minimal caffeine use as well.
- More than 250 mg of caffeine per day is associated with a decrease in fertility.
- More than 500 mg of caffeine per day is associated with an increase in spontaneous abortion.
- Dental disease is associated with a higher rate of premature birth and spontaneous abortion.
- Pseudoephedrine has the best safety record during pregnancy and is preferred over other decongestants.
- Acetaminophen is considered the nonnarcotic analgesic of choice because of its well-established safety profile in all trimesters.
- Recommend a multivitamin supplement with 400 mcg of folate to prevent neural tube defects.
- Advise women not to alter their regular exercise regimen.
- Live viruses should be administered 1 month prior to conception.

Resources

Johnson K, Posner SF, Biermann J, et al. Recommendations to improve preconception health and health care: United States—Report of the CDC/ATSDR Preconception Care Work Group and the Select Panel on Preconception Care. MMWR 55:1, 2006.

Lee RV, Rosene-Montella K, Barbour LA, et al. Medical care of the pregnant patient. American College of Physicians Women's Health Series. Philadelphia, 2000.

Chapter Self-Test Questions

Circle the correct answer. After you have responded to the questions, check your answers in Appendix A.

1. Which of these antihypertensives should not be prescribed for women who may become pregnant?

    a. Ramipril

    b. Metoprolol

    c. Hydrochlorothiazide

    d. Alpha methyldopa

2. Which of these drugs is least likely to cause fetal complications when used by a pregnant woman who has type 2 diabetes mellitus?

    a. Metformin

    b. Pioglitazone

    c. Glyburide

    d. Insulin

3. A 39-year-old primigravida at 8 weeks gestation and with no medical history develops a swollen leg. Noninvasive vascular Doppler imaging shows a thrombosis extending to the mid-femoral vein.

Which of these is the most appropriate treatment to prevent pulmonary embolism?

a. Warfarin adjusted to INR 2–3 for pregnancy duration

b. Warfarin adjusted to INR 2–3 for 6 weeks

c. Low molecular weight heparin for pregnancy duration

d. Inferior vena cava filter

 See the testbank CD for more self-test questions.

32 CHAPTER

HORMONE REPLACEMENT THERAPY

Jennifer A. Bierman, MD

I. Background

A. Hormone replacement therapy (HRT) consists of estrogen and/or progestin.

B. HRT is often used for treatment of menopausal complaints.

> Vasomotor symptoms or hot flashes are among the most common menopausal complaints and occur in up to 80% of women during their menopause transition. Of these women, 20% have disabling symptoms.

C. In the past estrogen/progestin was routinely used also for the prevention of chronic diseases such as osteoporosis and coronary heart disease (CHD).

   1. This was based on observational studies showing a beneficial effect of estrogen on bone and heart health.

   2. Most physicians recommended HRT to all menopausal women for chronic disease prevention.

   3. More recent randomized controlled trials including the Women's Health Initiative (WHI) trial have refuted the long-term benefits of HRT and have shown an increased risk of some chronic diseases such as CHD and strokes (Tables 32.1 and 32.2).

   4. Media stories abounded making it confusing for patients who were on HRT or considering this therapy for the treatment of menopausal symptoms.

   5. The WHI trial was a landmark study and changed how physicians and patients viewed HRT.

TABLE 32.1
Risk-Benefit: Estrogen and Progestin

10,000 women taking estrogen and progestin for 1 year might experience:

Risks	Benefits
• 7 more CHD events • 8 more strokes • 8 more pulmonary emboli (PEs) and 10 more deep venous thromboses (DVTs) • 8 more invasive breast cancers	• 6 fewer colorectal cancer deaths • 5 fewer hip fractures • 6 fewer vertebral fractures

Data from Women's Health Initiative (WHI) trial

> HRT is still the most effective therapy for the treatment of hot flashes; however, it should no longer be used for chronic disease prevention.

II. Epidemiology and Diagnosis of Menopause

   A. Menopause is a component of natural process of aging

      1. Early menopause is associated with:

         a. Lower body weight

         b. Nulliparity

         c. Smoking

         d. Absence of oral contraceptive use

         e. Lower socioeconomic status

TABLE 32.2
Risk-Benefit: Estrogen Alone

10,000 women taking estrogen alone for 1 year might experience:

Risks	Benefits
• 12 more strokes • 3 more PEs and 4 more DVTs	• 6 fewer hip fractures • 6 fewer vertebral fractures

No difference in CHD, breast, or colon cancer

Data from Women's Health Initiative (WHI) trial

B. Diagnosis

 Menopause is diagnosed after 12 consecutive months of amenorrhea not associated with a physiologic (pregnancy/lactation) or pathologic cause.

 The median age is 50 years plus or minus 2 years.

1. A high follicle-stimulating hormone (FSH) level is often used but not essential for diagnosis.
2. Premature ovarian failure is cessation of menses in a woman in her 30s or early 40s.

III. Symptoms of Menopause
A. Vasomotor symptoms—often called *hot flashes* or *flushes*
 1. Described as a sudden sensation of intense heat with sweating and flushing typically lasting 4–6 minutes
 2. Onset typically occurs 6–12 months prior to menopause when periods may still be present although irregular

 80% of women are affected by hot flashes; 10%–20% have severe symptoms.

 a. Severity ranges from mild, i.e., several per week, to severe, with more than six per day.
 b. Surgical- or chemotherapy-induced menopause leads to higher incidence and severity of hot flashes.
 3. Risk factors for more severe hot flashes
 a. Higher body mass index (BMI)
 b. Little or no exercise
 c. Smoking
 d. Ethnicity
   i. African Americans have higher incidence than whites
   ii. Whites have a higher incidence than Asians
   iii. May be cultural differences with respect to reporting symptoms
   iv. Diet may play role

4. Natural history

 For most women, hot flashes last for about 1 year and then resolve spontaneously.

a. 50% of women have symptoms that last up to 4 years.
b. 10% of women have symptoms that last up to 12 years.
5. Pathophysiology
a. Exact mechanism unknown
b. Believed to be secondary to thermoregulatory dysfunction
B. Vaginal dryness and painful intercourse
1. Low estrogen levels are associated with cellular changes in the vaginal epithelium, resulting in atrophy of the tissues.
C. Sleep disturbances
1. Common in men and women as they age but tied to menopausal transition in women
2. Vasomotor symptoms often contribute to sleep disturbance
D. Mood symptoms
1. Depression and anxiety may occur at the time of menopause.
2. It has been difficult to establish whether menopause is the cause of these symptoms as mood changes are often of multifactorial origin.
3. There is very little evidence that treatment with HRT results in improvement of mood symptoms associated with menopause.
4. Cognitive disturbances, somatic complaints, sexual dysfunction, and quality of life have been linked to the menopausal transition, but the majority of studies show no association between the prevalence of these symptoms and menopausal status.
E. Most studies limited to reduction of frequency and severity of hot flashes; little evidence on reduction of other symptoms.

IV. Benefits of HRT (see Tables 32.1 and 32.2)

 HRT improves hot flashes in 80%–90% of women.

A. Vaginal dryness and painful intercourse are reduced.

B. Hip and vertebral fractures due to osteoporosis are reduced.

    1. However, there are more focused treatments for osteoporosis without the HRT-associated risks of CHD and stroke. HRT should not be used as first-line management for osteoporosis treatment or prevention.

C. Colorectal cancer deaths are reduced; however, given the risks, HRT currently does not have a role in colon cancer prevention.

V. Risks of HRT (see Tables 32.1 and 32.2)

A. Endometrial hyperplasia and cancer

    1. Unopposed estrogen is linked to both.

 Women with an intact uterus need progestin when taking estrogen to minimize the risk of hyperplasia and cancer.

    2. Women who have undergone a hysterectomy may be given estrogen alone.

B. Venous thromboembolism (VTE) including deep venous thrombosis (DVT) and pulmonary embolus (PE)

    1. Users of HRT are at two to three times higher risk for VTE

C. CHD

    1. HRT users' risk increases 29%

    2. Of 10,000 women on HRT for 1 year, seven more CHD events expected

    3. Secondary analyses have evaluated risk of CHD by age and years since menopause; seems to be no increased risk in CHD or stroke in women age 50–59 years

D. Cerebrovascular accident (CVA)

    1. HRT users' risk increases 41%

    2. Of 10,000 women on HRT for 1 year, eight more strokes expected

E. Invasive breast cancer

    1. HRT users' risk increases 26%

F. Dementia

    1. Women's Health Initiative Memory Study (WHIMS) trial revealed increased risk of dementia after 4 years of HRT.

VI. Side Effects of HRT

A. Breast tenderness

B. Irregular vaginal bleeding

C. Headaches

    D. Nausea
    E. Weight gain
    F. Rare elevations in triglycerides

VII. Contraindications to HRT
    A. Breast cancer/ovarian cancer
    B. Undiagnosed vaginal bleeding
    C. History of VTE events
    D. Coronary artery disease
    E. Cerebrovascular disease

VIII. Formulations of HRT
    A. Oral estrogen preparations
      1. Low-dose and high-dose formulations available
      2. Advantage: ease of use and dosing
      3. Premarin, FemHRT, Estrace
    B. Progestin preparations
      1. Medroxyprogesterone acetate (Provera) most extensively studied and used
        a. Can be used in continuous or cyclical regimens
      2. Micronized progesterone (Prometrium)
      3. Drospirenone
    C. Cyclic versus continuous regimens
      1. Cyclic: daily estrogen and progestin on days 1 to 12–14
        a. Advantage: cyclical bleeding
        b. Often used in women near menopause to prevent irregular bleeding
        c. Example: Premphase, Ortho-Prefest
      2. Continuous regimen
        a. Advantage: more convenient
        b. May have irregular bleeding early although amenorrhea eventually results in most cases
        c. Examples: Prempro, Activella, FemHRT
    D. Transdermal patches
      1. Estrogen alone or combination patches
      2. Advantage: ease of use
    E. Estrogen vaginal ring
      1. Femrin delivers estradiol for 3 months
        a. Used for vasomotor and genitourinary (GU) symptoms
        b. Need to use with progestin if uterus intact

2. Estring
   a. Low-dose estrogen for treatment of GU symptoms
   b. No increases of serum estradiol levels or endometrial hyperplasia
   c. No need to use with progestin
   d. May be safe in women with breast cancer

F. Topical estrogen
   1. Estrasorb and EstroGel are foil patches and gel, respectively, applied to arm or leg daily
   2. Vaginal estrogen creams: most often used for GU symptoms of vaginal dryness
      a. May be used in low-dose or high-dose regimen
      b. If using high doses, need progestin also
      c. Lower doses do not need a progestin: estradiol serum levels not increased

IX. Alternatives to HRT

A. Most of these therapies aimed at reducing hot flashes
B. Behavioral
   1. Exercise, weight loss, tobacco cessation, paced respirations
   2. No good studies proving these therapies effective
C. Complementary and alternative medicine (CAM)

 46% of women use CAM therapies for menopausal symptoms.

 Most CAM users do not tell their physicians. Physicians should routinely ask about alternative treatments used.

   1. Many CAM therapies have not been studied well. Studies often do not have an adequate placebo arm.
   2. Many products are advertised for menopause, but most are without any evidence of benefit.
      a. Red clover, wild yam, dong quai, evening primrose oil, flaxseed
   3. Soy
      a. Postulated that dietary intake of soy may partly explain lower reporting of hot flashes by Asian women
      b. Most common plant containing phytoestrogens
      c. In 11 randomized controlled trials (RCTs)

i. Six demonstrated no difference

ii. Five demonstrated soy superior to placebo, with reduction of hot flashes by 45% compared with placebo of 30%

d. No significant side effects

e. Phytoestrogens may increase risk of breast cancer and antagonize antitumor effect of tamoxifen

f. Long-term use results in questions of safety; endometrial hyperplasia may be induced

g. Dosages: 50–100 mg/day

> Studies are contradictory and difficult to evaluate given variation in soy preparations; however, soy is probably safe in these doses.

4. Black cohosh

a. Most commonly used CAM therapy

b. Mechanism unclear

c. Indigenous North American rhizome

d. Five RCTs but results may not be conclusive: many without placebo arm

e. No adverse effects

f. Dose: 40–160 mg/day

g. Remifemin, Menofem

> No conclusive supportive data for use; however, German health authorities, World Health Organization, and North American Menopause Society recommend black cohosh as a treatment option for mild menopausal symptoms.

D. Bio-identical hormones

1. Often called *natural hormone therapy;* e.g., Biest, Triest

2. Individually compounded recipes of steroids in various dosage forms, including estrone, estradiol, estriol, progesterone, dehydroepiandrosterone (DHEA), testosterone, pregnenolone

3. Patients tested via salivary hormone level; steroid doses individualized to need

a. Salivary levels vary with time of day

b. Poor reproducibility of assays

c. No standardized or recognized recommendations based on salivary data

4. Dosages based and titrated on symptoms, not testing

5. Some formulations have more estrogen than conventional preparations

 There are no proven advantages over conventional or synthetic hormones and potentially the same risks.

E. Medications
1. Antidepressants
   a. Selective serotonin reuptake inhibitor (SSRI): best evidence with paroxetine
   b. Selective norepinephrine reuptake inhibitor (SNRI): venlafaxine
   c. Mechanism: two serotonin sites in hypothalamus associated with temperature control
   d. Studies show greater reduction in hot flashes 40%–65% versus placebo 14%–38%
2. Gabapentin
   a. Mechanism: may regulate calcium channels in hypothalamus that are involved in thermoregulation
   b. Modest reductions in hot flashes

X. Summary

A. HRT is very effective in alleviating menopausal symptoms.

B. Given the increased risk of CHD, CVA, breast cancer, and VTE, HRT should no longer be recommended for chronic disease prevention. It is not generally used for osteoporosis treatment or prevention.

C. Avoid use in women at risk for dementia, stroke, CHD, VTE, and breast or ovarian cancer.

D. Most women have spontaneous resolution of hot flashes within the first year.

E. Stop HRT after 6–12 months to reevaluate.

F. Use low-dose vaginal therapy for GU symptoms.

 When using oral hormone therapy, use the lowest dose possible for the shortest period of time.

MENTOR TIPS DIGEST

- Vasomotor symptoms or hot flashes are among the most common menopausal complaints and occur in up to 80% of women during their menopause transition. Of these women, 20% have disabling symptoms.
- HRT is still the most effective therapy for the treatment of hot flashes; however, it should no longer be used for chronic disease prevention.
- Menopause is diagnosed after 12 consecutive months of amenorrhea not associated with a physiologic (pregnancy/lactation) or pathologic cause.
- The median age is 50 years plus or minus 2 years.
- 80% of women are affected by hot flashes; 10%–20% have severe symptoms.
- For most women, hot flashes last for about 1 year and then resolve spontaneously.
- HRT improves hot flashes in 80%–90% of women.
- Women with an intact uterus need progestin and estrogen to minimize the risk of hyperplasia and cancer.
- 46% of women use CAM therapies for menopausal symptoms.
- Most CAM users do not tell their physicians. Physicians should routinely ask about alternative treatments used.
- Studies are contradictory and difficult to evaluate given variation in soy preparations; however, soy is probably safe in these doses.
- No conclusive supportive data for use; however, German health authorities, World Health Organization, and North American Menopause Society recommend black cohosh as a treatment option for mild menopausal symptoms.
- For bio-identical hormones, there are no proven advantages over conventional or synthetic hormones and potentially the same risks.
- When using oral hormone therapy, use the lowest dose possible for the shortest period of time.

Resources

Grady D, Herrington D, Bittner V, et al. Cardiovascular disease outcomes during 6.8 years of hormone therapy: Heart and estrogen/progestin replacement study follow-up. Journal of the American Medical Association 288:49–57, 2002.

Hickey M, Saunders CM, Stuckey BG. Nonhormonal treatments for menopausal symptoms. Maturitas 57:85–89, 2007.

Hulley S, Furberg C, Barrett-Connor E, et al. Noncardiovascular disease outcomes during 6.8 years of hormone therapy: Heart and estrogen/progestin replacement study follow-up. Journal of the American Medical Association 288:58–64, 2002.

Nelson, Heidi D. Postmenopausal estrogen for the treatment of hot flashes. Journal of the American Medical Association 291: 1621–1625, 2004.

NIH State of the Science Panel. Management of menopause-related symptoms. Annals of Internal Medicine 142:1003–1013, 2005.

Politi MC, Schleinitz MD, Col NF. Revisiting the duration of vasomotor symptoms: A meta-analysis. Journal of General Internal Medicine 9:1507–1533, 2008.

Rossouw JE, Anderson GL, Prentice RL, et al. Risks and benefits of estrogen plus progestin in healthy postmenopausal women: Principal results from the Women's Healthy Initiative Randomized Controlled Trial. Journal of the American Medical Association 288:321–333, 2002.

Chapter Self-Test Questions

Circle the correct answer. After you have responded to the questions, check your answers in Appendix A.

1. Postmenopausal estrogen replacement reduces long-term risk of which condition ?

a. Osteoporosis

b. Cardiac mortality

c. Breast cancer

d. Depression and anxiety

2. Estrogen replacement therapy is the preventive treatment of choice for which condition?

   a. Osteoporosis

   b. Endometrial cancer

   c. Colorectal cancer

   d. Prevention is not a use of estrogen

3. What is the most effective proven hormonal treatment for peri-menopausal depression and anxiety?

   a. Estrogen replacement

   b. Estrogen and progestin replacement

   c. Dietary soy

   d. There is no proven hormonal treatment

See the testbank CD for more self-test questions.

33

MENSTRUAL DISORDERS

Deborah L. Edberg, MD, Melissa Yvette Liu, MD, and Joseph P. Gibes, MD

I. Normal Menstrual Cycle

A. Normal cycle: mean interval between menses of 28 days (+/− 7 days); mean duration of 4 days; blood loss about 35 mL

B. Menstrual cycle has three phases

1. In the first part of the cycle, estrogen causes menstrual flow to stop and promotes endometrial proliferation.

2. In the second phase, after ovulation, progesterone stops endometrial proliferation and promotes maturation of the endometrium.

3. In the third phase, as the corpus luteum regresses, progesterone production falls, which causes the endometrium to shed its lining, resulting in menstrual bleeding.

II. Primary Amenorrhea

A. Definition

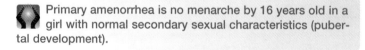
Primary amenorrhea is no menarche by 16 years old in a girl with normal secondary sexual characteristics (pubertal development).

1. May be defined as young as 14 years old in a girl with no secondary sexual characteristics

B. Evaluation

1. History: clarify if patient has any history of vaginal bleeding that may constitute menses; ask about sexual history and screen for abuse to evaluate for pregnancy

   2. Physical examination: assess for signs of secondary sexual characteristic (pubertal development)—breast development, pubic hair, underarm hair, body odor, acne.
C. Diagnostic tests

 Check pregnancy test.

   1. If no pregnancy and if patient has normal secondary sexual characteristics:
      a. Ultrasound uterus—if present, then evaluate for outflow obstruction
      b. Imperforate hymen
      c. Transverse vaginal septum
   2. If uterus is absent, then check karyotyping:
      a. If normal XX: mullerian agenesis
      b. If abnormal XY: androgen insensitivity
   3. If patient does not have secondary sexual characteristics:
      a. Check follicle-stimulating hormone (FSH) and luteinizing hormone (LH)
      b. If FSH >20 IU and LH >40 IU, then check karyotyping
         i. If normal XX: premature ovarian failure
         ii. If abnormal XO: Turner syndrome
      c. If FSH and LH <5, then work up for hypogonadism

 Constitutional delay in growth and puberty is most common explanation.

      i. Other possibilities:
         (1) Excessive exercise
         (2) Anorexia/bulimia
         (3) Malnutrition
         (4) Chronic illness (liver disease/renal disease)
         (5) Hypothalamic or pituitary destruction
         (6) Central nervous system tumor

III. Secondary Amenorrhea
A. Definition:

> Secondary amenorrhea is absence of menses for 3 months in women with previously normal menstruation or absence of menses for 9 months in women with previous oligomenorrhea.

B. Evaluation
1. History
   a. Determine frequency and duration of periods, amount of bleeding, and changes in character of period.
   b. Inquire about symptoms of metabolic disorders (e.g., galactorrhea, which suggests hyperprolactinemia, symptoms of thyroid disease), medications (e.g., tricyclic antidepressants, selective serotonin reuptake inhibitors, steroids, herbal substances), alcohol use, polycystic ovarian syndrome (signs of androgen excess such as acne, hirsutism, and obesity), hepatic disease, hypothalamic suppression (secondary to eating disorders, stress, excessive exercise).
   c. Inquire regarding possibility of pregnancy.
2. Physical examination
   a. Vital signs, body mass index (BMI), signs of androgen excess (such as acne and hirsutism), thyroid size, galactorrhea (suggests hyperprolactinemia, which can cause anovulation), visual field defects (may be caused by a pituitary tumor), signs of hepatitis, Pap smear, sexually transmitted disease (STD) screening, pelvic examination.
3. Diagnostic tests

 Check pregnancy test.

 Check thyroid-stimulating hormone (TSH) and prolactin levels.

   a. If both normal, then do progesterone challenge test (give patient Provera 10 mg daily for 7–10 days and expect withdrawal bleed)

b. If patient bleeds, there is ovarian malfunction (such as polycystic ovarian syndrome [PCOS])

c. If patient does not bleed, do estrogen/progesterone challenge (Premarin for 21 days)

  i. If patient bleeds, check follicle-stimulating hormone (FSH)/luteinizing hormone (LH) levels

   (1) If FSH/LH levels high, patient has ovarian failure (Turner syndrome)

   (2) If FSH low, check MRI to evaluate for pituitary tumor

  ii. If patient does not bleed, evaluate for outflow obstruction (i.e., cervical stenosis)

d. If TSH abnormal, treat thyroid disease

e. If TSH normal and prolactin level high

  i. If prolactin <100, consider medications, breastfeeding, hypothyroidism

  ii. If prolactin >100, check magnetic resonance imaging (MRI) to evaluate for prolactinoma

IV. Dysfunctional Uterine Bleeding (DUB)

A. Definitions

1. Abnormal uterine bleeding (AUB) is any bleeding that differs in regularity, frequency, duration, or volume from the patient's usual menses.

 DUB is abnormal uterine bleeding for which no systemic or anatomic cause has been identified.

a. Likely a disturbance of the hypothalamic-pituitary-ovarian axis that results in irregular, prolonged, and sometimes heavy menstrual bleeding

 DUB is a diagnosis of exclusion.

2. AUB can take many forms.

a. Polymenorrhea—uterine bleeding at regular intervals of fewer than 21 days

b. Oligomenorrhea—uterine bleeding at intervals of more than 35 days

    c. Menorrhagia—regularly occurring menstrual bleeding that is prolonged or excessive

    d. Metrorrhagia—bleeding at irregular intervals or between periods

    e. Menometrorrhagia—heavy or prolonged uterine bleeding occurring at irregular intervals

B. Impact of DUB

    1. Frequency: 5%–10% of outpatient complaints

    2. Morbidity/mortality:

        a. A single episode usually has no sequelae.

        b. Repetitive episodes increase the chance of iron deficiency anemia (up to 30% of cases).

        c. Up to 20% of adolescents with persistent menorrhagia have a concomitant bleeding disorder.

        d. Heavy flow can cause need for fluid management, blood transfusion, or intravenous (IV) hormone therapy (i.e., estrogen/progesterone).

        e. DUB can lead to unnecessary surgical evaluation (i.e., uterine curettage, endometrial ablation, hysterectomy).

        f. Continuous unopposed estrogen stimulation of the endometrium increases the risk for endometrial adenocarcinoma.

        g. Infertility is associated with chronic anovulation, particularly in patients with polycystic ovarian syndrome, obesity, and chronic hypertension.

C. Pathophysiology of DUB

    1. Most frequent:

 DUB usually represents anovulatory cycles.

        a. During a cycle in which ovulation does not occur, there is an absence of progesterone production, which in a normal ovulatory cycle acts to stop endometrial proliferation.

        b. The result is constant, noncycling estrogen stimulation of endometrial growth and proliferation, which causes the endometrium to outgrow its blood supply, and leads to irregular breakdown and sloughing.

    2. DUB occurs with ovulatory cycles, most often in adolescence and perimenopause; ovulatory dysfunctional bleeding may present as polymenorrhea, oligomenorrhea, midcycle spotting, menorrhagia

D. Differential diagnosis

 Because DUB is a diagnosis of exclusion, organic causes must be ruled out.

1. Systemic disease (coagulopathy, hypothyroidism, liver disease)
2. Pregnancy-related (implantation bleeding, threatened abortion, ectopic pregnancy)
3. Malignancy (endometrial or cervical cancer)
4. Anatomic abnormalities (endometrial hyperplasia, submucous myoma, cervical lesions)
5. Foreign bodies (e.g., intrauterine device [IUD])
6. Iatrogenic (e.g., medications, herbal substance)

E. Taking the history
1. Determine frequency and duration of periods, amount of bleeding, changes in character of period

 Rule out pregnancy.

2. Inquire about symptoms of metabolic disorders (e.g., galactorrhea, which suggests hyperprolactinemia; symptoms of thyroid disease), bleeding disorders (e.g., easy bruising, bleeding gums, epistaxis), medication causes (e.g., anticoagulants, tricyclic antidepressants, selective serotonin reuptake inhibitors, steroids, herbal substances), alcohol use, polycystic ovarian syndrome (signs of androgen excess such as acne, hirsutism, obesity), hepatic disease, hypothalamic suppression (secondary to eating disorders, stress, excessive exercise)

F. Physical examination
1. Vital signs, BMI, signs of androgen excess (such as acne and hirsutism), thyroid size, galactorrhea (suggests hyperprolactinemia, which can cause anovulation), visual field defects (may be caused by a pituitary tumor), ecchymosis and purpura (which suggest a bleeding disorder), signs of anemia, signs of hepatitis, Pap smear, sexually transmitted disease screening, pelvic examination

The hallmark of DUB is a negative pelvic examination (that is, no palpable uterine enlargement suggesting fibroids or polyps).

G. Diagnostic tests
   1. Laboratory
      a. Beta-HCG

 Most common cause of AUB is pregnancy-related.

      b. Complete blood count to evaluate for anemia, platelets, evidence of hematologic disease
      c. Pap smear to rule out cervical cancer (most common gynecologic cancer)
      d. Thyroid function tests, prolactin; abnormalities can cause ovulatory dysfunction and can be treated
      e. Liver function tests to evaluate for alcoholism or hepatitis, both of which can affect metabolism of estrogen
      f. Coagulation studies, hormone assays (such as FSH/LH)
      g. Endometrial evaluation with imaging or sampling recommended for women with risk factors for endometrial cancer, such as chronic anovulatory cycles, obesity, nulliparity, age older than 35 years, tamoxifen therapy
H. Imaging
   1. Consider transvaginal ultrasound in patients who cannot tolerate bimanual examination, obese patients, or if ovarian or uterine pathology is suspected.
   2. Ultrasound can identify endometrial hyperplasia, carcinoma, polyps, or uterine fibroids.
   3. Saline-infusion sonohysterography increases the diagnostic accuracy of ultrasonography.
I. Procedures to rule out endometrial carcinoma
   1. Endometrial sampling: aspiration, curetting, hysteroscopy or dilation and curettage (D&C)
   2. Ultrasound to measure the width of the endometrial stripe
J. Treatment
   1. Medical:

a. Acute, severe bleeding: conjugated equine estrogen (Premarin) 25 mg IV q4h for 24 hours, or orally in divided doses up to 10 mg/day; once acute bleeding stabilized, one monophasic oral contraceptive pill (OCP) twice a day until bleeding stops (usually 5–7 days); a withdrawal bleed usually occurs when pills stopped; on day 5 of bleeding, start regular regimen of OCPs

b. Less severe bleeding: OCPs two to four times daily until bleeding stops, then start regular regimen of OCPs

c. OCPs suppress endometrial development, reestablish cycle, decrease menstrual flow, lower risk of iron-deficiency anemia and endometrial carcinoma; first-line therapy in anovulatory DUB

d. Progestins suppress endometrial growth and mature endometrium so withdrawal bleeding organized; may be administered 5–10 mg/day for 21 days of the cycle or for the last 10 days of the cycle; especially useful for patients with anovulatory DUB for whom estrogen therapy is contraindicated (e.g., smokers over the age of 35 years, women at risk for thromboembolism)

e. Levonorgestrel-releasing intrauterine device (Mirena) releases low-level progestin, suppressing endometrial proliferation and reducing blood loss; useful in menorrhagic ovulatory DUB

f. Nonsteroidal anti-inflammatory drugs (NSAIDs) useful in menorrhagic ovulatory DUB; these are prostaglandin synthetase inhibitors: by blocking conversion of arachidonic acid to prostaglandins, they reduce prostaglandin levels, decreasing uterine bleeding

g. Antifibrinolytic agents (e.g., tranexamic acid [Cyklokapron]) reduce heavy bleeding by inhibiting breakdown of blood clots; most useful in women with menorrhagic ovulatory DUB; best to combine with OCP therapy (off-label use)

h. Androgens (Danazol) cause endometrial atrophy; seldom used due to side effects (including possibility of irreversible signs of masculinization)

i. Gonadotropic-releasing hormone (GnRH) agonists limited to women with severe blood loss who fail to respond to medical therapy and who do not want to resort to surgical intervention

2. Surgical (appropriate when medical therapy fails or is contraindicated):
   a. D&C: for those who fail hormonal management
   b. Hysterectomy: for those who fail or refuse hormonal therapy, have symptomatic anemia, or altered quality of life
   c. Endometrial ablation: less invasive and costly than hysterectomy; options include thermal balloon, rollerball, microwave, cryoablation, radiofrequency, electrocautery, laser

V. Dysmenorrhea
A. Definition

 Dysmenorrhea is painful menses in women with normal pelvic anatomy.

1. Crampy pelvic pain begins at or shortly before the onset of menses, lasting 1–3 days.
B. Prevalence

 It affects 20%–90% of adolescent women.

1. Of those, 15% say cramping severe enough to cause them to miss school.
C. Pathogenesis

 It is caused by release of prostaglandins in the menstrual fluid, which causes uterine contractions and menstrual pain.

1. Increased vasopressin also increases uterine contractility.
D. Risk factors
   1. Age younger than 20 years
   2. Attempts to lose weight—particularly in women 14–20 years of age
   3. Depression/anxiety
   4. Smoking
   5. Nulliparity
   6. Disruption of social networks

E. Diagnosis
  1. History: abnormal vaginal discharge, sexual activity, fever, pain not during time of menses, abnormal cycles, infertility, possibility of pregnancy
  2. Physical: evaluate for discharge, pelvic tenderness not during time of menses, enlarged ovaries, pelvic masses
  3. Laboratory: Pap smear, STD cultures, wet mount
  4. Imaging: for severe dysmenorrhea not responsive to treatment check ultrasound to rule out ovarian cyst
  5. Note: relationship between endometriosis and dysmenorrhea not clear
F. Treatment:
  1. NSAIDs—begin before onset of menstrual pain and flow to block prostaglandin release
  2. OCPs
  3. Depo-Provera injections
  4. Mirena IUD
  5. Intravaginal administration of normal birth control
  6. Lifestyle modification—low-fat vegetarian diet, exercise
  7. Alternative treatments (limited data):
     a. Thiamine
     b. Vitamin E
     c. Omega-3 polyunsaturated fatty acids
     d. Acupuncture/acupressure
     e. Transcutaneous electrical nerve stimulator (TENS)

MENTOR TIPS DIGEST

  • Primary amenorrhea is no menarche by 16 years old in a girl with normal secondary sexual characteristics (pubertal development).
  • Check pregnancy test.
  • Constitutional delay in growth and puberty is most common explanation.
  • Secondary amenorrhea is absence of menses for 3 months in women with previously normal menstruation or absence of menses for 9 months in women with previous oligomenorrhea.
  • Check thyroid-stimulating hormone (TSH) and prolactin levels.

- DUB is abnormal uterine bleeding for which no systemic or anatomic cause has been identified.
- DUB is a diagnosis of exclusion.
- DUB usually represents anovulatory cycles.
- Because DUB is a diagnosis of exclusion, organic causes must be ruled out.
- The hallmark of DUB is a negative pelvic examination (that is, no palpable uterine enlargement suggesting fibroids or polyps).
- Most common cause of AUB is pregnancy-related.
- Dysmenorrhea is painful menses in women with normal pelvic anatomy.
- It affects 20%–90% of adolescent women.
- It is caused by release of prostaglandins in the menstrual fluid, which causes uterine contractions and menstrual pain.

Resources

Albers H., et al. Abnormal uterine bleeding. American Family Physician 69:1915–1926, 2004 (available at www.aafp.org/afp/20040415/1915.html).

Behera M. Dysfunctional uterine bleeding. eMedicine. Available at www.emedicine.com/med/topic2353.html

French L. Dysmenorrhea. American Family Physician 71, 2005.

Gaunt AM, Mayeaux EJ Diagnosis and management of dysfunctional uterine bleeding. CME Bulletin 6, 2007 (available at www.aafp.org/online/en/home/cme/selfstudy/cmebulletin/dub.html).

Master-Hunter T, Heiman DL. Amenorrhea: Evaluation and treatment. American Family Physician, 2006, 73 (8): 1374-82.

Stenchever M, et al. Comprehensive gynecology, 4th ed., 1079–1098. St Louis: Mosby, 2001.

Chapter Self-Test Questions

Circle the correct answer. After you have responded to the questions, check your answers in Appendix A.

1. In the first phase of the menstrual cycle when the endometrium prolif- erates, what is the responsible hormone?

   a. Estrogen

   b. Progesterone

   c. Beta-hCG

   d. Prolactin

2. In the second phase of the menstrual cycle when endometrial proliferation stops and the endometrium matures, what is the responsible hormone?

   a. Estrogen

   b. Progesterone

   c. Beta-hCG

   d. Prolactin

3. The corpus luteum produces which hormone?

   a. Estrogen

   b. Progesterone

   c. Beta-hCG

   d. Prolactin

 See the testbank CD for more self-test questions.

FEMALE GENITAL SYMPTOMS

Marianne M. Green, MD

I. Pathophysiology
  A. Vulvar
  1. Dermatologic conditions
     a. *Lichen sclerosus:* benign, chronic inflammatory condition with epithelial thinning of unknown etiology
     b. *Lichen planus:* benign inflammatory condition that is more widespread; involves skin, nails, and mucous membranes
     c. *Contact dermatitis:* may be irritant (80%) or allergic (20%)
  2. Infectious conditions
     a. *Condyloma acuminatum:* sexually transmitted human papillomavirus (HPV), most commonly types 6 and 11
     b. *Genital ulcer disease (syphilis, herpes simplex [HSV]):* sexual transmission, e.g., HSV-1 and HSV-2 chancroid (Table 34.1)
  3. Unknown etiology
     a. *Vestibulitis:* inflammation of the minor vestibular glands
     b. *Vulvodynia:* possibly type of peripheral neuropathy
  B. Vaginal
  1. Infectious
     a. *Bacterial vaginosis:* a decrease in the normal lactobacillus leads to an overgrowth of gram-negative and variable rods in vaginal flora
     b. *Candida:* overgrowth of yeast after disruption of the vaginal ecosystem (85% *Candida albicans;* 15% other Candida spp.)
     c. *Trichomonas:* sexually transmitted infection with protozoan *Trichomonas vaginalis*

TABLE 34.1	Painful Versus Painless Genital Ulcers
Painful	Herpes simplex virus
	Chancroid
Painless	Chancre (primary syphilis)
	• *Condyloma latum* (secondary syphilis)
	Lymphogranuloma venereum
	Granuloma inguinale
	Molluscum contagiosum

   2. *Atrophic:* noninfectious form of vaginitis affecting the epithelium
      due to lack of estrogen
  C. Cervical
   1. Infectious
      a. *Chlamydia:* infection of the upper genital tract caused by
         obligate intracellular bacteria, *Chlamydia trachomatis*
      b. *Gonorrhea:* gram-negative diplococci infecting the columnar
         epithelium of the upper genital tract

II. Epidemiology

  A. Acute vulvovaginitis accounts for more than 10 million health-care
     visits per year.
   1. Bacterial vaginosis is the most common cause of acute vaginitis,
      accounting for 15%–50% of cases depending on the population
      studied.
   2. Women with bacterial vaginosis and trichomoniasis are at
      increased risk of infection with HIV.
   3. 75% of women have at least one candidal (yeast) infection in
      their lifetime, and 40%–45% have more than one.
   4. A single exposure to a partner infected with trichomonas will
      infect 85% of females.
  B. Vulvar syndromes and dermatologic conditions are less common
     causes of vaginal symptoms.
   1. Contact dermatitis accounts for a third to half of women's
      vulvar complaints.
  C. Cervicitis is a serious condition affecting millions of women,
     many of whom are asymptomatic, leading to infertility.

1. Chlamydia is the most common bacterial sexually transmitted disease (STD) in the United Sates, with nearly 3 million new cases every year.
2. The U.S. Centers for Disease Control (CDC) estimate at least 700,000 new cases of gonorrhea in the United States each year.

III. Patient History
A. Chief complaint
   1. Symptom and its duration

> Symptoms alone cannot be used to localize the site of infection and may not correlate with the presence of infection.

B. History of present illness
   1. Obstetric history, including past and current pregnancies
   2. Gynecologic history, including last menstrual period, sexual history, number of partners, new partners, and form of contraception if indicated
   3. Presence of pain, itching, irritation, discharge, lesions
      a. Discharge: describe color, texture, location, odor
      b. Lesions: describe number, size, location, whether painful or painless
   4. Include associated symptoms of dysuria, dyspareunia, abdominal or pelvic pain, fever, inguinal adenopathy
C. Past medical history
   1. Previous infections, diabetes, immunosuppression
D. Medications
   1. Recent antibiotic use, over-the-counter treatments, oral contraceptives
E. Allergies
   1. History of drug rash

IV. Physical Examination
A. Vital signs
   1. Note presence or absence of fever.
B. Abdominal examination
   1. Palpate for left or right lower quadrant tenderness.
   2. Palpate the inguinal area for adenopathy.

C. Pelvic examination
   1. Examine the external genitalia for lesions, erythema, or edema.
      a. About 25% of patients with vaginal candidiasis have excoriations on their external genitalia.
   2. With the speculum, examine the vagina and cervix, noting the presence, location (from the cervix or in the vagina only), and character of the discharge.
      a. The classic "strawberry cervix" represents erythematous punctuations on the cervix associated with *Trichomonas* infection but is only present in 2%–5% of cases.
   3. Obtain a vaginal pH from the side walls of the vagina with a cotton-tipped swab wiped onto commercially available pH paper.
      a. The normal vaginal pH is 4.0.
      b. Candidal vaginitis will not alter the normal pH.

 pH of >4.5 is present in over 95% of women with bacterial vaginosis and trichomoniasis.

      c. Trichomonas vaginitis and atrophic vaginitis are associated with the highest vaginal pH.
      d. The presence of sperm or blood raises the vaginal pH.
   4. Bimanual examination consists of the following.
      a. Determine if there is any cervical motion tenderness.
      b. Feel the uterus and adnexa for any tenderness or masses.

V. Differential Diagnosis
   A. Vulvar conditions
      1. *L. sclerosus*
         a. Symptoms include intense pruritus, dyspareunia, and burning pain.
         b. The skin appears thin and white.
         c. Biopsy reveals a thin epithelium with loss of rete ridges and inflammatory cells lining the basement membrane.
      2. *L. planus*
         a. Symptoms may include itching.
         b. Examination reveals slightly purple polygonal papules that have overlying fine white lines called Wickham striae.
      3. Vestibulitis
         a. Symptoms include severe dyspareunia at the introitus.

      b. On examination over the vestibula, there may be erythematous papules 1–4 mm that are extremely tender to touch with a cotton-tipped swab.

  4. Vulvodynia

      a. Symptoms include a nonspecific burning, itching, and pain involving some or all of the external genitalia.

      b. Examination results are usually normal.

  5. *C. acuminatum*

      a. Painless cauliflower-like growths on the vulva and vagina and sometimes involving the rectal mucosa.

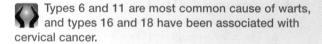

Types 6 and 11 are most common cause of warts, and types 16 and 18 have been associated with cervical cancer.

  6. Herpes simplex

      a. Symptoms include painful ulcerations on skin and mucosal surfaces. Vaginal discharge and dysuria may also be present. Burning pain may occur before outbreak of lesions. Primary infection may be accompanied by fever and flu-like symptoms.

      b. Examination reveals multiple painful grouped vesicles on an erythematous base. Vesicles erupt and form ulcerations. Inguinal adenopathy may be present.

      c. Viral shedding always occurs when lesions are present and may also occur when patients are asymptomatic.

      d. Diagnosis consists of the following.

        i. Viral culture of active lesion

        ii. Serologic tests for HSV-1 and HSV-2 antibodies may be helpful but do not differentiate present from past infection

B. Vaginal infections and conditions (Table 34.2)

  1. Bacterial vaginosis

      a. May occur in women who are not sexually active

      b. Symptoms sometimes include discharge with fish-like odor; usually no pruritus

      c. Examination reveals thin homogenous often gray or white vaginal discharge; vaginal pH >4.5

Diagnosis is by Amsel's criteria (Box 34.1).

TABLE 34.2 Diagnosis of Vaginitis

Diagnostic Study	Candida	Bacterial Vaginosis	Trichomonas	Atrophic Vaginitis
pH	3.8–4.2 (normal)	>4.5	>5.0	>5.0
Saline wet mount	Budding yeast	Clue cells No white blood cells (WBCs)	Flagellated organisms WBCs	Parabasal epithelial cells —
Potassium hydroxide (KOH) wet mount	Pseudohy-phae	—	—	
Culture	Candida spp.	Gram-negative	Trichomonas with Diamond media	—

Bacterial vaginosis is associated with an increased risk of upper genital tract infections, spontaneous abortion, and premature labor.

2. Candidiasis
   a. Risk is increased in patients with recent antibiotic use, diabetes mellitus, immunosuppression, and increased estrogen states (pregnancy and oral contraceptive use).

BOX 34.1 Amsel's Criteria for Bacterial Vaginosis

Three of four criteria should be met for diagnosis:
• Positive whiff (amine) test with application of 10% KOH
• Clue cells (epithelial cells with stippled borders due to adherent bacteria) present on saline wet mount
• Presence of thin, homogenous vaginal discharge
• Vaginal pH >4.5
• Absence of odor has strong negative likelihood ratio for bacterial vaginosis.

    b. Symptoms include itching and thick white cottage cheese–like discharge.

    c. Diagnosis consists of the following.

       i. Normal vaginal pH

      ii. KOH wet mount showing yeast elements (sensitivity around 60%)

      iii. Culture for *Candida*

      iv. Erythema found on examination increases likelihood of candidiasis

3. Trichomoniasis

Half of both males and females with trichomoniasis may be asymptomatic despite infection.

    a. Symptoms include thin, green frothy discharge, vulvovaginal irritation, and sometimes dyspareunia and dysuria.

    b. Physical examination may reveal hemorrhages on the endocervix (strawberry cervix).

    c. Diagnosis consists of the following.

      i. Saline wet mount reveals mobile flagellated organisms and a high number of WBCs (only 70% sensitive).

      ii. Culture should be performed when wet mount is negative (90% sensitive and specific).

4. Atrophic vaginitis

    a. Noninfectious form of vaginitis that occurs in postmenopausal females due to lack of estrogen

    b. Symptoms include vaginal soreness, discharge, dysuria, dyspareunia

    c. Physical examination reveals thin vaginal mucosa with diffuse erythema and lack of vaginal folds

    d. Vaginal pH elevated

C. Cervical infections (Table 34.3)

1. Chlamydia

    a. 40% of women are asymptomatic.

    b. Progression of the infection can lead to pelvic inflammatory disease and infertility.

    c. Symptoms may include vaginal discharge, dyspareunia, and postcoital bleeding.

TABLE 34.3	Diagnostic Tests for Cervical Infections
Diagnosis	**Test**
Herpes	*Culture, PCR, serologic studies, Tzanck smear
Chlamydia	*PCR of cervical discharge or urine
Gonorrhea	*Culture with chocolate agar, PCR of cervical discharge

*gold standard
  PCR = polymerase chain reaction

    d. Physical examination may reveal mucopurulent cervical discharge and a friable cervix.

    e. Diagnosis is made with nucleic acid amplification tests such as PCR (highly sensitive and specific) on cervical swabs and/or urine.

    f. Expert panels recommend screening for chlamydia for all women younger than 25 years, who have new or multiple sexual partners, or who use non-barrier contraceptives.

  2. Gonorrhea

    a. Up to 50% of women may be asymptomatic.

    b. Symptoms can occur up to 2 weeks post exposure and include vaginal discharge, dyspareunia, and vaginal irritation.

    c. Physical examination may reveal mucopurulent cervical discharge and a friable cervix.

    d. Untreated infections may develop pelvic inflammatory disease and infertility. Widespread dissemination may occur.

    e. Diagnosis is made with culture on chocolate agar or PCR of cervical discharge.

 If either chlamydia or gonorrhea is suspected, patients should be treated for both, as coinfection frequently occurs.

VI. Management

  A. Vulvar

    1. Dermatologic conditions such as *L. sclerosus* and *L. planus* should be referred to a dermatologist because biopsies may be necessary to distinguish these conditions from vaginal cancer.

Contact dermatitis may be treated with sitz baths and a low-potency topical steroid preparation.

2. *C. acuminatum* has the following profile.

   a. Cases may resolve spontaneously 20%–30% of the time.

   b. Medical therapies can be topical cryodestructive or immunoablative preparations.

   c. Surgical treatment may be necessary for more aggressive cases.

   d. Annual Pap smears are essential to detect early cervical dysplasia.

3. Herpes simplex has the following profile.

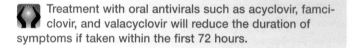

Treatment with oral antivirals such as acyclovir, famciclovir, and valacyclovir will reduce the duration of symptoms if taken within the first 72 hours.

   a. Treatment of the first outbreak may reduce the number of recurrent infections.

   b. Theses oral agents can be used as suppressive therapy for patients with frequent outbreaks and may reduce the rate of asymptomatic viral shedding.

   c. Topical treatments have little effect on the herpes virus.

4. Vestibulitis and vulvodynia have the following profile.

   a. Avoid vulvar irritants.

   b. Tricyclic antidepressants have been useful.

   c. Surgical treatment including vestibulectomy is controversial.

B. Vaginal

  1. Bacterial vaginosis

   a. Topical treatments are metronidazole gel 0.75% or clindamycin cream 2% applied intravaginally for 5 days.

   b. Oral treatment is metronidazole 500 mg twice daily for 7 days.

   c. There is no need to treat sexual partners.

  2. *Candida*

   a. Topical antimycotics cure more than 80% of all infections.

   b. A one-time dose of oral fluconazole (150 mg) can be used but has a lower rate of efficacy.

   c. A variety of treatments are available for recurrent candidiasis.

   d. There is no need to treat sexual partners.

3. *Trichomonas*
   a. The only treatment available is oral metronidazole.

   All sexual partners of patients with trichomoniasis should be treated, and both partners should be screened for other STDs.

4. Atrophic vaginitis
   a. Topical or oral estrogens are effective.

C. Cervical
   1. Chlamydia
      a. Treatment for the patient and her partner includes a single dose of azithromycin or a 1-week course of doxycycline. Alternate regimens include 1 week of erythromycin, levofloxacin, or ofloxacin.
      b. Patients should be treated for gonorrhea.
      c. All sexual partners should be treated.
      d. Patients should be tested for other STDs and counseled about HIV and safe sex practices.
   2. Gonorrhea
      a. A single dose of ceftriaxone 250 mg IM is effective.
      b. A variety of single-dose oral quinolone regimens is effective, but the resistance of gonorrhea to quinolones is increasing.
      c. The CDC considers gonorrhea in Hawaii and California to be quinolone-resistant.
      d. Patients should be treated empirically for chlamydia.
      e. All sexual partners should be treated, and patients should be counseled about safe sex and HIV as well as tested for other sexually transmitted infections.

MENTOR TIPS DIGEST

- In general, symptoms alone cannot be used to localize the site of infection and may not correlate with the presence of infection.
- pH of > 4.5 is present in over 95% of women with bacterial vaginosis and trichomoniasis.

- Condyloma acuminatum types 6 and 11 are most common cause of warts, and types 16 and 18 have been associated with cervical cancer.
- Bacterial vaginosis is diagnosed using Amsel criteria.
- Bacterial vaginosis is associated with an increased risk of upper genital tract infections, spontaneous abortion, and premature labor.
- Half of both males and females with trichomoniasis may be asymptomatic despite infection.
- If either chlamydia or gonorrhea is suspected, patients should be treated for both, as coinfection frequently occurs.
- In herpes simplex, treatment with oral antivirals such as acyclovir, famciclovir, and valacyclovir will reduce the duration of symptoms if taken within the first 72 hours.
- All sexual partners of patients with trichomoniasis should be treated, and both partners should be screened for other STDs.

Resources

Anderson MR, Klink K, Cohrssen A. Evaluation of vaginal complaints. Journal of the American Medical Association 291:1368–1379, 2004.

Beck WW. National medical series: Obstetrics and gynecology, 4th ed. Baltimore, Williams & Wilkins, 1997.
Excellent textbook that provides further details on vaginal symptoms.

Eckert LO: Acute vulvovaginitis. New England Journal of Medicine 355:1244–1252, 2006.
Excellent review with table on sensitivity and specificity of diagnostic tests as well as costs of treatment regimens.

Sobel JD: Vaginitis. New England Journal of Medicine 337:1896–1903, 1997.
Well-organized vaginitis review authored by a national expert.

Chapter Self-Test Questions

Circle the correct answer. After you have responded to the questions, check your answers in Appendix A.

1. Which of the following vulvovaginal conditions is infectious?

  a. *Lichen planus*

  b. *Lichen sclerosus*

  c. *Atrophic vaginitis*

  d. *Condyloma acuminatum*

2. What is the cause of *Lichen sclerosus?*

  a. Scleroderma (progressive systemic sclerosis)

  b. Estrogen deficiency

  c. *Trichomonas vaginalis*

  d. Unknown

3. Human papillomavirus (HPV) causes:

  a. *Condyloma acuminatum*

  b. Increased risk of spontaneous miscarriage

  c. Painless genital ulcers

  d. Painful genital ulcers

See the testbank CD for more self-test questions.

35

PAP SMEAR AND CERVICAL CANCER SCREENING

Ellen J. Gelles, MD

I. Pathophysiology of Cervical Cancer

A. Types include squamous cell carcinoma and adenocarcinoma; squamous by far most common

B. Role of human papillomavirus (HPV)

 HPV infections are believed to be the cause of most cervical cancers.

1. Serotypes 16, 18, 31, 33, and 35 are among the high-risk, or oncogenic, HPV strains; serotypes 6 and 11 are examples of the low-risk types.

2. Most HPV infections are transient; other factors are likely necessary for HPV to progress to dysplasia (Box 35.1).

BOX 35.1

Risk Factors for Cervical Cancer

Early onset of sexual activity (younger than 17 years)
Multiple sexual partners (more than two per lifetime)
History of herpes simplex virus or other sexually transmitted diseases
Immunosuppression, such as HIV infection or chemotherapeutic agents
Cigarette smoking
Low socioeconomic status
Radiation exposure
High-risk sexual partner
Prolonged use of contraceptive hormones
High parity

C. Cervical intraepithelial neoplasia (CIN)
  1. CIN pre-invasive stage of cervical cancer
  2. Precedes invasive cervical cancer by years to decades
  3. Biopsy specimens classified as CIN I–III, depending on how much cervical epithelium involved with dysplastic changes
    a. CIN I is known as low-grade dysplasia.
    b. CIN II and III are known as high-grade dysplasia.

II. Epidemiology of Cervical Cancer

A. Affects 10,000 women in the United States per year; more than 4000 U.S. women die from cervical cancer annually
B. Incidence higher in developing countries without access to screening
C. Median age of diagnosis 48 years; rarely occurs in women younger than 35 years
D. Risk factors listed in Box 35.1

III. Prevention of HPV and Cervical Cancer

A. Modifying risk factors
  1. Smoking cessation

 Smoking cessation can reduce the risk of cervical cancer two- to threefold.

  2. Limiting number of sexual partners, delaying onset of sexual activity, and using barrier contraception reduce HPV infection rates
B. Screening for cervical dysplasia and HPV
  1. Papanicolaou (Pap) smear
  2. Testing for high-risk HPV DNA
    a. Up to 95% sensitive for detecting cervical dysplasia
    b. Can be performed on same sample as liquid Pap smear; collected by people with little medical training or by patient

Disadvantages of HPV testing include its low specificity, particularly in young women. As most HPV infections are transient and never develop into cervical cancer, detection of every HPV infection is of questionable value.

    c. Not usually used alone as a primary screening tool; used to triage women with minor Pap smear abnormalities to decide whether further testing needed; also used in combination with Pap smear to decide which women are very low-risk for cervical cancer and can be screened less frequently; guidelines for this "combination Pap smear" being developed

C. HPV vaccine

> HPV vaccine targets four serotypes: 6, 11, 16, and 18. Types 16 and 18 cause the vast majority of cervical cancers; 6 and 11 are associated with genital warts.

    1. In women who have not yet been exposed to these serotypes, the vaccine has been shown to be highly effective in preventing high-grade cervical dysplasia.

    2. Three-dose vaccine is approved for use in females age 9–26 years and ideally should be given prior to the onset of sexual activity.

IV. Pap Smear

A. Features that make this a good screening test
    1. Inexpensive
    2. Easy to perform as part of a routine office visit
    3. Minimally uncomfortable to patients
    4. Targets a disease with a long, identifiable, precancerous stage, during which treatment and cure are possible

B. Current Pap smear screening guidelines
    1. Screening at some regular intervals is crucial; a single Pap smear may miss cervical dysplasia 30%–50% of the time.

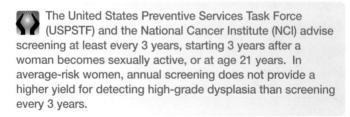

> The United States Preventive Services Task Force (USPSTF) and the National Cancer Institute (NCI) advise screening at least every 3 years, starting 3 years after a woman becomes sexually active, or at age 21 years. In average-risk women, annual screening does not provide a higher yield for detecting high-grade dysplasia than screening every 3 years.

2. After age 65–70 years (exact guidelines vary), Pap smear screening is no longer necessary, as long as the patient has undergone previous regular screening with normal test results.

3. Immunosuppressed women (those with HIV/AIDS and those on immunosuppressant drugs) should be screened more often as should those who have been sexually active and have not had regular screening in the past.

4. Women who have no cervix because they have undergone total hysterectomies for noncancerous conditions do not need Pap smears.

C. Tips and techniques for obtaining a good Pap smear

1. The patient should be made as comfortable as possible and draped appropriately. With newer liquid-based Pap smear collection systems (see later), use of small amounts of lubricants is fine and does not affect the adequacy of the specimen.

2. Avoid collecting specimens when the patient is menstruating or has an active vaginal or cervical infection.

3. Collect from best location.

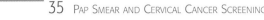 During the speculum examination, obtain the Pap smear sample from the transformation zone (the junction between the darker-colored columnar epithelium and the paler squamous epithelium), as this is where most cervical cancers arise.

a. Hormonal changes of pregnancy or hormonal contraceptives can cause the transformation zone to migrate outward, whereas in postmenopausal women it can be located inside the os where it is not visible to the examiner.

b. To maximize chances of getting transformation-zone cells on the specimen, both the endocervix and the ectocervix are sampled. An extended-tip spatula is used to sample the ectocervix, and a Cytobrush is used for the endocervix.

4. Conventional Pap smear is performed as follows.

a. Samples are spread directly on a slide in the examination room and fixed with a spray fixative.

b. This technique is more cumbersome and prone to sampling problems. Leaving the slide sitting in air before it is sprayed with fixative, the presence of blood or inflammatory vaginal discharge and use of examination lubricant can lower the sensitivity and lead to more unsatisfactory smears.

5. Liquid-based Pap smears are collected as follows.

    a. Cervical cells are collected in a container of liquid fixative rather than on a slide. In the laboratory, the specimen is filtered to remove blood and noncellular debris and transferred to a slide for interpretation.

    b. This method is more convenient, is higher-sensitivity for detecting cervical dysplasia, and fewer smears are deemed unsatisfactory for interpretation.

    c. This method is more expensive than the conventional Pap smear and has a longer processing time.

V. Interpretation and Management of Pap Smear Results

Pap smear cytology results are reported with a standardized system (the Bethesda System for Reporting Cervical/Vaginal Cytological Diagnoses).

A. Reports contain the following information:

    1. Assessment of specimen adequacy allows pathologist to comment if correct cell types (transformation zone) not present in specimen, smear not well labeled, or if blood or inflammatory cells comprise too much of the specimen for an adequate reading

    2. General categorization: (normal or other)

    3. Descriptive diagnosis that names any abnormalities on the smear

B. Squamous cell abnormalities and management

    1. Cervical carcinoma—immediate referral to gynecologist

    2. High-grade squamous intraepithelial lesion (HSIL)

        a. Cytologic equivalent to high-grade dysplasia (CINII-III); in practice, this correlation not always true: sometimes HSIL reading is false alarm and pathology more benign

        b. High rate of progression to invasive cervical carcinoma; patients should be referred for colposcopy with cervical biopsy

    3. Low-grade squamous intraepithelial lesion (LSIL)

        a. Correlates with mild dysplasia (CINI) and cellular changes associated with HPV infection

        b. Progression to invasive cervical cancer much lower than with HSIL

c. Management controversial; most experts advise referral for colposcopy

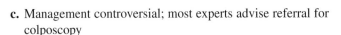 There is no role in testing for HPV in patients with LSIL, as nearly all test positive.

4. Atypical squamous cells (ASCs)

a. Cells appear abnormal but not severe enough to meet criteria for LSIL or HSIL

b. ASC not a clear step in progression from mild precancerous changes to cervical cancer

c. Can be caused by a variety of factors including non-HPV infections and postmenopausal atrophy

d. Subclassified into atypical squamous cells, favor high-grade dysplasia (ASC-H), and atypical squamous cells of uncertain significance (ASC-US); women with ASC-H should be referred for colposcopy

e. Management options for women with ASC-US

i. Send the same Pap smear specimen (if collected with a liquid-based collection system) for HPV (reflex HPV) testing. Only women who test positive for high-risk strains need to be referred for colposcopy. Women with ASC-US who are high-risk HPV-negative are at very low risk for having HSIL and can have their Pap smear repeated in 12 months. This approach limits the anxiety and cost of referring women unnecessarily for colposcopy and the inconvenience of needing to follow up for repeat Pap smears.

ii. Repeat serial Pap smears every 3–6 months, and refer for colposcopy only if the patient's Pap smear progresses in severity. This is a good plan for women younger than 30 years in whom HPV infection is often transient and high-grade dysplasia is extremely uncommon.

iii. Refer directly for colposcopy. For average-risk women, this strategy has become less desirable now that HPV testing is available. It is still a reasonable option when HPV testing is not available or when reliable follow-up for repeat Pap smears is not feasible.

Immunosuppressed women, including those who are HIV-positive, should always be referred for immediate colposcopy, with any epithelial cell abnormality on a Pap smear, including ASC-US.

C. Glandular cell abnormalities and their management

  1. All patients with glandular abnormalities seen on a Pap smear need referral for further evaluation; the Pap smear is designed to screen for squamous cell abnormalities.

  2. The glandular cells can originate from either the endocervix or endometrium, so adenocarcinoma of the cervix or endometrial cancer needs to be considered.

  3. Follow-up with serial Pap smears or reflex HPV testing alone is never appropriate for glandular abnormalities.

  4. Specific glandular abnormalities require the following.

  a. Adenocarcinoma in situ (AIS): immediate referral to gynecologist

  b. Atypical glandular cells (AGCs): referred for colposcopy; women older than 40 years should also be referred for endometrial biopsy to rule out endometrial cancer

  c. Endometrial cell abnormalities:

  i. Atypical endometrial cells: referred for endometrial biopsy, then colposcopy if the endometrial biopsy result abnormal

Specimens from postmenopausal women should not have endometrial cells. If endometrial cells are present, whether atypical or not, endometrial biopsy is indicated. The same holds true for any woman with endometrial cells present that do not correspond to the reported time of her last menstrual period and in women with irregular or heavy bleeding, suggesting endometrial abnormalities.

D. Other Pap smear results and their management

  1. Unsatisfactory for evaluation: repeat Pap smear in 3 months

  2. Satisfactory but limited:

  a. Repeat Pap smear in 3 months if the patient is at high risk for cervical cancer or in 1 year if average or low risk.

b. Treat any obvious causes of inflammation, such as infection, before repeating cytology.

c. If no endocervical cells are present, a good sample from the transformation zone was not obtained.

3. Benign cellular changes, inflammation/cellular repair: routine follow-up unless specimen unsatisfactory

4. Infection (chlamydia, herpes simplex virus, Trichomonas): with the exception of Trichomonas, which can be accurately diagnosed on a liquid-based Pap smear, infections should be clinically evaluated and treated.

 MENTOR TIPS DIGEST

- HPV infections are believed to be the cause of most cervical cancers.
- Smoking cessation can reduce the risk of cervical cancer two- to threefold.
- Disadvantages of HPV testing include its low specificity, particularly in young women. As most HPV infections are transient and never develop into cervical cancer, detection of every HPV infection is of questionable value.
- HPV vaccine targets four serotypes: 6, 11, 16, and 18. Types 16 and 18 cause the vast majority of cervical cancers; 6 and 11 are associated with genital warts.
- The United States Preventive Services Task Force (USPSTF) and the National Cancer Institute (NCI) advise screening at least every 3 years, starting 3 years after a woman becomes sexually active, or at age 21 years. In average-risk women, annual screening does not provide a higher yield for detecting high-grade dysplasia than screening every 3 years.
- During the speculum examination, obtain the Pap smear sample from the transformation zone (the junction between the darker-colored columnar epithelium and the paler squamous epithelium), as this is where most cervical cancers arise.
- Pap smear cytology results are reported with a standardized system (the Bethesda System for Reporting Cervical/Vaginal Cytological Diagnoses).
- There is no role in testing for HPV in patients with LSIL, as nearly all test positive.
- Immunosuppressed women, including those who are HIV-positive, should always be referred for immediate colposcopy, with any epithelial cell abnormality on a Pap smear, including ASC-US.

- Specimens from postmenopausal women should not have endometrial cells. If endometrial cells are present, whether atypical or not, endometrial biopsy is indicated. The same holds true for any woman with endometrial cells present that do not correspond to the reported time of her last menstrual period and in women with irregular or heavy bleeding, suggesting endometrial abnormalities.

Resources

A human papillomavirus vaccine. The Medical Letter on Drugs and Therapeutics 1241:65–66, 2006.

Naucler P, Ryd W, Törnberg S, et al: Human papillomavirus and Papanicolaou tests to screen for cervical cancer. New England Journal of Medicine 357:1589–1597, 2007.

Screening for Cervical Cancer in U.S. Preventive Services Task Force Guidelines. Available at http://www.ahrq.gov/clinic/uspstf/uspscerv.htm

Chapter Self-Test Questions

Circle the correct answer. After you have responded to the questions, check your answers in Appendix A.

1. Which type of cervical cancer is most common?

   a. Adenocarcinoma

   b. Squamous carcinoma

   c. Myosarcoma

   d. T-cell lymphoma

2. What is the cause of most or all cases of cervical carcinoma?

   a. Human immunodeficiency virus (HIV)

   b. Human papillomavirus (HPV)

   c. *Chlamydia trachomatis*

   d. Cigarette smoking

3. Which of the following statements accurately describes HPV and cervical cancer?

   a. All HPV strains are likely to lead to cervical cancer.

   b. Only some HPV serotypes are associated with high risk for cervical cancer.

   c. HPV serotypes that cause genital warts also have the highest risk of association with cervical cancer.

   d. HPV requires a co-infection to develop into cervical cancer.

See the testbank CD for more self-test questions.

36

OSTEOPOROSIS

Jordana Friedman, MD, and James J. Foody, MD

I. Definitions

A. Osteoporosis is a disease characterized by a decrease in bone mass and bone quality, which results in increased bone fragility and susceptibility to fracture (1993 consensus definition).

B. *Primary* osteoporosis is due to aging and menopause.

C. *Secondary* osteoporosis is due to underlying diseases or conditions.

 Fractures cause the morbidity and mortality associated with osteoporosis.

II. Pathophysiology

A. Remodeling, replacing old bone with new bone tissue maintains bone health.

  1. Active phases of remodeling are resorption and formation.

   a. Resorption: osteoclasts remove old bone tissue

   b. Formation: osteoblasts produce new bone matrix

B. If resorption exceeds formation, there is net loss of bone mass.

  1. Peak bone mass ages 20–30 years

  2. Age-related bone loss 0.5%–1% per year

  3. Menopausal estrogen deficiency accelerates bone loss 2%–5% annually for 5 years

 Bone loss is a normal part of aging that menopause accelerates.

III. Epidemiology

  A. U.S. prevalence is 10 million.

  B. Thirty four million people have low bone mass (osteopenia) with increased risk for osteoporosis.

  C. The cost of osteoporosis was $17 billion in 2001.

  D. Osteoporosis is responsible for more than 1.5 million fractures per year.

  E. Approximately half of 50-year-old women will sustain an osteoporotic fracture during their remaining life.

  F. Vertebral fractures are the most common type of osteoporotic fracture.

  G. Hip fractures are the second most common type of osteoporotic fracture and have the most serious consequences.

    1. 10%–25% of people with a hip fracture will die within the first year after the fracture.

      a. Increased risk for infection (urine, wound, pneumonia)

      b. Thromboembolic disease

    2. 25% of hip fracture survivors require institutionalization in long-term care facilities.

IV. Risk Factors

  A. The more risk factors from Box 36.1 a patient has, the higher the risk of osteoporosis.

V. History Key Components

  A. Medical conditions

  B. Medications

  C. Smoking history

  D. Alcohol history

  E. Prior fractures

  F. Loss of teeth (can indicate alveolar bone loss)

  G. Loss of height

  H. Activity level

  I. Loss of mobility

  J. Menstrual history (early menopause or amenorrhea)

  K. Calcium and vitamin D intake

  L. Family history

 Secondary causes of osteoporosis are common in post-menopausal women.

BOX 36.1

Risk Factors for Osteoporosis

Female:male 4:1
White or Asian
Advancing age
First-degree relative with low
    trauma fracture
Personal history of fracture after
    age 50 years
Thin body habitus or low body weight
Loss of estrogen
• Early menopause (younger than
    age 45 years)
• Previous amenorrhea
Medication
• Glucocorticoids
• Aromatase inhibitors
• Heparin
• Phenobarbital, phenytoin,
    carbamazapine, lithium
• Cyclosporine, tacrolimus,
    methotrexate
• Sustained progestins (e.g.,
    Depo-Provera)
• Excessive exogenous thyroid
    replacement, excessive vitamin A
• Antacids containing aluminum
Cigarette smoking
Excess alcohol intake
Sedentary lifestyle
Low calcium diet
Lack of vitamin D
• Low dietary intake
• Inadequate sunlight exposure

Endocrine diseases
• Primary hyperparathyroidism
• Hyperthyroidism
• Cushing syndrome
• Adrenal insufficiency
• Testosterone deficiency in men
• Hyperprolactinemia
Chronic kidney disease
Chronic liver disease
Malabsorption
• Celiac disease
• Inflammatory bowel disease
• Gastric or small bowel
    resection
Hematologic diseases
• Multiple myeloma
• Lymphoma
• Leukemia
• Pernicious anemia
Rheumatoid arthritis
Genetic diseases
• Glycogen storage diseases
• Marfan syndrome
• Ehler-Danlos syndrome
• Turner syndrome
• Hemochromatosis
Organ transplant
Immobilization

VI. Physical Examination Findings Suggesting Osteoporosis
A. Loss of height
B. Kyphosis
C. Fewer than 20 teeth
D. Forward head position

VII. Screening Guidelines

A. Many organizations publish screening guidelines; there is currently no set of consensus guidelines, but differences are minor.

B. United States Preventive Services Task Force, National Osteoporosis Foundation, American Academy of Clinical Endocrinology, North American Menopause Society, and International Society for Clinical Densitometry all recommend the following.

 Screen all women at age 65 years or older for osteoporosis. In women with increased risk, screen before age 65.

VIII. Diagnosis

A. Fragility fracture (occurs with less force than would be expected to cause a fracture [e.g., fall from a standing height]) can establish diagnosis of osteoporosis.

B. Decreased bone mineral density (BMD) measurement can diagnose osteoporosis.

  1. Dual energy x-ray absorption (DXA) is standard for measuring BMD.

  2. Central DXA measures density of proximal femur, lumbar spine, forearm, or total body.

Central DXA is the gold standard for evaluating bone density and is the only testing modality that can establish the diagnosis of osteoporosis.

  3. T-score represents the standard deviation from mean bone density of a healthy young adult population.

  4. Relative risk of fracture *increases* 1.5–2.5 for each T-score *decrease* in bone density.

  5. Z-score is the comparison of the patient's BMD with that of an age-matched population. Z-score of -2.0 or lower is below the expected range for age.

  6. The World Health Organization established definitions based on central DXA results in postmenopausal white women.

    a. T-score ≤-2.5 is *osteoporosis*

    b. T-score between -1.0 and -2.5 is *osteopenia*

7. Other modalities for measuring BMD that may be useful for screening but not diagnosis include the following.
   a. Peripheral DXA of wrist, heel or finger
   b. Quantitative ultrasound of calcaneus, tibia, or patella
   c. Quantitative computed tomography (CT) scan
C. Bone biomarkers have the following features.
   1. Biochemical markers of remodeling are markers of formation and resorption
   2. High levels of markers indicate high remodeling rate.
      a. High rate of remodeling usually indicates higher rate of *bone loss* as resorption exceeds formation with advancing age.
      b. Biomarkers are independent predictors for fracture.
   3. Changes in biomarkers typically precede changes in BMD.
   4. Biomarkers cannot diagnose osteoporosis.
   5. Potential uses of biomarkers are the following.
      a. Assessing rate of remodeling prior to starting therapy
      b. Selecting therapy
      c. Monitoring response to therapy

IX. Evaluation for Secondary Osteoporosis

A. Underlying secondary causes of osteoporosis occur in 20%–30% of postmenopausal women.
B. Consider the following secondary causes.
   1. Z-score <-2.0
   2. Premenopausal women with osteoporosis
   3. Men with osteoporosis
   4. Unexplained fragility fracture (e.g., fracture with normal BMD)
   5. Less than expected response to therapy
   6. High suspicion for secondary cause based on history and physical

> T-score compares BMD with that of healthy young adults. Z-score compares BMD with age- and sex-matched controls. Low Z-score raises alert to possibility of secondary osteoporosis.

C. Laboratory testing consists of the following.
   1. Routine laboratory testing
      a. Complete blood count (CBC)
      b. Chemistry panel (renal function, liver function, alkaline phosphatase, calcium, phosphorous, albumin)

c. Thyroid-stimulating hormone (TSH)
d. Parathyroid hormone (PTH)
e. 24-hour urinary calcium and creatinine
f. 25-hydroxy vitamin D
g. Testosterone level in males

2. Specialized testing
    a. Urine-free cortisol or overnight dexamethasone suppression test (for Cushing syndrome)
    b. Serum and urinary electrophoresis
    c. Sedimentation rate
    d. Celiac antibodies and small-bowel biopsy if needed (evaluate for celiac disease)
    e. Bone biopsy when needed to diagnose osteomalacia or renal osteodystrophy

X. Management

A. Nonpharmacologic treatment
    1. Calcium
        a. Best absorbed in doses of 500 mg or less
        b. Adequate calcium intake can slow rate of bone loss
        c. Recommended daily dose of calcium
            i. 1000 mg/day for premenopausal women and post-menopausal women on hormone replacement therapy
            ii. 1200–1500 mg/day for postmenopausal women not on hormone replacement therapy
    2. Vitamin D 800 IU/day
    3. Weight-bearing (e.g., walking) and resistance (e.g., weight-lifting) exercises
    4. Healthy lifestyle; avoid smoking and excess alcohol intake
    5. Monitoring home environment to decrease risk of falls

> Lifestyle factors, including supplemental calcium and vitamin D, exercise, tobacco cessation, and limiting alcohol, are both preventive for everyone and a component of treatment for persons with osteoporosis.

B. Pharmacologic treatment
    1. Antiresorptives decrease rate of bone remodeling
        a. Bisphosphonates

i. Decrease osteoporotic fractures 39%–56%
ii. Gastrointestinal (GI) side effects most common (e.g., abdominal pain, nausea/vomiting (N/V), acid reflux, dyspepsia, dysphagia, esophageal or gastric ulcer)
iii. Osteonecrosis of jaw (ONJ) rare side effect that can be associated with bisphosphonates
   (1) ONJ is the death of bone tissue in the jaw and typically presents as infection and necrosis in the mandible.
   (2) ONJ is less common with oral than IV bisphosphonates.
   (3) The estimated incidence is 7 cases per year for every million people taking oral bisphosphonates.
   (4) ONJ is seen after dental surgery or local infection.
   (5) Risk factors for ONJ include use of IV bisphosphonate, diagnosis of cancer (majority of patients with ONJ had either multiple myeloma or breast cancer), and dental surgery.
b. Selective estrogen receptor modulators (SERMs)
   i. Act as estrogen agonist or antagonist, depending on site (estrogen agonist at bone)
   ii. 30%–50% reduction in vertebral fractures; no reduction in nonvertebral fractures.

 Oral bisphosphonates and SERMs are the mainstay of osteoporosis treatment.

c. Nasal calcitonin
   i. 35% reduction in vertebral fracture; no reduction in nonvertebral fracture
   ii. May relieve fracture pain
2. Anabolic agent: teriparatide
   a. Recombinant parathyroid hormone
   b. Increases rate of bone formation
      i. Stimulates osteoblast function
      ii. Increases GI calcium absorption
      iii. Increases renal tubular reabsorption of calcium
   c. 65% decrease in new vertebral fracture, 53% decrease in risk of nonvertebral fragility fracture
   d. Daily subcutaneous injection; limited to 2 years because of oncogenic concern

Teriparatide is the only osteoporosis treatment that stimulates bone formation.

XI. Monitoring

A. Frequency of screening with DXA depends on the measurement site, type of therapy, patient factors, and precision of the testing center.

B. Gains in spine BMD with treatment usually occur within 1 year.

C. General recommendations for follow-up DXA comprise these guidelines.

   1. Recheck 1 year after starting or changing therapy; extend interval if BMD is stable or increasing.

   2. Monitor more often in patients on glucocorticoids (bone loss seen as soon as 6 months).

D. Appropriate response to therapy is stable or increasing BMD.

E. Significant decrease in BMD while on therapy merits investigation for secondary causes of osteoporosis.

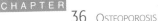

MENTOR TIPS DIGEST

- Fractures cause the morbidity and mortality associated with osteoporosis.
- Bone loss is a normal part of aging that menopause accelerates.
- Secondary causes of osteoporosis are common in post-menopausal women.
- Screen all women at age 65 years or older for osteoporosis. In women with increased risk, screen before age 65.
- Central DXA is the gold standard for evaluating bone density and is the only testing modality that can establish the diagnosis of osteoporosis.
- T-score compares BMD with that of healthy young adults. Z-score compares BMD with age- and sex-matched controls. Low Z-score raises alert to possibility of secondary osteoporosis.
- Lifestyle factors, including supplemental calcium and vitamin D, exercise, tobacco cessation, and limiting alcohol, are both preventive for everyone and a component of treatment for persons with osteoporosis.
- Oral bisphosphonates and SERMs are the mainstay of osteoporosis treatment.
- Teriparatide is the only osteoporosis treatment that stimulates bone formation.

Resources

Cummings S. A 55-year-old woman with osteopenia. Journal of the American Medical Association 296:2601–2610, 2006.

Renowned expert on osteoporosis discusses osteoporosis diagnosis, risk factors, and treatment in the framework of a case study; highlights the importance of individualizing treatment plans and provides a patient perspective on the disease.

Gass M, Dawson-Hughes B. Preventing osteoporosis-related fractures: An overview. American Journal of Medicine 119:3S–11S, 2006.

This article provides a concise overview of the pathophysiology, epidemiology, risk factors, and diagnosis of osteoporosis, followed by an in-depth discussion of osteoporosis treatment. The U.S. Surgeon General pyramidal approach to treatment of osteoporosis is used as the framework for approaching osteoporosis treatment. Level one is lifestyle changes; level two involves treating secondary causes of osteoporosis; level three is pharmacotherapy. The article reviews the role of each intervention in maintenance of bone health and fracture risk reduction.

Goroll H, Mulley A, eds. Prevention and management of osteoporosis. Primary care medicine, 5th ed. Lippincott, Williams & Wilkins, 2007.

Comprehensive textbook chapter that reviews bone physiology and pathophysiology as well as the risk factors, clinical presentation, diagnosis, prevention, and treatment of osteoporosis; briefly addresses the management of osteoporosis-related vertebral and hip fracture.

Stein E, Shane E. Secondary osteoporosis. Endocrinology and Metabolism Clinics 32:115–134, 2003.

Excellent, detailed discussion of secondary causes of osteoporosis including inherited disorders, hypogonadal states, endocrine disorders, GI diseases, hematologic disorders, rheumatologic conditions, medications, and organ transplantation. The article ends with overview of the diagnostic evaluation for secondary causes.

Chapter Self-Test Questions

Circle the correct answer. After you have responded to the questions, check your answers in Appendix A.

1. Which of the following is characteristic of osteoporosis?

    a. Most cases of osteoporosis in the United States result as a complication of a separate disease.

b. Most cases of osteoporosis in the United States result from vitamin D deficiency.

c. Most cases of osteoporosis in the United States result from calcium deficiency.

d. Most cases of osteoporosis in the United States result from accelerated age-related changes.

2. How does osteoporosis cause increased mortality?

   a. Fractures

   b. High output heart failure

   c. Chronic calcium depletion

   d. Nephrocalcinosis

3. Which statement describes osteoporosis?

   a. Bone remodeling stops, leading to increased bone fragility.

   b. Osteoclast activity decreases.

   c. Aging causes osteoclasts to be relatively more active than osteoblasts.

   d. Formation of new bone matrix exceeds resorption of bone.

 See the testbank CD for more self-test questions.

37

INTIMATE PARTNER VIOLENCE

Lenore F. Soglin, MD

I. Overview

A. Intimate partner violence (IPV) is an endemic problem. Medical providers are in a unique position to help identify and assist IPV victims.

B. This chapter helps providers identify victims of IPV, learn to screen for IPV, and teach intervention strategies.

II. Definition of IPV

> IPV is defined as a pattern of coercive behaviors that are designed to dominate and control an intimate partner through fear and intimidation.

A. Perpetrators use a variety of tactics to control their partners. These tactics may include:

1. Threats and intimidation

2. Isolation

3. Physical abuse

4. Forced sex

5. Economic deprivation

III. Demographics

A. IPV occurs in both heterosexual and homosexual relationships, but 90% of the victims are women and perpetrators are men. For discussion, IPV victims are called "her" or "she," and the perpetrators are called "he" or "him." (The author acknowledges that women are not the only victims nor are men the only perpetrators.)

B. IPV is the leading cause of injuries to women 15–44 years old.

C. In the emergency department, battering may account for 22%–35% of women seeking care for any reason. In the primary care setting, 10%–22% of women report physical assault by a partner in the last year, and 30%–40% have suffered abuse in their adult lifetime.

D. IPV occurs at all ages and in all socioeconomic strata of society.

IV. Description of Relationship Pattern in IPV

 The abusive relationship often involves a combination of physical, sexual, and psychological abuse.

A. The abuse is usually chronic and intensifies in a cyclic pattern.

  1. During the initial phase, the abuser exerts increasing control over his partner by using coercion, intimidation, and threats.

  2. The abuser often isolates the victim from family and friends and may withhold money to exert his power.

  3. The victim often has low self-esteem at the onset of the relationship, and her partner further undermines her self-confidence with his intimidating behavior.

  4. This initial phase may be followed by an episode of physical battering.

  5. This is followed by the "honeymoon phase," during which the abuser shows great remorse and promises to change his behavior.

  6. The cycle may begin again. Over time, the violent episodes may become more frequent and more severe.

V. Medical Presentation of IPV

A. Vague medical complaints, for which physical cause is hard to find, are common: e.g., dizziness, shortness of breath, headache

B. Specific medical complaints common to IPV

  1. Chronic abdominal pain/irritable bowel syndrome (IBS)

  2. Pelvic pain/dyspareunia

  3. Acute physical injuries

  4. Bilateral injuries in different stages of healing

  5. Multiple sites of injuries

  6. Contusions on ulnar surfaces of arms

  7. Injuries to the breasts and genitalia

    C. Common psychiatric presentations

      1. Depression

      2. Anxiety

      3. Panic attacks

      4. Suicidal ideation or attempts

      5. Substance abuse

    D. Behavioral clues during office visit

      1. Patient may be late for or miss appointment

      2. Abuser may accompany patient and answer questions for her or refuse to leave examination room

    E. Despite association between some specific medical conditions and a higher rate of IPV, *any* woman presenting to the medical setting may be struggling with IPV

VI. Barriers to IPV Identification

    A. Despite high prevalence rate of IPV, only 5%–7% of women have been queried about IPV by their physician; lack of disclosure compounded by physician discomfort and patients' reluctance to discuss; fewer than 25% of victims of IPV have brought up the issue with health-care providers

    B. Barriers to physician inquiry

      1. Fear of offending patient

      2. Sense of powerlessness to help patient

      3. Lack of physician education

      4. Lack of time

    C. Barriers to patient disclosure

      1. Fear of jeopardizing safety

      2. Shame and humiliation

      3. Feeling protective of partner

      4. Partner's promise to change

VII. Screening for IPV

    A. Screening for IPV important part of social history of all female patients

      1. Privacy essential; others asked to leave, including partners, family translators

      2. Screening questions should be asked calmly after establishing initial contact with patient

B. Approaching patient about IPV

   1. Frame the question by making a statement that makes your questions seem part of your routine.

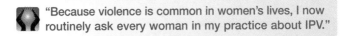

      "Because violence is common in women's lives, I now routinely ask every woman in my practice about IPV."

   2. The framing statement is followed by simple questions about IPV.

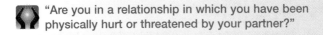

      "Are you in a relationship in which you have been physically hurt or threatened by your partner?"

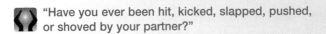

      "Have you ever been hit, kicked, slapped, pushed, or shoved by your partner?"

   3. Avoid words such as "abuse" or "violence" in your direct question because they mean something different to each person.

VIII. Assessing Safety

A. If the patient's response to the screening questions indicates abuse is present in her relationship, the provider or a social worker must assess the level of violence and the safety of the home by determining the following:

   1. Type and frequency of abuse

   2. Presence of weapons in the home

   3. Safety of the children

   4. Extent of patient's isolation

B. Determine if plans are in place for escaping from the home in an emergency.

C. Documentation in the medical record should be in the patient's own words.

D. Physical findings of injuries should be well described or depicted in sketches or photographs.

IX. Intervention Strategies

A. Treat injuries.

B. Physicians can play an invaluable role in helping patients change their lives.

1. Validate the patient's feelings by stating that IPV is wrong and that no one deserves such treatment.
2. Communicate empathy and concern; this lets patient know that her physician is a resource and confidante.
3. Provide referrals to social workers, shelters, and legal services.

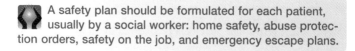

A safety plan should be formulated for each patient, usually by a social worker: home safety, abuse protection orders, safety on the job, and emergency escape plans.

X. Legal Concerns
A. Most states provide women with the right to confidentiality and do not require the reporting of partner abuse unless children are in danger or a firearm is involved.
B. Providers need to learn the legal requirements in their areas regarding reporting IPV.

XI. Summary
A. IPV is a common but under-recognized problem.
B. Routine screening and enhanced awareness among physicians can improve identification of victims of IPV.
C. Medical practitioners can help IPV victims transition to safer lives.

MENTOR TIPS DIGEST

- IPV is defined as a pattern of coercive behaviors that are designed to dominate and control an intimate partner through fear and intimidation.
- The abusive relationship often involves a combination of physical, sexual, and psychological abuse.
- Say, "Because violence is common in women's lives, I now routinely ask every woman in my practice about IPV."
- Ask, "Are you in a relationship in which you have been physically hurt or threatened by your partner?"
- Ask, "Have you ever been hit, kicked, slapped, pushed, or shoved by your partner?"
- A safety plan should be formulated for each patient, usually by a social worker: home safety, abuse protection orders, safety on the job, and emergency escape plans.

Resources

Eisenstat SA, Bancroft L. Intimate partner violence. New England Journal of Medicine 341:886–892, 1999.
Good review article on IPV.

McCauley J, Kern DE, et al. Relation of low severity violence to women's health. Journal of General Internal Medicine 13:687–691, 1998.
Clearly shows relationship between violence in the home and multiple medical complaints.

Warshaw C, Ganley AL. Improving the health care response to intimate partner violence: A resource manual for health care providers. Produced by The Family Violence Prevention Fund, San Francisco, CA 1996.
A practical guide for screening for IPV and developing a comprehensive response to the problem.

For self-test questions, see the testbank CD.

A

ANSWERS TO SELF-TEST QUESTIONS

Part I: Overview of Primary Care

Chapter 1: Office Management and the Principles of Diagnosis and Management of Ambulatory Patients

1. job change
   job loss
   marital difficulties
   illness of a family member
   being a caregiver
2. "Hi, my name is John Doe. I am a medical student working with Dr. X. Dr X asked me to get started and he/she will be in shortly."
3. Outpatient care is often focused on prevention and on longitudinal care of chronic illnesses, whereas inpatient care tends to focus on acute exacerbations.
   Outpatient care very often involves undifferentiated symptoms, which are often treated presumptively, whereas inpatient care more often involves a disease process that is already differentiated, and the focus is on treating that process.
   Outpatient care tends to involve serial testing, whereas inpatient care often involves parallel testing.

Chapter 2: Communicating With Patients

1. Set the stage
   Elicit information
   Give information
   Understand the patient's perspective (and show the patient that you understand)
   End the encounter

2. Leading question

3. Brain tumor/cancer

Chapter 4: Prevention and Screening

1. d. Rectal cancer

Response: Successful screening requires both effective treatment and to screen before a disease becomes untreatable. Lung, ovarian, and pancreatic cancer have not demonstrated either characteristic. Screening for rectal cancer enables detection before it becomes symptomatic. Surgical treatment of rectal cancer is highly successful.

2. b. Facilitate smoking cessation.

Response: Overwhelming evidence demonstrates cigarette smoking is the most important preventable cause of death. Lack of exercise is associated with increased mortality, but proof of benefit from encouraging more exercise is lacking. Mammography decreases mortality of breast cancer, and flexible sigmoidoscopy decreases mortality of colorectal cancer, but the benefit of smoking cessation exceeds them.

3. b. Colon.

Response: Breast cancer is the most common cause of cancer death in women. Colon cancer is almost half as common, but efficacy of colorectal cancer screening is superior to that of mammography for breast cancer. Screening for cervical cancer is very effective but has a lifetime incidence of 2%, which is one-fifth the incidence of breast cancer. No effective screening exists for ovarian cancer.

Chapter 5: Preoperative Evaluation

1. c. Discontinue warfarin 3–5 days before procedure; when INR <2 start heparin infusion until 4–6 hours before the procedure. Resume heparin infusion several hours after the procedure, and resume warfarin the night of procedure.

Response: Bridge anticoagulation is necessary when there is high risk of thrombosis and bleeding from the surgical procedure would be difficult to control. Atrial fibrillation and history of stroke are associated with high risk for thrombosis. Visceral organ biopsy can cause bleeding without a means of direct control.

2. d. Take measures to reduce perioperative risk.

Response: The preoperative consultant evaluates potential risks of surgery and makes recommendations to attenuate risk. The concept of "clearing" a patient for surgery is archaic because it ignores a comprehensive risk evaluation and does not include risk reduction. It is inappropriate to advise the anesthesiologist on the technique of anesthesia; it is better to advise about risks that warn of potential complications.

3. a. No testing.

Response: There is no general recommendation for any testing in general for low-risk surgery.

Part II: Diagnosis and Management of Common Outpatient Symptoms

Chapter 6: Headache

1. b. Primary headache describes neurogenic headache.

Response: Primary headache is the result of neurologic malfunction. Secondary headache has a definable anatomical origin.

2. b. Almost all people will experience headache.

Response: At least 90% of people experience headache. Most never seek medical attention. Although the female:male prevalence of migraine headache is 4:1, there is no gender difference for headache generally. Prevention is important for persons with frequent episodic headache.

3. c. Gradual onset of vision distortion that becomes progressively greater over 20 minutes.

Response: Aura is a spreading cortical depression preceding migraine headache that most often affects vision. Triptans have no effect on aura.

Chapter 7: Common Sleep Disorders

1. b. 15%–20%

Response: Chronic insomnia is not rare. More than twice as many people experience insomnia in a year, but most episodes are limited. Chronic insomnia lasts for 6 weeks or longer.

2. d. You can reassure her that her insomnia is very likely to remit spontaneously.

Response: Stressful life events may precipitate insomnia. Most insomnia remits within days or a couple of weeks. Reassurance is appropriate. Sometimes prescribing a short course of hypnotic sleeping medicine helps prevent habituation to sleeplessness. Benzodiazepine drugs are useful to decrease anxiety symptoms, but anxiety likely requires a higher dose to induce sleep than a person could tolerate all day. Polysomnogram is not indicated for acute insomnia; it is the diagnostic tool for obstructive sleep apnea

and periodic leg movement in sleep. Alcohol is a very inefficient sleep aide because it disrupts normal sleep rhythm and can become habituating quickly.
3. c. Fluoxetine.
Response: SSRI antidepressants can cause initial insomnia. Clopidogrel is an antiplatelet agent; atorvastatin is a lipid-lowering agent; and lisinopril is an ACE inhibitor. None of these has an association with insomnia.

Chapter 9: Chest Pain

1. b. Retrosternal pressure chest pain lasting for 2–15 minutes.
Response: There are many causes of retrosternal chest pain. Angina pectoris is chest pain resulting from ischemic coronary disease. If ischemic pain lasts much longer than 15 minutes, there will likely be some myocardial necrosis or infarction. Pain lasting seconds is more likely to be from a noncardiac cause. Although the usual description of typical angina is pressure pain, the type of pain is neither sensitive nor specific enough to be very helpful.
2. c. Retrosternal pressure chest pain lasting for hours to days, exacerbated by supine posture.
Response: The exacerbation of the pain by lying down suggests pericarditis because the source of the pain is friction of the pericardium against the epicardium. The long duration is inconsistent with other alternative diagnoses. Pericardial pain is seldom fleeting. Angina usually lasts minutes. Myocardial infarction can cause a pericarditis.
3. c. Obtain an ECG.
Response: He has two of the criteria for angina: squeezing retrosternal pain relieved by nitroglycerin. This description is also typical for esophageal reflux with spasm. Ischemic pain lasting more than an hour likely would cause infarction, so EEG is critical. Depending on clinical acumen and judgment, a physician might consider a normal EEG to be the most likely cause. If the description for a man this age meets one angina criterion, probability for ischemia is 6%; two criteria yield a 46% probability. Even a negative EEG might not be adequate reassurance to discharge the patient, but the EEG is the first test.

Chapter 10: Sinusitis, Bronchitis, and Pharyngitis

1. a. Hand washing.
Response: The common cold describes a syndrome resulting from one of a very large number of viruses. Studies demonstrate hand washing decreases person-to-person transmission. There is no evidence that a

paper face mask prevents transmission of respiratory viruses. Neither decongestants nor antibiotics have any effect.

2. c. Reassure and explain that sinus infections are not contagious.

Response: Sinusitis is a bacterial complication of sinus osteomeatal occlusion leading to effusion that is susceptible to infection with colonized nasopharyngeal bacteria. Sinusitis is not contagious. Preventive antibiotic therapy is ineffective.

3. b. *Streptococcus pneumoniae.*

Response: Chronic, not acute sinusitis, commonly involves *Staphylococcus aureus* and gram-negative rods. *Legionella pneumoniae* infects any part of the respiratory tract but much less commonly than *S. pneumoniae.*

Chapter 12: Diarrhea

1. c. More than three loose bowel movements in 24 hours.

Response: Flatus does not define diarrhea. Diarrhea must be loose or watery feces. Acute diarrhea lasts no more than 2 weeks.

2. b. Presence of white blood cells in feces.

Response: White blood cells in loose feces point to inflammation present in the gut. Malabsorption causes watery feces without white blood cells.

3. a. *Clostridium difficile* toxin.

Response: *C. difficile* typically does not invade colonic mucosa. It is often found in small numbers as one of the anaerobic flora of the colon. Antibiotic therapy can alter the normal flora, permitting *C. difficile* overgrowth. *C. difficile* secretes a toxin that causes watery diarrhea.

Chapter 13: Musculoskeletal Pain

1. d. Septic arthritis.

Response: Fever accompanying a joint or skeletal complaint suggests the possibility of infection. If there is joint effusion, it requires arthrocentesis and evaluation for infection. If the joint is normal, plain radiography or MRI scanning can identify osteomyelitis. Passive joint pain is a late finding of osteoarthritis. Rheumatoid arthritis rarely starts in the knee and has a strong predilection for women. Gout is possible, although it is typically extremely painful and more likely to occur initially in the first metatarsalphalangeal joint.

2. a. Malignancy.

Response: Unexplained weight loss in a middle-aged man raises the possibility of malignancy. Metastatic cancer, multiple myeloma, and osteosarcoma are the most common to invade the shaft of a long bone. The physical examination is not consistent with osteoarthritis and gout, which affect joints, or tenosynovitis, which is painful on active movement and palpation of a tendon.

3. d. No test.

Response: Low back pain is a common primary care complaint. As many as four out of five adults have low back pain at some time. The specific cause of pain can be difficult to identify unless there is a neurologic deficit; however, precise anatomical diagnosis is often not useful because a majority of cases of low back pain resolves without specific intervention. MRI scanning is the best test for herniated disc disease if there is a neurologic deficit that may require surgery. Plain radiographs are useful if cancer or vertebral fracture is suspected as the cause. EMG is useful in distinguishing upper from lower motor nerve involvement and defining the anatomical distribution of nerve injury.

Chapter 14: Dermatology in Primary Care

1. c. Basal cell carcinoma.

Response: Basal cell carcinoma is the most common skin cancer. It is also the least aggressive. It seldom metastasizes and locally invades slowly.

2. d. Melanoma.

Response: Although melanoma has a much lower incidence than basal cell or squamous cancer, it tends to metastasize early. Effective treatment is largely limited to surgical cure. Depth of invasion is the most important prognostic variable.

3. b. Acne vulgaris.

Response: Acne is almost universal at adolescence.

Chapter 15: Fatigue

1. c. Impaired cognitive performance.

Response: It is important to distinguish between fatigue and other subjective complaints such as weakness, hypersomnolence, dyspnea, or apathy. The examining provider should pay attention to impaired cognitive performance, which is most consistent with fatigue. Other supporting evidence is subjective and is part of the history.

2. b. 5%.

Response: As many as half of primary care patients report fatigue when questioned; 5% of primary care visits have fatigue as the chief complaint.

3. b. Unremitting weariness.
Response: It is important to distinguish hypersomnolence, apathy, and dyspnea from weariness.

Chapter 16: Erectile Dysfunction

1. b. Prevalence increases with age.
Response: Although prevalence of ED increases with age, it is not normal or inevitable.
2. b. Depression.
Response: Depression is a common cause of ED. Men may not complain of depression as the initial complaint, so screening for depression is important. Colorectal cancer does not cause ED. Hypogonadism causes ED and loss of libido, but it is not common. Occult *Chlamydia* infection can cause infertility.
3. c. Peripheral vascular disease.
Response: Peripheral vascular disease is the prime arteriogenic cause of ED. Colorectal cancer and osteoarthritis are common but do not cause ED. Hypogonadism causes ED and loss of libido, but it is not common.

Chapter 17: Anxiety and Depression

1. c. 1 in 5.
Response: Depression and anxiety affect 20%–35% of patients in primary care practice.
2. c. Most patients with mental illnesses are not recognized by primary care physicians.
Response: Primary care physicians recognize only a fraction of their patients with mental illness. Between one-fifth and one-third of primary care patients have mental illness. The most frequent are depression and anxiety. Most mental illness is unrecognized and not referred to psychiatrists. Much mental illness is amenable to treatment prescribed by primary care physicians.
3. d. Major depression.
Response: Major depression and anxiety are the most common mental illnesses seen in primary care. Obsessive-compulsive disorder and bipolar disorder are important not because of the prevalence but because of the need for psychiatric specialty consultation.

A P P E N D I X

Part III: Diagnosis and Management of Common Chronic Illnesses

Chapter 19: Congestive Heart Failure

1. a. Lethal arrhythmia.

Response: Approximately half the people who die of heart failure die as a result of sudden cardiac death. Heart failure has increased risk of embolic stroke. Acute pump failure can cause pulmonary edema. Chronic kidney disease can complicate heart failure. All increase mortality but much less than ventricular fibrillation.

2. d. Left bundle branch block.

Response: Disorganized myocardial tissue and fibrosis can disrupt the ventricular conduction system leading to bundle branch block.

3. d. Order transthoracic echocardiogram.

Response: The entire clinical picture fits heart failure. Because her clinical deterioration is gradual, symptomatic treatment before confirmed diagnosis is inappropriate for three reasons: (1) although the clinical presentation is classic for heart failure, it is not pathognomonic; (2) it is important to distinguish between systolic and diastolic dysfunction before treating if possible (some treatments that improve systolic dysfunction can exacerbate symptoms from diastolic dysfunction); and (3) it is always important to identify the cause of heart failure. The approaches to ischemic coronary disease, valvular disease, and cardiomyopathy are very different.

Chapter 20: Hypertension

1. b. 20%–30%.

Response: About 25% of adults in the United States have hypertension. Prevalence increases with age.

2. b. Pre-hypertension.

Response: Normal blood pressure is <120/<80. Pre-hypertension is 120–139/80–89. Stage 1 hypertension is 140–159/90–109. Stage 2 hypertension is <160/<100. The relative higher of systolic or diastolic pressures define the staging.

3. c. Stage 1 hypertension.

Response: Normal blood pressure is <120/<80. Pre-hypertension is 120–139/80–89. Stage 1 hypertension is 140–159/90–109. Stage 2 hypertension is >160/>100. The relative higher of systolic or diastolic pressures define the staging.

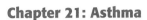

Chapter 21: Asthma

1. a. 5–10/100,000.
Response: Annual mortality in the United States is about 5.7/100,000 persons with asthma.
2. d. Over 30,000,000.
Response: Although it can be difficult to compare reported prevalence rates reliably (because of differing definitions), GINA's data put U.S. prevalence of asthma at 10.9%. That corresponds to over 30,000,000 Americans.
3. c. Inflammation of airways.
Response: Reversible airway obstruction describes the primary diagnostic criterion of asthma. However, it is important to recognize that asthma is an inflammatory disorder of the airway. Reversible airway obstruction is one of the consequences of this inflammation. The reason this distinction is crucial is that treatment of bronchial constriction without addressing inflammation leads to worse outcomes.

Chapter 22: Chronic Obstructive Pulmonary Disease

1. b. Airways obstruction that is not fully reversible with albuterol.
Response: Reversible airways obstruction is characteristic of asthma. COPD is an obstructive airway disease, not a restrictive lung disease. Alveolar infiltration with inflammatory cells is characteristic of pneumonia.
2. c. Productive cough for at least 3 months in 2 consecutive years.
Response: To make the diagnosis of COPD, it is necessary to fulfill requirements of both duration of productive cough and persistence in at least 2 consecutive years.
3. d. Among cigarette smokers, 15%–25% will develop COPD (85%–90% of COPD patients had been smokers).
Response: Although pipe smoking and COPD are associated, cigarette smoking is orders of magnitude more prevalent. About 15%–25% of long-term cigarette smokers develop COPD, but among persons with COPD 90% had been or are currently cigarette smokers.

Chapter 23: Diabetes

1. b. Progressive beta-cell insulin secretory failure associated with insulin resistance.
Response: More than 90% of Americans with diabetes have type 2 diabetes. Type 2 diabetes begins with insulin resistance, typically antedating

diagnosis by years. Insulin hypersecretion compensates to keep glucose normal until beta cells are unable to keep up with insulin demands. Type 1 diabetes occurs when autoimmune destruction of beta cells causes insulinopenia. A similar course follows pancreatectomy or pancreatic necrosis. Glucocorticoid, whether exogenous or the result of Cushing syndrome, interferes with glucose metabolism in a complicated fashion.

2. a. Non-fasting plasma glucose 215 mg/dL.

Response: Random plasma glucose >200 mg/dL combined with symptoms establishes the diagnosis of diabetes. In the absence of symptoms, fasting or 2-hour postprandial plasma glucose must exceed 200 mg/dL on at least 2 separate days. Hemoglobin A_{1c} is not part of the diagnostic criteria for diabetes but is demonstrably useful in monitoring treatment.

3. d. Initiate calorie-restricted diet and vigorous exercise at least three times weekly.

Response: Calorie-restricted diet to cause 5%–10% weight loss and 30–45 minutes of moderately vigorous exercise three times weekly is initial therapy for type 2 diabetes. Other types of diabetes or severe hyperglycemia may require initial insulin. Use of oral antidiabetic drugs should wait 3 months to allow assessment of therapeutic lifestyle changes.

Chapter 24: Hyperlipidemia

1. a. Subcutaneous cholesterol-filled nodules.

Response: Subcutaneous cholesterol-filled nodules, termed xanthalesma, occur in hyperlipidemia. Retinal hemorrhage can occur in hypertension and diabetes mellitus. Periarticular swelling of the distal phalangeal joints of hands is typical for osteoarthritis. S3 in adults suggests decreased myocardial compliance.

2. c. White-gray deposit around periphery of cornea.

Response: Arcus senilis is a white deposit in the periphery of corneal tissue. It is a normal part of the aging process, but premature arcus suggests hyperlipidemia. Cataracts are not the result of lipid abnormality. Keyser-Fleisher rings are a manifestation of Wilson disease. Blue sclerae are a manifestation of osteogenesis imperfecta. Aortic dilation and aortic valve regurgitation occur in osteogenesis imperfecta but not in lipid disorder.

3. d. TSH.

Response: Hypothyroidism, even mild disease, can cause severe hyperlipidemia. Idiopathic hypothyroidism is common among women over age 60 years. Diagnosis is critically important. It is tempting to treat with a statin, but lipids may normalize once euthyroid state returns. Apo-B

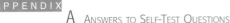

metabolism is abnormal in hyperlipidemia, but measurement is not useful. Except in rare circumstances, calculate LDL rather than measure directly. Direct LDL measurement is an expensive and complicated test. Cushing's disease is rare.

Chapter 25: Obesity

1. c. Polycystic ovarian syndrome.
Response: Polycystic ovarian syndrome is one of several chronic disorders associated with insulin resistance. Adiposity, particular visceral adiposity, is the most important factor in insulin resistance. Type 1 diabetes mellitus and diabetes insipidus are unrelated to weight. Restrictive lung disease in obesity is the result of extrinsic chest and diaphragmatic forces, not lung parenchyma changes seen in pulmonary fibrosis.
2. d. Myocardial infarction.
Response: Obesity, particularly visceral adiposity, contributes to athero-sclerosis. Hypertrophic cardiomyopathy is an inherited heart disease. There is no connection between obesity and valvular heart disease.
3. a. Obesity.
Response: Along with increasing prevalence of obesity, there is an explosion of nonalcoholic fatty liver disease (NAFLD). Considered benign in the past, NAFLD is a frequent cause of liver cirrhosis, often presenting as variceal hemorrhage. Transaminases are often normal in cirrhosis because they represent hepatocellular injury rather than scarring. It is important to consider alcohol or high-dose acetaminophen use despite denial, but not to assume, especially when there is a likely alternative explanation. The liver is not very vulnerable to atherosclerotic disease.

Part IV: Diagnosis and Management of Age-Related Conditions

Chapter 26: Well-Child Visit

1. c. You need to observe the child's activity and socialization development.
Response: Urgent care visits are not substitutes for well-child visits. It is important to observe children's social development and their activity directly. Reliance on parents' observations is not adequate. Many families face financial barriers to obtaining care for their children. It is important to recognize these obstacles and provide assistance. Although anyone can look up immunization recommendations on the Internet, the

reason for well-child visits is not limited to immunizations. The schedule for immunizations is a convenience for organizing well-child visits.
2. a. Suffocation.
Response: Suffocation is a leading cause of death in infants. Intussusception, volvulus, and retinoblastoma occur in this age group, but they are uncommon.
3. c. The family lives in a 100-year-old home undergoing extensive renovation.
Response: Lead accumulates in the body. It can cause anemia, mental retardation, and other illnesses. Lead-containing paint was sold in the United States until 1978. Although 30 years have passed, lead-containing paint is still a risk because existing paint coatings did not disappear from the walls and window frames of pre-1978 homes. Lead has also recently appeared in foreign-manufactured toys. The greatest concern for lead ingestion is children eating chips of old paint. Passive cigarette smoke exposure is a risk for asthma and other chronic diseases but not for lead toxicity. The United States outlawed lead additives in gasoline in 1976. Smog is unhealthy but does not cause lead toxicity. Lead is not an important groundwater contaminant.

Chapter 28: Otitis Media in Children

1. b. Complication of antecedent viral upper respiratory infection.
Response: Eustachian tubes open to permit pressure equalization between the middle ear and the ambient atmosphere. Viral upper respiratory infections can occlude eustachian tubes because of mucosal edema. Children are more susceptible, likely the result of smaller anatomy. When the middle ear becomes a closed chamber, oxygen depletion creates a negative pressure, leading to transudation. The middle ear fluid is a good culture medium for nasopharyngeal bacteria. Suppurative middle ear infections are the result of this process. Chronic bacterial otitis media is unusual. The common process is repeated suppurative infection of chronic middle ear effusion. The source of bacteria is the individual's own nasopharyngeal organisms. Tympanic membrane trauma can cause perforation, not otitis media.
2. b. Increased risk compared with breastfed infants.
Response: Bottle-fed babies have increased risk of acute otitis media. Sterilizing bottle nipples in boiling water is an out-of-date practice.
3. b. 2–3 years of age.
Response: The greatest risk of acute otitis media occurs between 6 months and 3 years of age.

Chapter 29: Geriatric Conditions

1. b. Living conditions, including stairs, floor coverings, and bathing facilities.
Response: Fall risk increases with age. Information about the home environment is a critical part of the geriatric assessment. This includes whether there are stairs; throw rugs, which can trip or slide; and grab bars and slip-resistant flooring in bath or shower.

2. c. Jaeger or Snellen test.
Response: It is unnecessary to send every older person for ophthalmologic evaluation, but checking visual acuity is important. Jaeger and Snellen charts provide a reasonable way of determining need for referral. Funduscopic and extraocular muscle examination do not assess acuity.

3. a. Depression.
Response: Depression often causes a decline in cognitive function. An older term for this is pseudodementia. Antidepressant therapy often improves cognition as depression improves.

Part V: Women's Health

Chapter 30: Benign Breast Disease

1. b. Reassurance that this is common; return for breast examination in 2 weeks.
Response: An isolated tender breast nodule in a menstruating woman is likely to be a functional change as the result of the menstrual cycle. If the nodule regresses in midcycle, no further evaluation is necessary. On first inspection, it is not possible to be certain the nodule is benign. Waiting 3 months would not permit assessment of menstrual cycle change. Imaging is not appropriate because it does not contribute to diagnosis; it does pose some risk for false-positive findings.

2. b. Fine-needle aspiration of nodule.
Response: On presentation, the tender nodule might have been the result of cyclic hormonal changes. If the nodule does not regress at a different part of the menstrual cycle, that merits evaluation. Imaging would not ascertain the diagnosis. Biopsy would not be necessary if the nodule is a cyst that resolved with fine-needle aspiration.

3. d. Reassurance and observation only.
Response: Aspiration of a cyst that causes it to resolve confirms that the cyst is benign. No further evaluation is necessary. Cytology of the

aspirated fluid does not contribute at all. If the aspirate were to be bloody or the cyst not resolve, benign cytology would not permit avoiding a biopsy. Tamoxifen serves as chemoprevention for women at high risk of developing cancer. Imaging does not aid in diagnosis. Moreover, screening implies normal disease risk rather than investigate an abnormality.

Chapter 31: Preconception Care

1. a. Ramipril.
Response: Angiotensin-converting enzyme inhibitors (ACEIs) cause fetal birth defects. FDA classification is D. Pregnant women should not take ACEI drugs. No antihypertensive is totally without risk; however, the decision on treatment depends on the relative balance between risk to the fetus and benefit to the mother. There are substantial anecdotal data to suggest that thiazide diuretics are relatively safe. Accordingly, the FDA rates them class B. There is similar extensive experience with beta blockers; the FDA regards most of them (except atenolol) as class C. Alphamethyldopa had been the antihypertensive of choice in pregnancy for many years. Although it is a class B drug because there have been no prospective studies, there are no confirmed reports of fetal injury. Use is rare because side effects are more prominent than with newer drugs.
2. d. Insulin.
Response: Oral antihyperglycemic agents are class C drugs, but recommendations are strong that they should not be used in pregnancy. Insulin is the treatment of choice for diabetes in pregnancy.
3. c. Low molecular weight heparin for pregnancy duration.
Response: Warfarin causes fetal defects. Its use in pregnancy is contraindicated. Because pregnancy is a predisposing condition for venous thromboembolism, treatment needs to encompass all of pregnancy and 6 weeks beyond delivery. Low molecular weight heparin is the most convenient anticoagulant. Change to standard unfractionated heparin is necessary at the time of delivery to permit rapid adjustment. Interruption of the IVC prevents embolization in the short term. Studies show no advantage in long-term risk of pulmonary embolism or mortality. It carries an increased risk of recurrent DVT. Moreover, insertion requires significant radiation exposure for the fetus.

Chapter 32: Hormone Replacement Therapy

1. a. Osteoporosis.
Response: Estrogen replacement therapy used to be standard preventive treatment for osteoporosis. Although it has a proven benefit, prospective

controlled trials have demonstrated that adverse risks exceed the benefit. Cardiac mortality and possible breast cancer are among those adverse consequences. There is no evidence showing estrogen is useful at preventing or treating depression and anxiety that can occur with menopause.

2. d. Prevention is not a use of estrogen.

Response: Estrogen replacement therapy used to be standard preventive treatment for osteoporosis. Although it has a proven benefit, prospective controlled trials have demonstrated that adverse risks exceed the benefit. Therefore, it is no longer a viable approach to prevention. Estrogen without progestin increases risk of endometrial cancer, whereas adding progestin appears to lower the risk. Colorectal cancer has a small decrease in risk with estrogen therapy. Adverse risk outweighs all the potential benefits.

3. d. There is no proven hormonal treatment.

Response: Depression and anxiety often complicate early menopause. Estrogen, soy, or other hormone replacements have no effect on development or treatment of affective disorders.

Chapter 33: Menstrual Disorders

1. a. Estrogen.
Response: Estrogen causes proliferation and thickening of the endometrium.
2. b. Progesterone.
Response: Progesterone secreted by the corpus luteum after ovulation maintains the prepared endometrium prior to implantation.
3. b. Progesterone.
Response: Progesterone secreted by the corpus luteum after ovulation maintains the prepared endometrium prior to implantation.

Chapter 34: Female Genital Symptoms

1. d. *Condyloma acuminatum.*
Response: Condyloma acuminatum is the result of HPV infection.
2. d. Unknown.
Response: The cause of lichen sclerosis is unknown. Biopsy is necessary to confirm the diagnosis. Scleroderma is not associated with vaginal conditions. Estrogen deficiency causes atrophic changes.
3. a. *Condyloma acuminatum.*
Response: HPV is the most frequent female sexually transmitted disease in the United States. It causes external warts (condyloma acuminatum) and cervicitis. HPV does not cause ulcerations. Bacterial vaginosis and miscarriage are associated.

Chapter 35: Pap Smear and Cervical Cancer Screening

1. b. Squamous carcinoma.
Response: Squamous cell carcinoma is by far the most common cervical cancer. Adenocarcinoma can arise only from the endocervix or endometrium. Neither myosarcoma nor lymphoma is a primary cervical cancer.
2. b. Human papillomavirus (HPV).
Response: The association of HPV, most often serotypes 16 and 18, with infection and cervical cancer risk is close to or is 100%. Co-infection and cigarette smoking increase the risk that HPV infection will develop into cancer.
3. b. Only some HPV serotypes are associated with high risk for cervical cancer.
Response: Serotypes 16 and 18 have the highest rate of developing into cervical cancer. Serotypes 6 and 11, which are responsible for genital warts, have low risk of developing into cancer. Co-infection with a different sexually transmitted disease increases the risk of cancer, but HPV does not require co-infection to cause cancer.

Chapter 36: Osteoporosis

1. d. Most cases of osteoporosis in the United States result from accelerated age-related changes.
Response: Most osteoporosis occurs in postmenopausal women. Estrogen deficiency in menopause accelerates age-related bone loss. Secondary osteoporosis occurs in 20%–30% of women who have postmenopausal age-related osteoporosis. Calcium and vitamin D deficiency are common. Slowing bone loss is largely ineffective unless deficiencies are corrected.
2. a. Fractures.
Response: Osteoporosis makes bones more fragile, leading to fracture. High-output heart failure in bone disease is a complication of Paget disease. Osteoporosis does not cause calcium depletion or precipitate calcium in kidneys.
3. c. Aging causes osteoclasts to be relatively more active than osteoblasts.
Response: Osteoclasts resorb bone. Osteoblasts create bone matrix. The balance between their activities determines the rate of bone growth or loss. Osteoblast activity predominates until ages 20–30 years. After that, osteoclast activity predominates.

ABBREVIATIONS

Abbreviation	Meaning
AAA	abdominal aortic aneurysm
AAFP	American Academy of Family Physicians
AAP	American Academy of Pediatrics
ABCDs	airway, breathing, circulation, disability (priorities in emergency situations)
	asymmetry, border, color, diameter (malignant melanoma recognition)
ABG	arterial blood gas
AC	acromioclavicular
ACC	American College of Cardiology
	associated clinical conditions
ACE	angiotensin-converting enzyme
ACEI	angiotensin converting enzyme inhibitor
ACL	anterior cruciate ligament
ACS	acute coronary syndrome
	American Cancer Society
ACTH	adrenocorticotropic hormone
AD	atopic dermatitis
ADA	American Diabetes Association
ADHD	attention deficit–hyperactivity disorder
ADP	adenosine diphosphate
AGC	atypical glandular cells
AGS	American Geriatrics Society
AHA	American Heart Association
AHI	apnea/hypopnea index
AICD	automated implantable cardioverter-defibrillator
AIS	adenocarcinoma in situ
AK	actinic keratoses
ALT	alanine transaminase
AOM	acute otitis media
AR	absolute risk (difference)
ARB	angiotension receptor blocker
ARR	absolute risk reduction
ASA	American Society of Anesthesiologists

ASC	atypical squamous cell
ASC-US	atypical squamous cell of uncertain significance
AST	aspartate transaminase
ATP	adenosine triphosphate
AUB	abnormal uterine bleeding
BDZ	benzodiazepine
bid	twice a day *(bis in die)*
BMD	bone mineral density
BMI	body mass index
BODE index	body mass index, airflow obstruction, dyspnea, and exercise capacity
BP	blood pressure
	benzoyl peroxide
BPH	benign prostatic hyperplasia
	benign prostatic hypertrophy
BPV	benign positional vertigo
BRAT diet	bananas, rice, apples/applesauce, toast
BUN	blood urea nitrogen
CABG	coronary artery bypass graft (surgery)
CAD	coronary artery disease
CAM	complementary and alternative medicine
CBC	complete blood count
CBT	cognitive behavioral therapy
CCU	coronary care unit
CD	contact dermatitis
CDC	U.S. Centers for Disease Control and Prevention
CFS	chronic fatigue syndrome
cGMP	cyclic guanosine monophosphate
CHD	coronary heart disease
CHF	congestive heart failure
CIN	cervical intraepithelial neoplasia
CKD	chronic kidney disease
CNS	central nervous system
CO	carbon monoxide
CO_2	carbon dioxide
COPD	chronic obstructive pulmonary disease
COX	cyclooxygenase
CPAP	continuous positive airway pressure
CPK	creatine phosphokinase
CPPD	calcium pyrophosphate deposition
Cr	chromium
	creatinine
CRF	chronic renal failure

CSF	cerebrospinal fluid
CT	computed tomography
CV	cardiovascular
CVA	cerebrovascular accident
	costovertebral angle
CVD	cardiovascular disease
CVS	chorionic villus sampling
CXR	chest x-ray
DASH diet	Dietary Approaches to Stop Hypertension (diet rich in fruits, vegetables, and whole grains)
DBP	diastolic blood pressure
DCCT	Diabetes Control and Complication Trial
DEXA	dual energy x-ray absorptiometry
DHE	dihydroergotamine
DHEA	dehydroepiandrosterone
DIC	disseminated intravascular coagulation
DIP	distal interphalangeal (joints)
DLCO	diffusing capacity of the lung for carbon monoxide
DM	diabetes mellitus
DNA	deoxyribonucleic acid
DPP-4	dipeptidyl peptidase-4
DSM-IV-TR	*Diagnostic and Statistical Manual of Mental Disorders,* 4th edition, text revision
DTaP	diphtheria, tetanus, acellular pertussis (vaccine)
DUB	dysfunctional uterine bleeding
DVT	deep venous thrombosis
EBV	Epstein-Barr virus
ECG	electrocardiogram
ED	erectile dysfunction
EDS	excessive daytime sleepiness
EEG	electroencephalogram
EF	ejection fraction
EGD	esophagogastroduodenoscopy
EMG	electromyography
ERCP	endoscopic retrograde cholangiopancreatography
ESR	erythrocyte sedimentation rate
ETOH	ethanol
FDA	U.S. Food and Drug Administration
FEV_1	forced expiratory volume in 1 second
FPG	fasting plasma glucose
FSH	follicle-stimulating hormone
FUO	fever of unknown origin
FVC	forced vital capacity

FWLS	fever without localizing sign
GAS	group A streptococcus
GBS	group B streptococcus
GERD	gastroesophageal reflux disease
GI	gastrointestinal
GINA	Global Initiative for Asthma
GIP	gastric inhibitory polypeptide
GLP-1	glucagon-like peptide-1
GnRH	gonadotropin-releasing hormone
GOLD	Global Initiative of Obstructive Lung Disease
GU	genitourinary
hCG	human chorionic gonadotropin
HDL	high-density lipoprotein
HEENT	head, eyes, ears, nose, throat
Hgb	hemoglobin
HIB	*Haemophilus influenzae* type B (vaccine)
HLA	human leukocyte antigen
HPA	hypothalamic-pituitary-adrenal (axis)
HPI	history of present illness
HPV	human papillomavirus
HRT	hormone replacement therapy
HSIL	high-grade squamous intraepithelial lesion
HSV	herpes simplex virus
HTN	hypertension
IBD	inflammatory bowel disease
IBS	irritable bowel syndrome
ICS	inhaled corticosteroids
ICU	intensive care unit
Ig	immunoglobulin
IIEF	international index of erectile function
IL	interleukin
IM	intramuscular
INR	International Normalized Ratio
IPV	inactivated poliomyelitis vaccine
	intimate partner violence
IUD	intrauterine device
IV	intravenous
IVIG	intravenous immunoglobulin
JNC	Joint National Committee (on Prevention, Detection, Evaluation, and Treatment of High Blood Pressure)
JRA	juvenile rheumatoid arthritis
JVD	jugular vein distention
KOH	potassium hydroxide

LABA	long-acting beta agonist
LASGB	laparoscopic adjustable silicone gastric banding
LBBB	left bundle branch block
LDL	low-density lipoprotein
LH	luteinizing hormone
LMWH	low molecular weight heparin
LR	likelihood ratio
LSIL	low-grade squamous intraepithelial lesion
LTOT	long-term oxygen therapy
LUTS	lower urinary tract symptom
LVH	left ventricular hypertrophy
MAO	monoamine oxidase
MAOI	monoamine oxidase inhibitor
MEE	middle ear effusion
MET	metabolic equivalent
MI	myocardial infarction
MM	malignant melanoma
MMR	measles, mumps, rubella (vaccine)
MRI	magnetic resonance imaging
MRSA	methicillin-resistant *Staphylococcus aureus*
MUSE	medicated urethral system for erection
NAFLD	nonalcoholic fatty liver disease
NAION	nonarteritic anterior ischemic optic neuropathy
NCEP	U.S. National Cholesterol Education Program
NCI	U.S. National Cancer Institute
NCV	nerve conduction velocity
NHANES	U.S. National Health and Nutrition Examination Survey
NHLBI	U.S. National Heart, Lung, and Blood Institute
NIH	U.S. National Institutes of Health
NIPPV	noninvasive positive pressure ventilation
NNH	number needed to harm
NNT	number needed to treat
NO	nitric oxide
NSAID	nonsteroidal anti-inflammatory drug
NSVD	normal spontaneous vaginal delivery
OA	osteoarthritis
OR	odds ratio
	operating room
OCP	oral contraceptive pill
OME	otitis media with effusion
ONJ	osteonecrosis of the jaw
OSA	obstructive sleep apnea
OTC	over-the-counter (drugs)

PAI-1	plasminogen activator inhibitor 1
PCN	penicillin
PCOS	polycystic ovarian syndrome
PCR	polymerase chain reaction
PDE	phosphodiesterase (various types: 5, 6, 11, etc.)
PE	pulmonary embolism
PEFR	peak expiratory flow rate
PFT	pulmonary function test
PICA	posterior inferior cerebellar artery
PIP	proximal interphalangeal (joint)
PLMD	periodic leg movement disorder
PLMI	periodic leg movement index
PMI	point of maximum impulse
p.o.	by mouth *(per os)*
PPC	postoperative pulmonary complication
PPI	proton pump inhibitor
prn	as necessary *(pro re nata)*
PSA	prostate specific antigen
PT	prothrombin time
PTCA	percutaneous transluminal coronary angioplasty
PTH	parathyroid hormone
PTT	partial thromboplastin time
PUD	peptic ulcer disease
PUVA	psoralen + ultraviolet A light (treatment)
qid	four times a day *(quater in die)*
RA	rheumatoid arthritis
RAST	radioallergosorbent test
RBC	red blood cell
RCRI	Revised Cardiac Risk Index
RCT	randomized controlled trial
RICE protocol	rest, ice, compression, and elevation
RLS	restless legs syndrome
ROC	receiver operating characteristic (curve)
ROS	review of systems
RR	relative risk
RRR	relative risk reduction
RSV	respiratory syncytial virus
RV	residual volume
RYGB	Roux-en-Y gastric bypass
S3	third heart sound
SBI	serious bacterial infection
SBP	systolic blood pressure
SCC	squamous cell carcinoma

SD	seborrheic dermatitis
SEGUE	Set the stage
	Elicit information
	Give information
	Understand the patient's perspective (and show the patient you understand)
	End the encounter
SERM	selective estrogen receptor modulator
SITS (mnemonic)	supraspinatus, infraspinatus, teres minor, and subscapularis
SLE	systemic lupus erythematosus
SNASI	areas of guidance for parents: safety, nutrition, activity, socialization, immunizations
SNRI	serotonin-norepinephrine reuptake inhibitor
SOB	shortness of breath
SQ	subcutaneous
SSRI	selective serotonin reuptake inhibitor
STD	sexually transmitted disease
TB	tuberculosis
TCA	tricyclic antidepressant
TENS	transcutaneous electrical nerve stimulation
TIA	transient ischemic attack
tid	three times a day *(ter in die)*
TLC	total lung capacity
TM	tympanic membrane
TMP-SMZ	trimethoprim-sulfamethoxazole
TNF	tumor necrosis factor
TOD	target organ damage
TSH	thyroid-stimulating hormone
tTGA	tissue transglutaminase
TZD	thiazolidinedione
UKPDS	United Kingdom Prospective Diabetes Study
URI	upper respiratory infection
USDA	U.S. Department of Agriculture
USPSTF	U.S. Preventive Services Task Force
UTI	urinary tract infection
UV	ultraviolet (light) (UVA, UVB, etc.)
VAT	visceral adipose tissue
VTE	venous thromboembolism
WBC	white blood cell
WHI	Women's Health Initiative
WHO	World Health Organization

Key Contacts and Notes

Physician Contacts

NAME	CONTACT
Dr	Home phone:
	Mobile phone:
	Pager:
	Other:
Dr	Home phone:
	Mobile phone:
	Pager:
	Other:
Dr	Home phone:
	Mobile phone:
	Pager:
	Other:

Community Resources and Phone Numbers

NAME/PROGRAM	PHONE NUMBERS
Sexual and Physical Abuse	
Substance Abuse	
Communicable Diseases (HIV, Hepatitis, Others)	
Homeless Shelters	
Child/Adolescent Hotlines	
Suicide Hotlines	
Hospitals (General, Veterans, Psychiatric)	
Medicare	
Medicaid	
Other	

Facility Phone Numbers

NAME/PROGRAM	PHONE NUMBERS
Main	Phone:
	Fax:
Laboratory	Phone:
	Fax:
Radiology	Phone:
	Fax:
Physical therapy	Phone:
	Fax:
ECG/EEG	Phone:
	Fax:
Outpatient Scheduling	Phone:
	Fax:
Emergency	Phone:
	Fax:
Operating Suite	Phone:
	Fax:
Admissions	Phone:
	Fax:
Billing	Phone:
	Fax:
Medical Records	Phone:
	Fax:
Medical Staff Office	Phone:
	Fax:
Other important numbers	Phone:
	Fax:

Formulary Notes Specific to Your Facility

Other Important Information

INDEX